Management and Treatment of Eating Disorders

Management and Treatment of Eating Disorders

Edited by Caden Knight

hayle medical

New York

Hayle Medical,
750 Third Avenue, 9th Floor,
New York, NY 10017, USA

Visit us on the World Wide Web at:
www.haylemedical.com

ISBN: 978-1-63241-460-1

The publisher's policy is to use permanent paper from mills that operate a sustainable forestry policy. Furthermore, the publisher ensures that the text paper and cover boards used have met acceptable environmental accreditation standards.

Printed in China.

Cataloging-in-Publication Data

Management and treatment of eating disorders / edited by Caden Knight.
p. cm.
Includes bibliographical references and index.
ISBN 978-1-63241-460-1
1. Eating disorders. 2. Eating disorders--Prevention. 3. Eating disorders--Treatment.
I. Knight, Caden.
RC552.E18 M36 2017
616.852 6--dc23

Table of Contents

Preface

This book was inspired by the evolution of our times; to answer the curiosity of inquisitive minds. Many developments have occurred across the globe in the recent past which has transformed the progress in the field.

Eating disorders adversely impact a person's mental and physical health. They are characterised by abnormal eating habits. Some of the most popular eating disorders include anorexia nervosa, bulimia nervosa and binge eating disorder. This book unravels the recent studies in the field of eating disorders. It provides significant information of this discipline to help develop a good understanding. It provides incredible insights into the diagnosis and treatment of eating disorders. This book will serve as a reference to a board spectrum of readers including students, researchers, experts and professionals associated with this field.

This book was developed from a mere concept to drafts to chapters and finally compiled together as a complete text to benefit the readers across all nations. To ensure the quality of the content we instilled two significant steps in our procedure. The first was to appoint an editorial team that would verify the data and statistics provided in the book and also select the most appropriate and valuable contributions from the plentiful contributions we received from authors worldwide. The next step was to appoint an expert of the topic as the Editor-in-Chief, who would head the project and finally make the necessary amendments and modifications to make the text reader-friendly. I was then commissioned to examine all the material to present the topics in the most comprehensible and productive format.

I would like to take this opportunity to thank all the contributing authors who were supportive enough to contribute their time and knowledge to this project. I also wish to convey my regards to my family who have been extremely supportive during the entire project.

Editor

1

A review of the psychological and familial perspectives of childhood obesity

Yael Latzer[1,2*] and Daniel Stein[3]

Abstract

Childhood obesity is on the rise in both industrialized and developing countries. The investigation of the psychosocial aspects of childhood obesity has been the focus of long- standing theoretical and empirical endeavor. Overweight in children and adolescents is associated with a host of psychological and social problems such as reduced school and social performance, less favorable quality of life, societal victimization and peer teasing, lower self-and body-esteem, and neuropsychological dysfunctioning. Whereas community samples of obese youngsters usually do not show elevated psychopathology, clinically-referred overweight children show elevated depression, anxiety, behavior problems, attention deficit hyperactivity disorder and disordered eating. Parents' perceptions of their child's overweight highly influence the well-being of obese children and the way in which they perceive themselves.

The present review paper aims to broaden the scope of knowledge of clinicians about several important psychosocial and familial dimensions of childhood obesity: the psychosocial functioning, self and body esteem and psychopathology of overweight youngsters, the influence of children's perceptions of overweight, including those of the obese children themselves on their well being, and the influence of parental attitudes about weight and eating on the psychological condition of the obese child.

Keywords: Adolescence, Childhood, Familial obesity, Overweight, Psychological psychosocial

Review

The investigation of the psychological and familial aspects of childhood obesity has been the focus of long-standing theoretical and empirical effort [1,2]. In this review paper we aim to describe the main psychosocial dimensions of childhood obesity: overall psychosocial functioning, cognitive performance, self and body esteem and psychopathology in overweight youngsters, the influence of children's perception of overweight on their well being, and the influence of parental attitudes about weight and eating on the psychological condition of the obese child.

The current review focuses on an updated analysis of the most relevant psychiatric and psychosocial issues in childhood overweight. In order to identify the relevant articles on this topic, we conducted a comprehensive systematic computerized literature search of the Cochrane, PUBMED, PSYCHLIT, PSYCHINFO, and ERIC databases from 1991–2012 using the following terms: "childhood obesity," "childhood overweight" "pediatric obesity" "pediatric overweight" "overweight and obesity in youngsters and in adolescents,". We also combined the terms: "overweight" and "obesity' with "family", "familial", "prevalence", "psychoeducation", "psychiatric", "psychopathology", "psychosocial", and "socio-cultural". Lastly, in order to provide a more clinically oriented review, we included in our analysis not only controlled and randomized controlled trails (RCTs), but also findings of open studies.

* Correspondence: latzer@zahav.net.il
[1]Faculty of Social Welfare & Health Sciences, Haifa University, Haifa, Israel
[2]Eating Disorders Clinic, Psychiatric Division, Rambam Medical Center, Haifa, Israel
Full list of author information is available at the end of the article

Definitions

Obesity is a well-defined term in adults but in children and adolescents its definition is less consistent. The US Center for Disease Control (CDC) growth charts include gender-specific body mass index (BMI)-for age growth charts for ages 2 to 19 years [3]. Obesity among individuals 2–19 years old is defined as the 95th percentile or greater of BMI–for age, and overweight is defined as the 85th percentile or greater, but less than the 95th percentile of BMI-for age [3]. Because of the likelihood of stigmatization associated with the term "obesity", several leading authorities in the field have suggested to define a "risk for overweight" as BMI between 85-95%, and overweight as a BMI > 95% (see for example [4,5]. An international forum of consensus development, the International Obesity Task Force (IOTF) [6], has recently recommended adopting the risk-related cut-off concept of Cole et al. [7], who developed age and sex specific cut-off points using the BMI. These charts extrapolate risk from the adult experience to children. The IOTF defines childhood overweight as a BMI of approximately 91% or greater and obesity as a BMI of approximately 99% or greater [6].

Prevalence

Childhood obesity is epidemic around the globe, and has increased in prevalence over the past 2 decades in both industrialized and developing countries. Thus, whereas the prevalence of child and adolescent obesity has been relatively stable during the 1960th and early 1970th, it has begun to accelerate since the late 1970th [8,9]. Accordingly, in the US, the prevalence of overweight has doubled among youngsters 6 to 11 years of age and tripled among those 12 to 17 years of age between 1976–1980 and 1999–2002, respectively [8]. The prevalence of overweight in the United States around the end of the 1990th has been estimated around 10.4%, 15.3% and 15.5% for children 5–10, 6–11, and 12–19 years old, respectively [10]. In 2007–2008, 9.5% of American infants and toddlers have been at or above the 95th percentile of the weight-for-recumbent-length growth charts. Among American children and adolescents aged 2 through 19 years, 11.9% have been at or above the 97th percentile of the BMI-for-age growth charts; 16.9% have been at or above the 95th percentile; and 31.7% at or above the 85th percentile of BMI for age [11].

In the UK, the rate of overweight, including obesity, has risen from 17 to 22% and from 20 to 25% in 2–5 years old boys and girls, respectively, between the early 1990th and early 2000th [12]. Similarly high rates of childhood obesity have been also found recently in other Western countries. Thus, a recent review summarizes data showing that in the beginning of the 21st century, for the European region as a whole, around 20% of children aged 5–9 years are overweight (of which 6% are obese), and 16% of children aged 13–17 years are overweight (of which 4% are obese) [13]. Moreover, data from 11 countries of the European Union show that the annual increases in prevalence of overweight (including obesity) have risen from typically below 0.5 percentage points in the 1980s, to over 1.0 percentage points in the late 1990s, and it is still in the rise in the first years of the 21st century [13].

High rates of pediatric obesity have been observed also in non-Western countries in recent years. For example, in China, the overall prevalence of overweight and obesity for children aged 2–6 years has been 10.7% and 4.2%, respectively in the first years of the 21st century [14]. Interestingly, studies in some countries have found stabilization in the rate of pediatric overweight and obesity in recent years. This has been noted, for example, in the USA from 2000 to 2008 [11], and in France from 2000 to 2007 [15]. Still it is predicted that by the year 2025, childhood obesity will be the world's number one health problem [16].

Genetic factors account for around 50% of the risk for overweight and obesity among children [17], whereas specific genetic or endocrine diseases account for less than 10% of all cases, and hypothalamic injuries and drug-induced obesity are even less common. As the gene pool has likely not changed during the past 2–3 decades, environmental, social and psychological factors are largely thought to account for the high prevalence of overweight and obesity in recent years. It is important to note that while the individual effect sizes of most environmental factors are likely to be small and the validation of their causality is not straight-forward [17], the simultaneous change in many socio-environmental risk factors from the second half of the 20th century may explain the parallel changes in the prevalence of childhood obesity [10,18].

The psychosocial perspective

Educational achievements

Overweight in children and adolescents may be associated with a host of psychological and social problems, which can have a considerable deleterious impact on the psychological development and quality of life of the overweight youngster. In addition, the school and social performance of obese children are often [19,20], although not always [21,22], less favorable in comparison to normal weight youngsters. One explanation for this finding is that overweight children are absent form school significantly more than normal-weight children. Thus, the obese category remains a significant contributor to the number of days absent from school even after adjusting for age, race/ethnicity, and gender [23]. Obese children are in addition at increased risk of psychosocial distress relative to their non-obese peers [24], and their overall quality of life [20,25,26] and emotional well-being [27,28] are often less favorable. Lastly, lower school performance during childhood and adolescence is an important predictor for the development of obesity in later life [29]. Psychosocial factors such as global self-concept, body dissatisfaction [25] and weight-based teasing [19,30], may mediate in the influence of overweight/obesity on the performance of children and adolescents in their required age-specific developmental tasks and their well-being.

Interestingly, lower childhood IQ scores may be associated with an increased prevalence of adult obesity, this relation largely mediated via lower educational achievements and less adoption of healthy diets in later life [31]. From a different perspective, children and adolescents whose diets are nutritious and whose participation in physical activity is high have been found to perform better on various measures of cognitive performance and academic achievement [32]. Thus, in one cross- sectional study of school children in Iceland, body mass index (BMI), diet and physical activity have explained up to 27% of the variance in academic achievement when controlling for gender, parental education, family structure, absenteeism, depressed mood, and self-esteem [32]. Moreover, an association has been recently found between overweight/obesity and decreased visuospatial organization in 8–16 years old [21], and reduced motor, verbal, cognitive and social skills in 4–9 years old [33], and even in 2–3 years old [34] children, particularly, although not exclusively, in boys. The finding of less than normal visuospatial functioning in obese youngsters retains its significance after adjusting for confounding variables such as parental/familial characteristics, sports participation, physical activity, hours spent watching TV, psychosocial development, blood pressure, and serum lipid profile [21]. Although these studies do not provide causal explanations for their findings. The liklihood of the reduced skill attainment during infency and childhood to decrease the academic performance of overwiet adolescents and adults is of considereble concern (33,34).

Self and body esteem

The association between overweight and global self-esteem in youngsters is not straightforward. Thus, some studies have indicated that overweight youngsters have lower self-esteem than non-obese teens [7,21,22,35-39], whereas other studies have shown no difference in the self-esteem of overweight and normal weight youngsters [1,40,41]. Still other studies have found that self-esteem is no longer lower in overweight children when controlling for the influence of body image and body dissatisfaction [42].

Self-esteem in overweight children and adolescents varies with gender, with females; may be at a greater risk of developing low self-esteem than males [43,44]. The influence of age on self-esteem is not clear cut. Thus, some studies have shown that young overweight children are at particular risk for lower self-esteem [27], whereas in others, adolescents are more vulnerable than younger children [42,43].

The association between the severity of overweight and self-esteem in overweight and obese children is not straightforward. Still, although some studies have shown no association in obese youngsters between BMI levels and self-esteem [43] and others have suggested that many obese youngsters assessed in the community are not concerned with their weight [9], most studies do show a greater concern with weight in obese vs. normal weight children and adolescents, likely influencing their sense of self-esteem [45-47].

The socio-cultural status and region of residence may also have an influence on self-esteem. For example, overweight may influence self-esteem in Caucasian and Latin American but not in African-American girls) [2,48], or in Australian as opposed to Hong Kong youngsters [41]. In addition, low self-esteem in overweight youngsters may be related to the presence of disturbed eating [49], dieting behavior, and preoccupation with weight and shape [22,42,48], and to an overall inactive lifestyle [22], particularly among overweight females, these being in some cases even more influential than the actual overweight. Lastly, bullying has been found a worldwide factor in decreasing the sense of self-esteem of obese youngsters, irrespective of their age and gender [49].

The findings concerning the association of body image with overweight are more consistent in comparison to self-esteem. Favorable body image and perception have been found to be inversely correlated with the actual weight, and overweight youngsters usually show more body image disturbances and more body-related negative attitudes than their normal weight counterparts [1,2,38,41,50-52]. In some studies [21,38,42], body dissatisfaction has been found to mediate the association between obesity and self-esteem, with obese children with greater body dissatisfaction having significantly lower self-esteem. Still other studies have shown no mediating effect of body image on self-esteem [41].

Children's perceptions of childhood obesity

Adiposity is very visible to youngsters, and even young children tend to rate disease and minor deformities as less detrimental than obesity, and to ascribe more negative attitudes to overweight than normal-weight youngsters [5]. Studies assessing attributes related by children to obesity emphasize primarily those of laziness, selfishness, lower intelligence, social isolation, poor social functioning and low academic success [50]. Overweight children are also perceived by their normal weight peers as being less healthy, eating less well, and exercising significantly less [50]. This stigmatization may stem from children's beliefs that weight is under one's own personal control [5].

In addition, children as young as five years old are very aware of their own overweight, which has a considerable influence on the more derogatory manner in which they perceive their own appearance, athletic ability, physical competence, social competence, self-worth, and general health [5,28,53-55]. These findings support the notion that independent of their own weight status or gender, children share the overall negative parental and societal perceptions towards those who are overweight or obese.

Considering the issue of popularity, overweight preadolescent girls are significantly less likely to be considered pretty, although they may not differ in popularity [56]. A considerable decrease in popularity occurs during adolescence, as weight teasing in these age groups is highly correlated with actual weight. Weight-related teasing is greater in girls than in boys and in adolescents than in younger children [57]. Moreover, overweight girls may report more victimization compared with their average-weight peers and are less likely to date than their peers [5,58]. Similarly, overweight children and adolescents are often less liked, and less chosen as friends, and are more rejected, isolated and peripheral to social networks than their normal-weight peers [5,59]. Indeed, large scale community-based studies have shown a greater prevalence of overweight and obesity in preschool children showing problematic relations with their peers in comparison to children with adaptive peer relationships [60].

There is currently growing literature showing that overweight and obese children and adolescents are targets of societal stigmatization and teasing by peers, educators, and even parents [5,16,19,30,56,57,61-63]. Puhl and Latner [5] have recently critically analyzed the findings about the association between obesity, teasing, and health among youth. According to these authors and others [63], higher BMI is associated with more frequent and intense stigmatization in children and adolescents of both sexes. Internalization of this weight stigma in overweight and obese youth has been found to be associated with lower self-esteem, decreased physical activity, and elevated depression, anxiety, suicidality, and body dissatisfaction. Among the socio-cultural factors affecting children's weight-related attitudes, greater media use, in particular magazine and videogame use, is significantly correlated with more negative reactions to obese girls and boys among 10–13 years old youngsters [64].

Psychiatric and psychological disturbances

Childhood obesity per se is not considered a behavioral or psychiatric disturbance [65,66], and most overweight young individuals do not show significant psychiatric morbidity [67]. Accordingly, in most studies of non-clinical overweight populations, the psychological condition of the youngster is found to be within normal ranges of healthy behavior [16,54,68,69], and overweight is usually not associated with elevated depression and anxiety [38,51].

Still, in several community-based studies [61,70], overweight boys and girls have been more likely to report the presence of emotional problems as compared with normal-weight adolescents, already at a very young age (3–5 years) [71] This recent study, conducted in the UK, has shown that by the ages of 3–5 years, obese boys have more conduct problems, hyperactivity, inattention problems and peer relation problems than normal weight children. Interestingly, obese girls of these respective ages present only with more peer relation problems in comparison to normal weight girls, suggesting obese boys to be at a greater risk for the development of emotional and behavioral problems already at an early age [71]. Lastly, another study has found that 23% of non-referred obese youngsters (mean age around 14 years) meet criteria for at least one mental disorder (in comparison to 37.5% of youngsters referred for overweight treatment; [72]).

In contrast to community populations, elevated rates of psychopathological disturbances, primarily depression, anxiety, somatoform disorders and eating disorders, are usually reported in clinical populations of overweight youngsters [16,24]. It is not surprising thus to find that in many studies [73], although not all [20], clinical samples of obese children have a less favorable quality of life and self-esteem than community samples. One explanation for the difference between referred and non-referred obese youngsters is that the former are significantly more overweight [72]. Putatively, neuroendocrine changes associated with stress, depression, and anxiety in clinically-referred obese children may cause metabolic changes that further increase the severity of obesity in these populations [16]. Research has shown that between 30-60% of overweight children aged 5 to 18 years referred for treatment show at least one internalizing or externalizing mental disorder [16,24,72]. This rate is higher in comparison with children with many other chronic physical disorders [24].

Specifically, between 30-50% of clinical samples of obese children and adolescents show moderate to severe depression, and around a third have high levels of anxiety [74]. Conversely, latency children and adolescents suffering from depression and anxiety are at greater risk to develop elevated BMI [75], including obesity [76], in later life in comparison to healthy controls, although other studies have not found such an association [77]. Depression in obese children is associated with the magnitude of BMI in preadolescent girls but not in boys, this relationship likely explained by an excess of overweight concerns among girls [45]. In addition, overweight boys and girls have been found to engage in significantly more unhealthy risk-taking behaviors, and to experience psychosocial distress to a greater extent than their non-overweight peers [63]. In particular, overweight girls may attempt suicide to a greater extent than normal-weight girls.

Psychopathology in overweight children is associated with gender (girls report more problems than boys), ethnicity (African-American youngsters report more problems than Caucasians), peer teasing, obesity-induced distress, body dissatisfaction and parental overweight and overall psychopathology [24,44,63,78]. Interestingly, actual BMI is found less influential than these parameters in inducing psychological disturbances in obese and overweight youngsters. Reduction of physical activity may also mediate in the association of depression with childhood overweight [79].

Behavioral problems

Behavioral problems are also found to a greater extent in overweight youngsters compared with normal-weight peers, particularly in prepubertal children [52]. Moreover, youngsters with disruptive disorders are found to have a higher BMI than subjects without disruptive disorders [75], and behavioral problems during childhood and early adolescence may be associated with a greater risk to develop overweight and obesity in early adulthood [80-82]. These associations remain consistent also after adjusting for a variety of parental characteristics (i.e., demographics and life style), child dietary patterns, family meals, television watching, and participation in sports and exercise during childhood (81). For the most part, the behavioral problems of overweight children do not reach the intensity of full-blown behavioral disorders. Nevertheless, some studies have shown greater rates of full blown attention deficit hyperactivity disorder (ADHD) in obese clinically-referred school-age children vs. normal-weight children of similar ages [82-85]. Furthermore, overweight children show a greater preponderance of ADHD symptoms of both inattention, for example deficits in set shifting and attention abilities, and impulsivity in comparison to normal-weight youngsters [86,87].

Several lines of investigation have been suggested to account for the association of ADHD during childhood with overweight and obesity in adolescence or young adulthood.

1. More children with ADHD have a BMI that is greater than the mean BMI for their respective age in comparison to children with no ADHD [88].
2. A greater prevalence of ADHD has been found in obese children who also show binge eating behaviors [89]. Similarly, overrepresentation of binge eating behavior has been shown in adolescents and adults diagnosed with ADHD during childhood [90,91].
3. Binge eating behavior may be associated with impulsivity [92], considered one of the diagnostic requirements of ADHD, as well as with specific elements of impulsivity, including the urgency element [93], and the need for immediate gratification [90].
4. The presence of hyperactivity in girls with ADHD has been found to predict the development of elevated weight [94].
5. The development of overweight and obesity in children with ADHD may be associated with disturbances in several neuro-cognitive tasks that are characteristic of ADHD, partly mediated by elevated risk for binge eating. These include regulation, restraint, working memory set-shifting and perseverative modes of thinking and behavior [95,96].
6. The presence of ADHD has been found do be associated with more difficulties in the process of weight reduction and the maintenance of reduced weight in obese children [84] and adults [97].

Eating disorders

The lifetime rates of eating disorders (EDs), mainly bulimia nervosa (BN), binge eating disorder (BED), and/or ED not otherwise specified (ED-NOS), is significantly greater in clinical samples of overweight youngsters compared with population-based overweight groups [72,98,99]. Moreover, clinically-referred obese patients with childhood-onset obesity have a significantly higher lifetime prevalence of EDs in general, and BN in particular, than adult-onset obesity patients [100]. Still, although psychological traits associated with disordered eating, for example pursuit of thinness and body dissatisfaction, appear among community samples of obese patients, being close in this respect to young ED patients, these obese youngsters do not usually show clinically full-blown EDs [101]. Furthermore, if an overweight youngster has an ED, its course and outcome are less favorable if the ED develops in the context of premorbid normal weight, in comparison to premorbid overweight [102].

Although obesity per se is not classified as an ED, it shares important psychosocial antecedents of EDs. Accordingly, peer teasing, disturbed self- and body-esteem, and self-directed and naturalistic dieting may be all precursors for the development of both disturbances [5,77,103]. Furthermore, elevated weight may increase the risk for the development of an ED [62], conversely, disturbed eating, in children in particular binge eating, may predict an increase in body fat [77]. It is, thus, not surprising that prevention programs targeted for both problems are similar in many cardinal aspects [62], and programs aimed toward reducing the risk of one, may often improve also the condition of the other [104].

Binge eating disorder (BED)

BED is defined as a subcategory of the ED-NOS diagnosis in which uncontrolled binge eating episodes occur at least twice a week for a period of no less than three consecutive months, with no evidence of weight-reduction compensatory behaviors [105]. Two patterns of BED have been identified in both adults and adolescents, in that the onset of binge eating may occur either before or after the onset of dieting. Whereas in the dieting-associated BED subtype, binge eating usually appears in late adolescence, non-dieting BED may appear as early as 11–13 years of age [64,106-108].

BED is currently considered a major clinical problem in overweight individuals [51,109], as 20–40% of severely obese adults [106,110] and adolescents [51,68,98,111-113] seeking treatment report significant binge eating symptomatology. The prevalence of BED and sub-threshold BED among adult overweight individuals in the general community is much lower (5-8%) [114,115]. Although the findings for children and adolescents are still inconclusive [106], some studies have shown that up to 5.3% of overweight children 6–10 years of age may be diagnosed with BED [116].

Studies that have associated binge eating only with eating a large amount of food have shown that boys report more binges and recurrent bingeing behaviors, but girls are more embarrassed and self-critical about their binges [117]. By contrast, studies that define binge eating as including loss of control over eating as well, have found a greater extent of bingeing behaviors among girls, in keeping with findings in adults [118-122]. With respect to age, binge eating has been found to increase with age for Caucasian youngsters and decrease with age for African-American youngsters, independent of gender [123]. Compensatory weight reduction purging and non-purging restricting behaviors occur only infrequently in overweight youngsters.

For both children and adolescents, a personal and family history of obesity likely increases the risk for the development of binge eating in the context of adverse childhood experiences, problematic family relationships, maladaptive parental eating-related attitudes, weak social support, and elevated psychiatric morbidity (particularly depression, but also emotional disinhibition) [124,125]. It is not yet clear whether binge eating or BED in childhood and adolescence continuous to BED in adulthood [106].

The implications of binge-eating behavior have been repeatedly investigated in overweight adults, but only a few studies have evaluated this behavior in overweight children and adolescents. The presence of binge eating behavior in overweight individuals signifies the likelihood of greater eating-related and non-eating related lifetime morbidity in comparison to non-binge eating overweight, although an inclination towards more severe overweight has been found only in adult [126] but not in adolescent binge eaters. Non-bingeing severely overweight adults [1] and adolescents [51] report relatively few psychological difficulties, although they do score low on self-esteem, and may show considerable social difficulties. By contrast, overweight children and adolescents with binge eating behavior and BED, characterized by loss of control over eating above and beyond overeating, show problematic eating behaviors, particularly eating in the absence of hunger and in secrecy [46,125,127]. These youngsters eat significantly more, have greater weight and shape concerns, as well as significantly elevated levels of depressive and anxiety symptoms and significantly lower self-esteem, in comparison to non-bingeing overweight youngsters [46,51,116,128]. In addition, the greater the severity of bingeing behavior among overweight youngsters, the more are these youngsters at risk to develop depression, anxiety, and self-and body esteem problems [51,128].

Both adult and adolescent overweight binge eaters do not usually compensate for bingeing episodes by restricting food intake between episodes [54], and loss of control over eating in childhood binge eating is usually not associated with dieting [116]. Dieting behavior is usually not a necessary factor for the development of binge eating in overweight children [106], whereas adult overweight binge-eating individuals do diet more frequently than overweight non-binge eaters. From a different perspective, studies in adults have shown that BED and BN represent different syndromes on a continuum of disturbed eating that are likely associated with different etiological factors [106]. Accordingly, patients with BN show greater eating related and non-eating related psychopathology than BED patients [129]. This phenomenon has not been investigated yet in adolescents, but apparently BED in youngsters does not develop into BN in later life [106].

Binge eating behavior can be identified early in childhood [116,120], is relatively frequent among young overweight individuals, and can lead to considerable emotional distress and psychiatric morbidity [46,106,128]. Nevertheless, although binge eating is defined identically in children, adolescents and adults, converging evidence indicates that it is difficult to systematically diagnose BED in young children with accepted adult criteria [105,130]. Factors considered of particular relevance for this diagnostic ambiguity are the inclination of children either not to understand the meaning of loss of control when it comes to binge-eating, or to frankly deny such behaviors when asked, out of shame and embarrassment [46,109,127]. Moreover, parents also tend to deny binge-eating in their children for similar reasons. Large scale community studies applying broad, less stringent and developmentally-appropriate criteria for the characterization of BED (for example, inclusion of food seeking in the absence of hunger, and sneaking or hiding food), using age appropriate interview techniques for both children and parents, are required to improve the characterization of BED in younger age groups [106,120,130].

Parental influences and attitudes

The likelihood of the family to be involved in the predisposition to obesity in their children and in the well-being of their obese children may be associated with a host of familial variables. These include the knowledge and involvement of the parents in the selection of food, control over food and the patterns of eating at home (e.g., the provision of healthy food, the insistence on breakfast, and the family's meals patterns), the acting of the parents as role models and their overall impact on healthy eating and physical activity, and issues related to family dieting, satisfaction with one's body, and weight teasing at home [131-133].

Another important factor in the well-being of obese children relates to the influence of parental psychopathology and distress on the emotional condition of the overweight child. For example, maternal anxiety may predict the overweight child's severity of depression and anxiety (134). Still, the presence of adequate coping strategies in the child may considerably reduce the impact of the mother's mental state on his/her well-being [134]. In addition, child neglect has been found a specifically important factor in the predisposition to obesity at young ages [135].

Thirdly, several parenting styles have been found more prevalent than others in families of obese children in comparison to normal weight children [133]. Parenting style is defined as the combination of attitudes and the emotional climate created by parents through which parental behaviors or practices are expressed. The parenting style defined as authoritarian seems to be specifically prevalent in families of obese children [133]. This style is high in parental demanding and control and low in responsiveness, i.e. low in fostering individuality and self-assertion. As such, it may interfere with teaching the child how to chose the appropriate food and regulate food choice. In addition, parenting styles defined by low demanding and high responsiveness (permissive) and by low demanding and low responsiveness (neglectful) increase the odds of having an overweight child [136]. By contrast, the authoritative parenting style, which is high in both demanding and responsiveness, sets the structure for adequate food choice at home, and supports the child in learning how to handle effectively issues related to food choice both at home and outside of home. As such, it has been found prevalent in families of normal weight children and infrequent in obese children [133,136].

Attitudes of parents toward their child's overweight

Parents of overweight/obese children may be either not worried [137-143] about their child's weight, or, alternatively, be over-concerned with and critical about it [143,144]. Not surprisingly, ignoring weight may be considerable in parents of overweight children (above 80%), than in parents of obese children (less but not 20%) [138,141,145]. Furthermore, parents are more concerned about their young children being underweight than overweight [146]. Accordingly, one study has shown that more than 50% of mothers perceiving their child to be overweight or obese are not concerned about it [139].

One explanation for the inconsistencies in parental perceptions of their child's overweight likely relates to the tendency of parents to be unaware [138], misperceive [147,148], or disconnect between the perceived and actual weight of their child [145,149]. For example, over 70% of mothers of overweight children see them as being of similar weight to their peers, as being equally or more active than other children, and as having a diet at least as healthy as their peers [150]. Parents mostly underestimate their child's weight, with more than 50% of parents of obese and overweight children being unable to recognize when their child is overweight [138,145,151-154]. Still, in some studies, parents have been found to overestimate their overweight child's weight [147].

The inclination for misperception is greater for boys than for girls [147]. In addition, parents of young overweight children misperceive their child's weight to a greater extent than parents of overweight adolescents (65% vs. 51% respectively, [145]. Interestingly, parents tend to perceive their child's weight significantly less accurately than their own [139,155]. There is some debate whether the inaccuracy in the perception of the child's weight is related to parental overweight. Whereas some studies have found no association between parental perceptional inaccuracy and parental overweight [145,152], others have shown a significant difference in the proportion of distorted perception of shape between mothers of normal-weight children vs. those of overweight and obese children (17 vs. 87.5%, respectively, see [153]). This inaccuracy in perception is not related to socioeconomic status and education level in some studies [145,152], whereas others [139] have shown greater misperception in families with lower education levels. In addition, African-American parents have been found twice as likely to underestimate as Caucasians [145]. BMI screening and feedback, may improve parental perception to some extent [145].

In addition to parental misperception about overweight, mothers may exhibit poor overall ability to estimate the way their overweight and obese children eat [137,139]. A significant difference may, thus, be found in the proportion of distorted perception of eating habits between mothers of normal-weight children vs. those of overweight and obese children (36.3 vs. 90.8%, see [153]). Eighty-four and 96% of mothers of obese and overweight children, respectively, in that study, have actually thought that their children ate right or little [153]. Most importantly, mothers' distorted perceptions of shape and eating habits of their overweight children [153], found already during infancy [156], may become significant independent risk factors for the prediction of frank obesity in later life.

Parental attitudes toward obesity in their children may be associated with the child' gender and age, as well as with their own ethnic background and/or level of education. For example, parents of boys [150], or of African-American descent, or with less education [157], have been shown to associate lower risk to their child's overweight. Parents with less education are also less inclined to take action to prevent unhealthy weight gain in their children [138]. Parents of overweight children tend not to include weight in their distinction of health, and have been found to be more concerned with their child's health than with his/her weight [158].

Unfortunately, not only parental lack of concern [153], but also their overconcern [144], may be associated with elevated BMI and adiposity in their children. Factors increasing parental weight concern include higher child BMI, less parental underestimation of child body size, and lower child health-related quality of life [141]. In other studies, parents have been found to be concerned about overweight among children and adolescents in general, but are reluctant to address it with their own children [159]. Conversely, some researchers have reported no difference in the manner in which parents of normal and overweight children estimate their weight, with both groups likely inclining toward underestimation [137,160].

One of the most important factors affecting parental attitude toward their child's overweight is the manner in which parents perceive and are preoccupied with their own weight. Accordingly, parents are more likely to worry about their child's potential for future overweight if they or the other parent are, or have been, overweight [137]. In addition, parents may become over-concerned with their child's overweight as the result of problematic consultations they have had with health care professionals [161]. Lastly, although parents appreciate the role of diet and inactivity in the causation of overweight, they tend to underestimate the difficulties involved in their children's attempts to change maladaptive eating behaviors [140,162,163].

Parents may endorse and transmit weight based stereotypes to their children [5]. Moreover, children's' perceptions about their own overweight have been found to be influenced to a greater extent by the manner in which their parents relate to their overweight than by their actual BMI. For example, for overweight girls, their mothers' weight-related over-reacting, likely leading to restriction of food, and their fathers' overt criticism about their weight, are among the factors that have the most detrimental influence on their self-perception [53,164], and well-being [165]. By contrast, lack of parental criticism with respect to the child's overweight may be a protective factor for the child's self-esteem [44]. The latter youngsters tend to use adaptive compensatory methods for the regulation of self-esteem, such as reducing the importance of areas in which they are less competent and increasing the importance of domains in which they perform well [37,50].

Limitations

The main limitation of the present review is inherent in its design, as we have specifically decided to relate to open studies in addition to controlled and randomized controlled trials (RCTs). This has been done with the purpose of broadening our scope of information and providing the clinician with relevant findings that are not addressed in RCTs. Still, this can cause doubt about the validity of some of the findings described in this review.

Conclusions

Several important findings are highlighted in the present review paper. The school and social performance of obese children and their overall quality of life are often less favorable compared to their normal weight peers. This is a multi-faceted problem, related to greater school absenteeism and overall psychosocial stress, less nutritious diet and physical activity, more behavioral problems, and less favorable neuropsychological functioning.

Not all obese youngsters show low self esteem, and the association between the extent of overweight and global self-esteem is not straightforward. By contrast, negative body esteem is usually correlated with the severity of overweight. Normal weight children tend to show negative attitudes towards their overweight peers. Obese adolescents are usually considered less popular than normal-weight teens, and overweight during childhood and adolescence may be associated with considerable societal victimization and peer teasing. Moreover, obese children themselves perceive negatively many of their own characteristics and attach them to their overweight.

In many studies, although not in all, overweight children in community-based samples do not show a greater extent of psychiatric morbidity in comparison to normal weight populations. By contrast, clinically-referred youngsters show elevated rates of depression, anxiety, behavioral disturbances, attention deficit hyperactivity disorder, and eating disorders. BED in youngsters does not usually follow a course of dieting. Its presence in overweight children increases the likelihood of overall psychopathology. BED may be difficult to diagnose during childhood, and adult criteria are often not suitable for children.

Parents may not show concern with their child's overweight, as they tend to underestimate its severity and to misperceive what their children actually eat. In the same token, parents tend also to underestimate the difficulties involved in their children's attempts to change their maladaptive eating behaviors. Still, other parents may be overconcerned with their child' overweight Whereas lack of parental criticism about the child's overweight may be a protective factor for the child's self-esteem and overall coping and well-being, parental criticism may negatively influence the well-being of overweight children to a greater extent than their actual BMI.

Critical comments, clinical implications and recommendations for future research

The present review sought to evaluate both the psychosocial factors potentially associated with the predisposition to childhood obesity, and those that may account for the well-being of the obese child. Not surprisingly, both sets of factors can be divided to three dimensions: the child, the family, and the overall surroundings of the child and family.

Two points are often emphasized with respect to the obese child. The first is that obese children show greater distress and more psychopathology than overweight children. The second is that obese children in community samples seem to be less affected psychologically than clinically-referred obese children. Still, there are studies showing that greater weight by itself is not always directly indicative of greater distress and psychopathology, and that other factors have to be involved. These relate, first and foremost, to greater weight concern, both of the obese child and of the family. Another factor that seems to be of considerable importance in interfering with the functioning and well being of at least some obese children, irrespective of their actual weight, is their less favorable neurocognitive constellation.

With respect to the differentiation of community and clinical samples of obese children, it is important to note that there are studies showing considerable psychological distress and elevated psychopathology of different types in community samples of obese children. Still, it is still not clear why in some community studies obese children and adolescents show greater psychopathology than normal weight youngsters, whereas in other studies there are no differences in the psychopathology of non-clinically referred obese children and their normal weight peers.

When considering the place of the family in the life of the obese child, it seems plausible that the attitudes of the family towards the child's weight and eating and toward weight and eating-related issues in general, have a considerable role both in the predisposition to obesity and in the well-being of the obese child. Not surprisingly, a very influential societal influence on the well-being of the obese child relates to similar aspects of weight discrimination, weight teasing, and bullying.

In line with the main findings presented in the present review, we recommend that the psychological assessment of overweight/obese young individuals should be performed with age and developmentally appropriate criteria and tools. Any psychological assessment should relate to the parents' and children attitudes with respect to overweight, and assess the children's overall well-being psychological functioning and psychiatric condition, their strengths as well as their weaknesses.

Future research requires the design of prospective and longitudinal studies with appropriate sample sizes, age-appropriate assessment techniques, inclusion of the families and social organizations in the interventions, and adequate long-term follow-up.

It is further recommended to encourage primary health care professionals to integrate the relevant psychosocial issues described in this review paper and in others in their evaluation procedures and intervention strategies. In particular, the use of adult psychosocial assessment tools, adult psychiatric diagnoses, and adult intervention strategies should not be the practice in younger populations.

Competing interests

None of the authors have any conflicts of interest, financial or non-financial, to disclose.

Authors' contributions

Both authors read and approved the final manuscript.

Authors' information

This paper in based on a paper published as a book chapter and approved by the publisher: Stein, D., Latzer, Y., Fennig, S., Golan, M., Gur, E., Levin-Zamir, D., Zuberi, E., Edmunds, L., Speisser, P., & Hochberg, Z. (2011) Psychiatric, psychological, & familial parameters in childhood obesity. In Vinai Dott Piergiuseppe (Eds). *Pathways to obesity and main roads to recovery.* New York: Nova publisher (Pp: 59–82).

Author details

[1]Faculty of Social Welfare & Health Sciences, Haifa University, Haifa, Israel. [2]Eating Disorders Clinic, Psychiatric Division, Rambam Medical Center, Haifa, Israel. [3]Pediatric Psychosomatic Department, the Edmond and Lily Safra Children's Hospital, The Chaim Sheba Medical Center, Tel Hashomer, affiliated with The Sackler Faculty of Medicine, Tel Aviv University, Tel Aviv, Israel.

References

1. Renman C, Engstrom I, Silfverdal SA, Aman J: **Mental health and psychosocial characteristics in adolescent obesity: a population-based case-control study.** *Acta Paediatr* 1999, **88**(9):998–1003.
2. Strauss RS: **Childhood obesity and self-esteem.** *Pediatrics* 2000, **105**(1):e15.
3. Hedley AA, Ogden CL, Johnson CL, Carroll MD, Curtin LR, Flegal KM: **Prevalence of Overweight and Obesity Among US Children, Adolescents, and Adults, 1999-2002.** *JAMA* 2004, **291**(23):2847–2850.
4. Ogden CL, Carroll MD, Curtin LR, McDowell MA, Tabak CJ, Flegal KM: **Prevalence of overweight and obesity in the United States, 1999–2004.** *JAMA* 2006, **295**(13):1549–1555.
5. Puhl RM, Latner JD: **Stigma, obesity, and the health of the nation's children.** *Psychol Bull* 2007, **133**(4):557–580.
6. Bellizzi MC, Dietz WH: **Workshop on childhood obesity: summary of the discussion.** *Am J Clin Nutr* 1999, **70**(1):173S–175S.
7. Cole TJ, Bellizzi MC, Flegal KM, Dietz WH: **Establishing a standard definition for child overweight and obesity worldwide: international survey.** *BMJ* 2000, **320**(7244):1240–1243.
8. Institute of Medicine (U.S.): *Committee on Food Marketing and the Diets of Children and Youth. Food marketing to children and youth: threat or opportunity?* Washington, D.C.; Oxford: National Academies; Oxford Publicity Partnership distributor; 2006.
9. Sweeting H, West P, Young R: **Obesity among Scottish 15 year olds 1987–2006: prevalence and associations with socio-economic status, well-being and worries about weight.** *BMC Public Health* 2008, **8**:404.
10. Ogden CL, Troiano RP, Briefel RR, Johnson CL: **Prevalence and Trends in Overweight Among US Children and Adolescents, 1999–2000.** *JAMA* 2002, **288**:1728–1732.
11. Ogden CL, Carroll MD, Curtin LR, Lamb MM, Flegal KM: **Prevalence of high body mass index in US children and adolescents, 2007–2008.** *JAMA* 2010, **303**(3):242–249.
12. Hawkins SS, Cole TJ, Law C: **Maternal employment and early childhood overweight: findings from the UK Millennium Cohort Study.** *Int J Obes (Lond)* 2008, **32**(1):30–38.
13. Jackson-Leach R, Lobstein T: **Estimated burden of paediatric obesity and co-morbidities in Europe. Part 1. The increase in the prevalence of child obesity in Europe is itself increasing.** *Int J Pediatr Obes* 2006, **1**(1):26–32.
14. Jiang J, Rosenqvist U, Wang H, Greiner T, Ma Y, Toschke AM: **Risk factors for overweight in 2- to 6-year-old children in Beijing, China.** *Int J Pediatr Obes* 2006, **1**(2):103–108.
15. Salanave B, Peneau S, Rolland-Cachera MF, Hercberg S, Castetbon K: **Stabilization of overweight prevalence in French children between 2000 and 2007.** *Int J Pediatr Obes* 2009, **4**(2):66–72.
16. Vaidya V: **Psychosocial aspects of obesity.** *Adv Psychosom Med* 2006, **27**:73–85.
17. Hebebrand J, Hinney A: **Environmental and genetic risk factors in obesity.** *Child Adolesc Psychiatr Clin N Am* 2009, **18**(1):83–94.
18. Speiser PW, Rudolf MC, Anhalt H, Camacho-Hubner C, Chiarelli F, Eliakim A, *et al*: **Childhood obesity.** *J Clin Endocrinol Metab* 2005, **90**(3):1871–1887.
19. Krukowski RA, Smith West D, Philyaw Perez A, Bursac Z, Phillips MM, Raczynski JM: **Overweight children, weight-based teasing and academic performance.** *Int J Pediatr Obes* 2009, **4**(4):274–280.
20. Pinhas-Hamiel O, Singer S, Pilpel N, Fradkin A, Modan D, Reichman B: **Health-related quality of life among children and adolescents: associations with obesity.** *Int J Obes (Lond)* 2006, **30**(2):267–272.
21. Li YP, Ma GS, Schouten EG, Hu XQ, Cui ZH, Wang D, *et al*: **Report on childhood obesity in China (5) body weight, body dissatisfaction, and depression symptoms of Chinese children aged 9–10 years.** *Biomed Environ Sci* 2007, **20**(1):11–18.
22. Wang F, Veugelers PJ: **Self-esteem and cognitive development in the era of the childhood obesity epidemic.** *Obes Rev* 2008, **9**(6):615–623.
23. Geier AB, Foster GD, Womble LG, McLaughlin J, Borradaile KE, Nachmani J, *et al*: **The relationship between relative weight and school attendance among elementary schoolchildren.** *Obesity (Silver Spring)* 2007, **15**(8):2157–2161.
24. Janicke DM, Harman JS, Kelleher KJ, Zhang J: **Psychiatric diagnosis in children and adolescents with obesity-related health conditions.** *J Dev Behav Pediatr* 2008, **29**(4):276–284.
25. Wallander JL, Taylor WC, Grunbaum JA, Franklin FA, Harrison GG, Kelder SH, *et al*: **Weight status, quality of life, and self-concept in African American, Hispanic, and white fifth-grade children.** *Obesity (Silver Spring)* 2009, **17**(7):1363–1368.
26. Yackobovitch-Gavan M, Nagelberg N, Phillip M, Ashkenazi-Hoffnung L, Hershkovitz E, Shalitin S: **The influence of diet and/or exercise and parental compliance on health-related quality of life in obese children.** *Nutr Res* 2009, **29**:397–404.
27. Cornette R: **The emotional impact of obesity on children.** *Worldviews Evid Based Nurs* 2008, **5**(3):136–141.
28. Wille N, Erhart M, Petersen C, Ravens-Sieberer U: **The impact of overweight and obesity on health-related quality of life in childhood–results from an intervention study.** *BMC Public Health* 2008, **8**:421.
29. Alatupa S, Pulkki-Raback L, Hintsanen M, Ravaja N, Raitakari OT, Telama R, *et al*: **School performance as a predictor of adulthood obesity: a 21-year follow-up study.** *Eur J Epidemiol* 2010, **25**(4):267–274.
30. Kestila L, Rahkonen O, Martelin T, Lahti-Koski M, Koskinen S: **Do childhood social circumstances affect overweight and obesity in early adulthood?** *Scand J Public Health* 2009, **37**(2):206–219.
31. Chandola T, Deary IJ, Blane D, Batty GD: **Childhood IQ in relation to obesity and weight gain in adult life: the National Child Development (1958) Study.** *Int J Obes (Lond)* 2006, **30**(9):1422–1432.
32. Sigfusdottir ID, Kristjansson AL, Allegrante JP: **Health behaviour and academic achievement in Icelandic school children.** *Health Educ Res* 2007, **22**(1):70–80.
33. Mond JM, Stich H, Hay PJ, Kraemer A, Baune BT: **Associations between obesity and developmental functioning in pre-school children: a population-based study.** *Int J Obes (Lond)* 2007, **31**(7):1068–1073.
34. Cawley J, Spiess CK: **Obesity and skill attainment in early childhood.** *Econ Hum Biol* 2008, **6**(3):388–397.
35. French SA, Story M, Perry CL: **Self-esteem and obesity in children and adolescents: a literature review.** *Obes Res* 1995, **3**(5):479–490.
36. Harris JL, Pomeranz JL, Lobstein T, Brownell KD: **A crisis in the marketplace: how food marketing contributes to childhood obesity and what can be done.** *Annu Rev Public Health* 2009, **30**:211–225.
37. Manus HE, Killeen MR: **Maintenance of self-esteem by obese children.** *J Child Adolesc Psychiatr Nurs* 1995, **8**(1):17–27.
38. Shin NY, Shin MS: **Body dissatisfaction, self-esteem, and depression in obese Korean children.** *J Pediatr* 2008, **152**(4):502–506.
39. Wang F, Wild TC, Kipp W, Kuhle S, Veugelers PJ: **The influence of childhood obesity on the development of self-esteem.** *Health Rep* 2009, **20**(2):21–27.
40. Gortmaker SL, Must A, Perrin JM, Sobol AM, Dietz WH: **Social and economic consequences of overweight in adolescence and young adulthood.** *N Engl J Med* 1993, **329**(14):1008–1012.
41. Marsh HW, Hau KT, Sung RY, Yu CW: **Childhood obesity, gender, actual-ideal body image discrepancies, and physical self-concept in Hong Kong children: cultural differences in the value of moderation.** *Dev Psychol* 2007, **43**(3):647–662.
42. Pesa JA, Syre TR, Jones E: **Psychosocial differences associated with body weight among female adolescents: the importance of body image.** *J Adolesc Health* 2000, **26**(5):330–337.
43. Nowicka P, Hoglund P, Birgerstam P, Lissau I, Pietrobelli A, Flodmark CE: **Self-esteem in a clinical sample of morbidly obese children and adolescents.** *Acta Paediatr* 2009, **98**(1):153–158.
44. Zametkin AJ, Zoon CK, Klein HW, Munson S: **Psychiatric aspects of child and adolescent obesity: a review of the past 10 years.** *J Am Acad Child Adolesc Psychiatry* 2004, **43**(2):134–150.
45. Erickson SJ, Robinson TN, Haydel KF, Killen JD: **Are overweight children unhappy? Body mass index, depressive symptoms, and overweight concerns in elementary school children.** *Arch Pediatr Adolesc Med* 2000, **154**(9):931–935.
46. Tanofsky-Kraff M, Yanovski SZ: **Eating disorder or disordered eating? Non-normative eating patterns in obese individuals.** *Obes Res* 2004, **12**(9):1361–1366.
47. Allen KL, Byrne SM, Blair EM, Davis EA: **Why do some overweight children experience psychological problems? The role of weight and shape concern.** *Int J Pediatr Obes* 2006, **1**(4):239–247.
48. Maynard MJ, Baker G, Rawlins E, Anderson A, Harding S: **Developing obesity prevention interventions among minority ethnic children in schools and places of worship: the DEAL (DiEt and Active Living) study.** *BMC Public Health* 2009, **9**:480.
49. Danielsen YS, Stormark KM, Nordhus IH, Maehle M, Sand L, Ekornas B, *et al*: **Factors Associated with Low Self-Esteem in Children with Overweight*.** *Obes Facts* 2012, **5**(5):722–733.
50. Israel AC, Ivanova MY: **Global and dimensional self-esteem in preadolescent and early adolescent children who are overweight: age and gender differences.** *Int J Eat Disord* 2002, **31**(4):424–429.

51. Phillips RG, Hill AJ: **Fat, plain, but not friendless: self-esteem and peer acceptance of obese pre-adolescent girls.** *Int J Obes Relat Metab Disord* 1998, **22**(4):287–293.
52. Stradmeijer M, Bosch J, Koops W, Seidell J: **Family functioning and psychosocial adjustment in overweight youngsters.** *Int J Eat Disord* 2000, **27**(1):110–114.
53. Davison KK, Birch LL: **Weight status, parent reaction, and self-concept in five-year-old girls.** *Pediatrics* 2001, **107**(1):46–53.
54. Epstein LH, Klein KR, Wisniewski L: **Child and parent factors that influence psychological problems in obese children.** *Int J Eat Disord* 1994, **15**(2):151–158.
55. McCullough N, Muldoon O, Dempster M: **Self-perception in overweight and obese children: a cross-sectional study.** *Child Care Health Dev* 2009, **35**(3):357–364.
56. Neumark-Sztainer D, Falkner N, Story M, Perry C, Hannan PJ, Mulert S: **Weight-teasing among adolescents: correlations with weight status and disordered eating behaviors.** *Int J Obes Relat Metab Disord* 2002, **26**(1):123–131.
57. Krukowski RA, West DS, Siddiqui NJ, Bursac Z, Phillips MM, Raczynski JM: **No change in weight-based teasing when school-based obesity policies are implemented.** *Arch Pediatr Adolesc Med* 2008, **162**(10):936–942.
58. Pearce MJ, Boergers J, Prinstein MJ: **Adolescent obesity, overt and relational peer victimization, and romantic relationships.** *Obes Res* 2002, **10**(5):386–393.
59. Strauss RS, Pollack HA: **Social marginalization of overweight children.** *Arch Pediatr Adolesc Med* 2003, **157**(8):746–752.
60. Boneberger A, Von Kries R, Milde-Busch A, Bolte G, Rochat MK, Ruckinger S, *et al*: **Association between peer relationship problems and childhood overweight/obesity.** *Acta Paediatr* 2009, **98**(12):1950–1955.
61. Falkner NH, Neumark-Sztainer D, Story M, Jeffery RW, Beuhring T, Resnick MD: **Social, educational, and psychological correlates of weight status in adolescents.** *Obes Res* 2001, **9**(1):32–42.
62. Levine MP, Smolak L: **"What exactly are we waiting for?" The case for universal-selective eating disorders prevention programs.** *Int J Child Adolesc health* 2008, **1**:295–304.
63. Young-Hyman D, Tanofsky-Kraff M, Yanovski SZ, Keil M, Cohen ML, Peyrot M, *et al*: **Psychological status and weight-related distress in overweight or at-risk-for-overweight children.** *Obesity (Silver Spring)* 2006, **14**(12):2249–2258.
64. Latner JD, Rosewall JK, Simmonds MB: **Childhood obesity stigma: association with television, videogame, and magazine exposure.** *Body Image* 2007, **4**(2):147–155.
65. Epstein LH, Roemmich JN, Raynor HA: **Behavioral therapy in the treatment of pediatric obesity.** *Pediatr Clin North Am* 2001, **48**(4):981–993.
66. World Health Organization: *The ICD-10 Classification of Mental and Behavioral Disorders.* Geneva, Switzerland: World Health Organization; 1992.
67. Whitaker RC, Wright JA, Pepe MS, Seidel KD, Dietz WH: **Predicting obesity in young adulthood from childhood and parental obesity.** *N Engl J Med* 1997, **337**(13):869–873.
68. Ackard DM, Neumark-Sztainer D, Story M, Perry C: **Overeating among adolescents: prevalence and associations with weight-related characteristics and psychological health.** *Pediatrics* 2003, **111**(1):67–74.
69. Wadden TA, Brown G, Foster GD, Linowitz JR: **Salience of weight-related worries in adolescent males and females.** *Int J Eat Disorders* 1991, **10**:407–414.
70. Mellin AE, Neumark-Sztainer D, Story M, Ireland M, Resnick MD: **Unhealthy behaviors and psychosocial difficulties among overweight adolescents: the potential impact of familial factors.** *J Adolesc Health* 2002, **31**(2):145–153.
71. Griffiths C, Gately P, Marchant PR, Cooke CB: **Cross-sectional comparisons of BMI and waist circumference in British children: mixed public health messages.** *Obesity (Silver Spring)* 2012, **20**(6):1258–1260.
72. Van Vlierberghe L, Braet C, Goossens L, Mels S: **Psychiatric disorders and symptom severity in referred versus non-referred overweight children and adolescents.** *Eur Child Adolesc Psychiatry* 2009, **18**(3):164–173.
73. Flodmark CE: **The happy obese child.** *Int J Obes (Lond)* 2005, **29**(Suppl 2):S31–S33.
74. Isnard P, Michel G, Frelut ML, Vila G, Falissard B, Naja W, *et al*: **Binge eating and psychopathology in severely obese adolescents.** *Int J Eat Disord* 2003, **34**(2):235–243.
75. Anderson SE, Cohen P, Naumova EN, Must A: **Relationship of childhood behavior disorders to weight gain from childhood into adulthood.** *Ambul Pediatr* 2006, **6**(5):297–301.
76. Rofey DL, Kolko RP, Iosif AM, Silk JS, Bost JE, Feng W, *et al*: **A longitudinal study of childhood depression and anxiety in relation to weight gain.** *Child Psychiatry Hum Dev* 2009, **40**(4):517–526.
77. Tanofsky-Kraff M, Faden D, Yanovski SZ, Wilfley DE, Yanovski JA: **The perceived onset of dieting and loss of control eating behaviors in overweight children.** *Int J Eat Disord* 2005, **38**(2):112–122.
78. Park CM, Kim MD, Hong SC, Kim Y, Hyun MY, Kwak YS, *et al*: **Effects of obesity and obesity-induced stress on depressive symptoms in Korean elementary school children.** *Int J Soc Psychiatry* 2009, **55**(4):322–335.
79. Gray WN, Janicke DM, Ingerski LM, Silverstein JH: **The impact of peer victimization, parent distress and child depression on barrier formation and physical activity in overweight youth.** *J Dev Behav Pediatr* 2008, **29**(1):26–33.
80. Duarte CS, Sourander A, Nikolakaros G, Pihlajamaki H, Helenius H, Piha J, *et al*: **Child mental health problems and obesity in early adulthood.** *J Pediatr* 2010, **156**(1):93–97.
81. Mamun AA, O'Callaghan MJ, Cramb SM, Najman JM, Williams GM, Bor W: **Childhood behavioral problems predict young adults' BMI and obesity: evidence from a birth cohort study.** *Obesity (Silver Spring)* 2009, **17**(4):761–766.
82. White B, Nicholls D, Christie D, Cole TJ, Viner RM: **Childhood psychological function and obesity risk across the lifecourse: findings from the 1970 British Cohort Study.** *Int J Obes (Lond)* 2012, **36**(4):511–516.
83. Agranat-Meged AN, Deitcher C, Goldzweig G, Leibenson L, Stein M, Galili-Weisstub E: **Childhood obesity and attention deficit/hyperactivity disorder: a newly described comorbidity in obese hospitalized children.** *Int J Eat Disord* 2005, **37**(4):357–359.
84. Altfas JR: **Prevalence of attention deficit/hyperactivity disorder among adults in obesity treatment.** *BMC Psychiatry* 2002, **2**:9.
85. Fleming JP, Levy LD, Levitan RD: **Symptoms of attention deficit hyperactivity disorder in severely obese women.** *Eat Weight Disord* 2005, **10**(1):e10–e13.
86. Braet C, Claus L, Verbeken S, Van Vlierberghe L: **Impulsivity in overweight children.** *Eur Child Adolesc Psychiatry* 2007, **16**(8):473–483.
87. Cserjesi R, Molnar D, Luminet O, Lenard L. **Is there any relationship between obesity and mental flexibility in children?** *Appetite* 2007, **49**(3):675–678.
88. Cortese S, Angriman M, Maffeis C, Isnard P, Konofal E, Lecendreux M, *et al*: **Attention-deficit/hyperactivity disorder (ADHD) and obesity: a systematic review of the literature.** *Crit Rev Food Sci Nutr* 2008, **48**(6):524–537.
89. Cortese S, Bernardina BD, Mouren MC: **Attention-deficit/hyperactivity disorder (ADHD) and binge eating.** *Nutr Rev* 2007, **65**(9):404–411.
90. Davis C, Levitan RD, Smith M, Tweed S, Curtis C: **Associations among overeating, overweight, and attention deficit/hyperactivity disorder: a structural equation modelling approach.** *Eat Behav* 2006, **7**(3):266–274.
91. Biederman J, Ball SW, Monuteaux MC, Surman CB, Johnson JL, Zeitlin S: **Are girls with ADHD at risk for eating disorders? Results from a controlled, five-year prospective study.** *J Dev Behav Pediatr* 2007, **28**(4):302–307.
92. Keel PK, Striegel-Moore RH: **The validity and clinical utility of purging disorder.** *Int J Eat Disord* 2009, **42**(8):706–719.
93. Combs JL, Pearson CM, Smith GT: **A risk model for preadolescent disordered eating.** *Int J Eat Disord* 2011, **44**(7):596–604.
94. Holtkamp K, Konrad K, Muller B, Heussen N, Herpertz S, Herpertz-Dahlmann B, *et al*: **Overweight and obesity in children with Attention-Deficit /Hyperactivity Disorder.** *Int J Obes Relat Metab Disord* 2004, **28**(5):685–689.
95. Tchanturia K, Anderluh MB, Morris RG, Rabe-Hesketh S, Collier DA, Sanchez P, *et al*: **Cognitive flexibility in anorexia nervosa and bulimia nervosa.** *J Int Neuropsychol Soc* 2004, **10**(4):513–520.
96. Bosanac P, Kurlender S, Stojanovska L, Hallam K, Norman T, McGrath C, *et al*: **Neuropsychological study of underweight and "weight-recovered" anorexia nervosa compared with bulimia nervosa and normal controls.** *Int J Eat Disord* 2007, **40**(7):613–621.
97. Kaplan AS, Howlett AL, Yilmaz Z, Levitan R: **Attention Deficit Hyperactivity Disorder and Binge Eating: Shared Phenomenology, Genetics and Response to Treatment.** *Int J Child Health Adolescents Health* 2009, **2**:165–174.

98. Britz B, Siegfried W, Ziegler A, Lamertz C, Herpertz-Dahlmann BM, Remschmidt H, *et al*: **Rates of psychiatric disorders in a clinical study group of adolescents with extreme obesity and in obese adolescents ascertained via a population based study.** *Int J Obes Relat Metab Disord* 2000, **24**(12):1707–1714.
99. Schuetzmann M, Richter-Appelt H, Schulte-Markwort M, Schimmelmann BG: **Associations among the perceived parent–child relationship, eating behavior, and body weight in preadolescents: results from a community-based sample.** *J Pediatr Psychol* 2008, **33**(7):772–782.
100. Guerdjikova AI, McElroy SL, Kotwal R, Stanford K, Keck PE Jr: **Psychiatric and metabolic characteristics of childhood versus adult-onset obesity in patients seeking weight management.** *Eat Behav* 2007, **8**(2):266–276.
101. Lundstedt G, Edlund B, Engstrom I, Thurfjell B, Marcus C: **Eating disorder traits in obese children and adolescents.** *Eat Weight Disord* 2006, **11**(1):45–50.
102. Bean P, Loomis CC, Timmel P, Hallinan P, Moore S, Mammel J, *et al*: **Outcome variables for anorexic males and females one year after discharge from residential treatment.** *J Addict Dis* 2004, **23**(2):83–94.
103. Field AE, Austin SB, Taylor CB, Malspeis S, Rosner B, Rockett HR, *et al*: **Relation between dieting and weight change among preadolescents and adolescents.** *Pediatrics* 2003, **112**(4):900–906.
104. Neumark-Sztainer D, Wall M, Haines J, Story M, Eisenberg ME: **Why does dieting predict weight gain in adolescents? Findings from project EAT-II: a 5-year longitudinal study.** *J Am Diet Assoc* 2007, **107**(3):448–455.
105. American Psychiatric Association Committee on Nomenclature,and Statistics: *Diagnostic and Statistical Manual of Mental Disorders (DSM-IV)*. Fourthth edition. Washington, DC: American Psychiatric Association; 1994.
106. Marcus MD, Kalarchian MA: **Binge eating in children and adolescents.** *Int J Eat Disord* 2003, **34**(Suppl):S47–S57.
107. Tzischinsky O, Latzer Y: **Sleep-Wake cycles in obese adolescents with and without Binge Eating Episodes.** *European Eating Disorders Review* 2006, **14**(2):111–117.
108. Tzischinsky O, Latzer Y: **Sleep-wake cycles in obese children with and without binge-eating episodes.** *J Paediatr Child Health* 2006, **42**(11):688–693.
109. Spitzer RL, Yanovski SZ, Wadden T: **Binge eating disorder: Its further validation in a multisite study.** *Int J Eat Disorder* 1993, **13**:137–153.
110. Yanovski SZ, Nelson JE, Dubbert BK, Spitzer RL: **Association of binge eating disorder and psychiatric comorbidity in obese subjects.** *Am J Psychiatry* 1993, **150**(10):1472–1479.
111. Berkowitz R, Stunkard AJ, Stallings VA: **Binge-eating disorder in obese adolescent girls.** *Ann N Y Acad Sci* 1993, **699**:200–206.
112. Decaluwe V, Braet C, Fairburn CG: **Binge eating in obese children and adolescents.** *Int J Eat Disord* 2003, **33**(1):78–84.
113. Severi F, Verri A, Livieri C: **Eating behavior and psychological profile in childhood obesity.** *Adv Biosci* 1993, **90**:329–336.
114. Stice E, Marti CN, Rohde P: **Prevalence, Incidence, Impairment, and Course of the Proposed DSM-5 Eating Disorder Diagnoses in an 8-Year Prospective Community Study of Young Women.** *J Abnorm Psychol* 2012, Epub ahead of print.
115. Marcus M: **Binge Eating and Obesity.** In *Eating disorders and obesity, a comprehensive book.* 1st edition. Edited by Brownell KD, Fairburn CG. New York: The Guilford Press; 1995:441–444.
116. Morgan CM, Yanovski SZ, Nguyen TT, McDuffie J, Sebring NG, Jorge MR, *et al*: **Loss of control over eating, adiposity, and psychopathology in overweight children.** *Int J Eat Disord* 2002, **31**(4):430–441.
117. Whitaker A, Davies M, Shaffer D, Johnson J, Abrams S, Walsh BT, *et al*: **The struggle to be thin: a survey of anorexic and bulimic symptoms in a non-referred adolescent population.** *Psychol Med* 1989, **19**(1):143–163.
118. Croll J, Neumark-Sztainer D, Story M, Ireland M: **Prevalence and risk and protective factors related to disordered eating behaviors among adolescents: relationship to gender and ethnicity.** *J Adolesc Health* 2002, **31**(2):166–175.
119. Goldschmidt AB, Jones M, Manwaring JL, Luce KH, Osborne MI, Cunning D, *et al*: **The clinical significance of loss of control over eating in overweight adolescents.** *Int J Eat Disord* 2008, **41**(2):153–158.
120. Tanofsky-Kraff M, Goossens L, Eddy KT, Ringham R, Goldschmidt A, Yanovski SZ, *et al*: **A multisite investigation of binge eating behaviors in children and adolescents.** *J Consult Clin Psychol* 2007, **75**(6):901–913.
121. Goossens L, Braet C, Decaluwe V: **Loss of control over eating in obese youngsters.** *Behav Res Ther* 2007, **45**(1):1–9.
122. Tanofsky-Kraff M, Yanovski SZ, Schvey NA, Olsen CH, Gustafson J, Yanovski JA: **A prospective study of loss of control eating for body weight gain in children at high risk for adult obesity.** *Int J Eat Disord* 2009, **42**(1):26–30.
123. Johnson WG, Rohan KJ, Kirk AA: **Prevalence and correlates of binge eating in white and African American adolescents.** *Eat Behav* 2002, **3**(2):179–189.
124. Johnson JG, Cohen P, Kotler L, Kasen S, Brook JS: **Psychiatric disorders associated with risk for the development of eating disorders during adolescence and early adulthood.** *J Consult Clin Psychol* 2002, **70**(5):1119–1128.
125. Fisher JO, Birch LL: **Eating in the absence of hunger and overweight in girls from 5 to 7 y of age.** *Am J Clin Nutr* 2002, **76**(1):226–231.
126. French SA, Jeffery RW, Sherwood NE, Neumark-Sztainer D: **Prevalence and correlates of binge eating in a nonclinical sample of women enrolled in a weight gain prevention program.** *Int J Obes Relat Metab Disord* 1999, **23**(6):576–585.
127. Eddy KT, Tanofsky-Kraff M, Thompson-Brenner H, Herzog DB, Brown TA, Ludwig DS: **Eating disorder pathology among overweight treatment-seeking youth: clinical correlates and cross-sectional risk modeling.** *Behav Res Ther* 2007, **45**(10):2360–2371.
128. Goossens L, Braet C, Van Vlierberghe L, Mels S: **Weight parameters and pathological eating as predictors of obesity treatment outcome in children and adolescents.** *Eat Behav* 2009, **10**(1):71–73.
129. Salvemini V, Berna G, Foca F, Indrimi M, Sammartino F, Spinosa L, *et al*: **Differences and similarities in the personality structure of 327 women with eating disorders.** *Eat Weight Disord* 2000, **5**(2):108–115.
130. Goldschmidt AB, Doyle AC, Wilfley DE: **Assessment of binge eating in overweight youth using a questionnaire version of the Child Eating Disorder Examination with Instructions.** *Int J Eat Disord* 2007, **40**(5):460–467.
131. Golan M, Crow S: **Parents are key players in the prevention and treatment of weight-related problems.** *Nutr Rev* 2004, **62**(1):39–50.
132. Neumark-Sztainer D: **Preventing obesity and eating disorders in adolescents: what can health care providers do?** *J Adolesc Health* 2009, **44**(3):206–213.
133. Hughes SO, O'Connor TM, Power TG: **Parenting and children's eating patterns: Examining control in a broader context.** *Int J Child Adolesc health.* 2008, **1**:323–330.
134. Roth B, Munsch S, Meyer A, Isler E, Schneider S: **The association between mothers' psychopathology, childrens' competences and psychological well-being in obese children.** *Eat Weight Disord* 2008, **13**(3):129–136.
135. Lissau I, Sorensen TI: **Parental neglect during childhood and increased risk of obesity in young adulthood.** *Lancet* 1994, **343**(8893):324–327.
136. Rhee KE, Lumeng JC, Appugliese DP, Kaciroti N, Bradley RH: **Parenting styles and overweight status in first grade.** *Pediatrics* 2006, **117**(6):2047–2054.
137. Campbell MW, Williams J, Hampton A, Wake M: **Maternal concern and perceptions of overweight in Australian preschool-aged children.** *Med J Aust* 2006, **184**(6):274–277.
138. Crawford D, Timperio A, Telford A, Salmon J: **Parental concerns about childhood obesity and the strategies employed to prevent unhealthy weight gain in children.** *Public Health Nutr* 2006, **9**(7):889–895.
139. Genovesi S, Giussani M, Faini A, Vigorita F, Pieruzzi F, Strepparava MG, *et al*: **Maternal perception of excess weight in children: a survey conducted by paediatricians in the province of Milan.** *Acta Paediatr* 2005, **94**(6):747–752.
140. Jain A, Sherman SN, Chamberlin LA, Carter Y, Powers SW, Whitaker RC: **Why don't low-income mothers worry about their preschoolers being overweight?** *Pediatrics* 2001, **107**(5):1138–1146.
141. Lampard AM, Byrne SM, Zubrick SR, Davis EA: **Parents' concern about their children's weight.** *Int J Pediatr Obes* 2008, **3**(2):84–92.
142. Hood MY, Moore LL, Sundarajan-Ramamurti A, Singer M, Cupples LA, Ellison RC: **Parental eating attitudes and the development of obesity in children. The framingham children's study.** *Int J Obes* 2000, **24**(10):1319–1325.
143. Baughcum AE, Chamberlin LA, Deeks CM, Powers SW, Whitaker RC: **Maternal perceptions of overweight preschool children.** *Pediatrics* 2000, **106**(6):1380–1386.
144. Burdette HL, Whitaker RC, Hall WC, Daniels SR: **Maternal infant-feeding style and children's adiposity at 5 years of age.** *Arch Pediatr Adolesc Med* 2006, **160**(5):513–520.

145. West DS, Raczynski JM, Phillips MM, Bursac Z, Heath Gauss C, Montgomery BE: **Parental recognition of overweight in school-age children.** *Obesity (Silver Spring)* 2008, **16**(3):630–636.
146. Pagnini DL, Wilkenfeld RL, King LA, Booth ML, Booth SL: **Mothers of pre-school children talk about childhood overweight and obesity: the weight of opinion study.** *J Paediatr Child Health* 2007, **43**(12):806–810.
147. Dubois L, Girad M: **Accuracy of maternal reports of pre-schoolers' weights and heights as estimates of BMI values.** *Int J Epidemiol* 2007, **36**(1):132–138.
148. Watkins MG, Clark KM, Foster CM, Welch KB, Kasa-Vubu JZ: **Relationships among body mass index, parental perceptions, birthweight and parental weight after referral to a weight clinic.** *J Natl Med Assoc* 2007, **99**(8):908–913.
149. Doolen J, Alpert PT, Miller SK: **Parental disconnect between perceived and actual weight status of children: a metasynthesis of the current research.** *J Am Acad Nurse Pract* 2009, **21**(3):160–166.
150. Campbell KJ, Crawford DA, Ball K: **Family food environment and dietary behaviors likely to promote fatness in 5–6 year-old children.** *Int J Obes (Lond)* 2006, **30**(8):1272–1280.
151. Adams AK, Quinn RA, Prince RJ: **Low recognition of childhood overweight and disease risk among Native-American caregivers.** *Obes Res* 2005, **13**(1):146–152.
152. Hackie M, Bowles CL: **Maternal perception of their overweight children.** *Public Health Nurs* 2007, **24**(6):538–546.
153. Hirschler V, Gonzalez C, Talgham S, Jadzinsky M: **Do mothers of overweight Argentinean preschool children perceive them as such?** *Pediatr Diabetes* 2006, **7**(4):201–204.
154. Parry LL, Netuveli G, Parry J, Saxena S: **A systematic review of parental perception of overweight status in children.** *J Ambul Care Manage* 2008, **31**(3):253–268.
155. Nazario Rodriguez IJ, Figueroa WI, Rosado J, Parrilla IC: **Perception of parents regarding their children's weight.** *Boletin- Asociacion Medica de Puerto Rico* 2008, **100**:33–38.
156. Kroke A, Strathmann S, Gunther AL: **Maternal perceptions of her child's body weight in infancy and early childhood and their relation to body weight status at age 7.** *Eur J Pediatr* 2006, **165**(12):875–883.
157. Nsiah-Kumi PA, Ariza AJ, Mikhail LM, Feinglass J, Binns HJ, Pediatric Practice Research Group: **Family history and parents' beliefs about consequences of childhood overweight and their influence on children's health behaviors.** *Acad Pediatr* 2009, **9**(1):53–59.
158. Goodell SL, Pierce MB, Bravo CM, Ferris AM: **Parental perceptions of overweight during early childhood.** *Qual Health Res* 2008, **18**:1548–1555.
159. Booth ML, King LA, Pagnini DL, Wilkenfeld RL, Booth SL: **Parents of school students on childhood overweight: the Weight of Opinion Study.** *J Paediatr Child Health* 2009, **45**(4):194–198.
160. Kersey M, Lipton R, Quinn MT, Lantos JD: **Overweight in Latino preschoolers: do parental health beliefs matter?** *Am J Health Behav* 2010, **34**(3):340–348.
161. Edmunds LD: **Parents' perceptions of health professionals' responses when seeking help for their overweight children.** *Fam Pract* 2005, **22**(3):287–292.
162. Cullen KW, Baranowski T, Rittenberry L, Olvera N: **Social-environmental influences on children's diets: results from focus groups with African-, Euro- and Mexican-American children and their parents.** *Health Educ Res* 2000, **15**(5):581–590.
163. Rainey CJ, Kemper KA, Poling R, Tucker S: **Parents' perceptions of influences on child eating behaviors: An attitudinal approach.** *J Health Educ* 1998, **29**:223–229.
164. Birch LL, Fisher JO, Davison KK: **Learning to overeat: maternal use of restrictive feeding practices promotes girls' eating in the absence of hunger.** *Am J Clin Nutr* 2003, **78**(2):215–220.
165. Rumpel C, Harris TB: **The influence of weight on adolescent self-esteem.** *J Psychosom Res* 1994, **38**(6):547–556.

2

A systematic review of the frequency, duration, type and effect of involuntary treatment for people with anorexia nervosa, and an analysis of patient characteristics

Loa Clausen[1*] and Allan Jones[2]

Abstract

Objective: Involuntary treatment of anorexia nervosa is controversial and costly. A better understanding of the conditions that determine involuntary treatment, as well as the effect of such treatment is needed in order to adequately assess the legitimacy of this model of care. The aim of the present study was to investigate the frequency and duration of involuntary treatment, the characteristics of this group of patients, the kind of involuntary actions that are applied and the effect of such actions.

Review: Relevant databases were systematically searched for studies investigating the involuntary treatment of individuals diagnosed with anorexia nervosa.

Results: The studies included in the review contained people treated in an inpatient setting for severe or severe and enduring anorexia nervosa. People that were treated involuntarily were characterised by a more severe psychiatric load. The levels of eating disorder pathology between involuntary and voluntary groups were similar and the outcome of involuntary treatment was comparable in terms of symptom reduction to that of voluntary treatment.

Conclusion: Despite inconsistent findings, the comparable levels of eating disorder pathology observed between involuntary and voluntary patient-groups together with findings of higher co-morbidity, more preadmissions, longer duration of illness and more incidences of self-harm for involuntary patients suggest that involuntary treatment is not a reaction to the severity of eating disorder symptoms alone, but is most likely a response to the complexity of the patient's situation as a whole.

Keywords: Anorexia nervosa, Forced treatment, Involuntary treatment, Coercion, Compulsory treatment, Tube feeding, Treatment outcome

Introduction

Anorexia nervosa (AN) is a serious illness with the highest mortality of all psychiatric diseases [1]. Treatment usually consists of at least one year of therapy and even the most effective treatment-results still leave around 50% of patients unremitted after 5 years [2,3]. People with severe or severe and enduring anorexia nervosa often need inpatient treatment and some are treated involuntary, either under formal coercion, persuasion by relatives or professionals, or through parental consent (for children and some adolescents - due to differences in parental consent laws). Involuntary treatment in relation to patients with anorexia nervosa is usually characterised by involuntary admission or detention following voluntary admission. Involuntary treatment may in some cases involve procedures such as forced feeding, restraint or referral to a locked ward.

Several articles have been published discussing the ethical, clinical or legal aspects of involuntary treatment including case reports exploring the consequences of

* Correspondence: loaclaus@rm.dk
[1]Centre of Child- and Adolescent Psychiatry, Aarhus University Hospital, Skovagervej 2, DK-8240 Risskov, Denmark
Full list of author information is available at the end of the article

either using or not using involuntary treatment; some advocate for the use of involuntary treatment [4,5], while others take a more critical stance to the practice [6,7].

A study by Guarda et al. [8] reported that patients admitted to inpatient and day-care programmes perceived a high level of coercion even though the treatment was not categorized as involuntary. One third of the patients sampled (N = 139) had a perception of not endorsing treatment upon admission, however, after two weeks of nutritional rehabilitation nearly half (43%) of the "coerced" patients perceived the treatment as necessary. Two other studies surveyed attitudes of patients and mothers of patients diagnosed with anorexia nervosa and found that the majority of those interviewed deemed the use of involuntary treatment as appropriate when risk of mortality is high [9,10].

In order to better understand and adequately assess the utility and legitimacy of involuntary treatment of patients with anorexia nervosa, a systematic evaluation of the conditions that determine involuntary treatment and the effect of such treatment is needed. A systematic evaluation of the effect of involuntary treatment is however lacking. Previous reviews of involuntary treatment have not focused specifically on the frequency, type and effect of involuntary treatment [11-13]. The review by Russell [13] provides an overview of ethical and legal aspects of involuntary treatment along with a brief summary of three studies published at the time [14-16]. The review by Thiel and Paul [11] is written in German and includes three studies published in English and one study published in German [14-17], with a brief English version published by Thiels [12]. The three articles review part of the research in the area of involuntary treatment, however, a systematic and updated review of all studies evaluating the frequency, type, and effect of involuntary treatment as well as patient characteristics is needed.

Aim of study

The aim of the present study is to systematically review the eating disorder literature in order to evaluate the frequency, duration, type and effect of involuntary treatment of people with anorexia nervosa as well as the characteristics of this group of patients.

Review

PubMed, Embase, and Cinahl databases were searched using the following search strategy: ((("Coercion" OR"Treatment Refusal") OR (Coercion[Mesh] OR Treatment Refusal [Mesh] OR"involuntary treatment" OR"forced treatment" OR"compulsory treatment" OR"forced feeding"))) AND ("Anorexia Nervosa"[Mesh] OR"Anorexia Nervosa"). No restrictions on date of publication were applied, with all studies published up until August 2013 included in the search. Articles published in the following languages were included: English, Danish, Swedish, and Norwegian. In addition, reference lists of relevant articles were searched for any articles that may have been missed by the initial search. Studies were included if they reported the effect (change in eating disorder symptoms e.g. BMI) of involuntary treatment of patients with anorexia nervosa. Single case studies were excluded.

Results

The initial search resulted in 191 articles. Figure 1 provides a flowchart of the process of study selection. Nine articles meeting the inclusion criteria were retrieved from the databases and an additional article was identified by searching the reference lists of relevant articles. Three out of the ten articles included for review contained the same sample, making a total of eight samples included in the review.

Table 1 provides a description of the eight studies including the following information: patient data (including type, age and number of patients), treatment type, treatment length, admission data, discharge data and follow-up data. Differences between involuntary and voluntary groups on all measures are shown in Table 2, and an assessment of the methodological quality of each study is presented in Table 3.

The N of the eight samples ranged between 11 and 397 patients, with a combined total of 873 patients (231 treated involuntary and 642 voluntary). One study examined the outcome of involuntary patients only [23], while the remaining studies compared patients treated involuntary with patients treated voluntary.

Six studies reported the frequency of involuntary treatment in total inpatient samples, with frequencies ranging from 13-44%. When comparing treatment duration between involuntary and voluntary patients, five out of seven studies reported significantly longer treatment durations for involuntary patients [14-16,18,22]. The type of involuntary treatment applied was also examined, with forced tube feeding used in four of the studies [17-19,23]. Two of the studies evaluated the frequency of tube feeding, finding a significantly higher frequency among involuntary treated patients [18,19]. Only one study reported the non-use of forced tube feeding or of physical restraint [15]. Finally, the study by Carney et al. found use of locked wards and episodes of re-feeding syndrome to be significantly higher for involuntary patients [19].

Involuntary and voluntary patient characteristics at treatment admission

All of the studies reported BMI at admission (see Table 2). However, BMI was not found to characterise group affiliation. Only the studies by Ayton et al. [18]

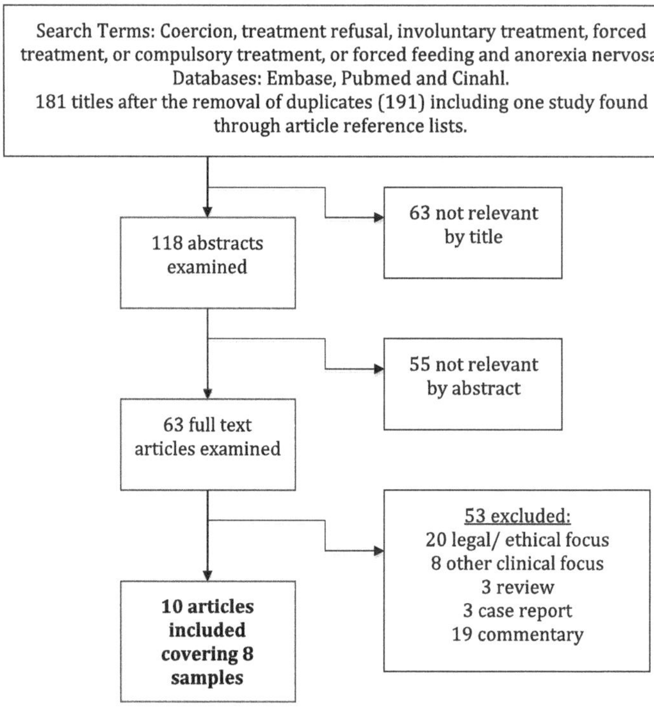

Figure 1 A flowchart of the process of study selection.

and Carney et al. [19] found significant differences between involuntary and voluntary treated patient groups, with the two studies reporting diverging results (see Table 2). Involuntary treated patients displayed a more severe psychiatric load compared to voluntary treated patients. For example, four out of six studies found significantly more preadmissions among patients treated involuntary [15,16,18,19], two out of four studies reported significantly higher co-morbidity in involuntary patients at baseline [18,19], and duration of illness was found to be significantly higher for involuntary patients in the study by Ayton et al. [18] Involuntary patients measured significantly higher on episodes of self-harm in two of the studies [15,18], physical or sexual abuse in one study [15], and significantly lower on age at illness onset [18], CGAS [18], IQ [16], and socioeconomic status (SES) [14].

Involuntary and voluntary patient characteristics at treatment discharge

All of the included studies reported patient data on weight at discharge, with overall findings indicating more similarities than differences between groups. No significant differences between groups on discharge BMI were observed in any of the studies (see Table 2), although the study by Watson et al. [16] found involuntary patients reported significantly greater increases in weight at discharge, and number of days needed to restore weight was found to be significantly longer for patients treated involuntary in the Ramsey et al. study [15].

Involuntary and voluntary patient characteristics at follow-up

Only three out of the eight studies included follow-up data. The study by Serfaty & McCluskey reported that 45% of involuntary patients sustained their weight above BMI 17.5, however no data were available for voluntary patients in this study [23]. The study by Ayton et al. found that patients treated involuntary reported significantly better outcome at follow-up compared to voluntary patients, including better general functioning and normalisation of weight [18]. Finally, Ramsey et al. reported a significant difference in mortality between groups, with a 13% mortality rate for the involuntary group compared to 3% for the voluntary group [15].

Discussion

Frequency, duration and type of involuntary treatment

The frequency of involuntary treatment was reported in six of the studies reviewed and ranged from 13-44% of patients treated for anorexia nervosa. The differences between studies in the percentage of patients treated involuntary may partly be explained by differences between patient populations in eating disorder symptom-

Table 1 Description and results of studies included in the review

Study	Patients/Age/N	Treatment type	Treatment length	Admission data	Discharge data	Follow-up data
1. Ayton et al. [18] **UK** **Naturalistic 3 years inclusion**	Adolescents	16 detained under section 3: 7/16 patients detained under VT, 9/16 before transfer to the clinic.	IT: 14 months	BMI: IT 16.6 ± 2.6, VT 14.2 ± 1.9	BMI: IT 19.6 ± 18.5 VT 18.5 ± 1.6	1 year follow-up
	Total N = 50	Nasogastric feeding:	VT: 8 months	Duration of illness: IT 3.8, VT 1.9	Menstrual period: 69% vs. 17%	N =41 (IT: 12/16 and VT: 29/34)
	IT: 16 (32%)	IT:69%, VT:12%		Age at onset: IT 12.5, VT 14.3	Overall ED outcome on M-R: IT 5.3 ± 3.1, VT 4 ± 2	Good outcome on weight and general functioning: IT 50%, VT 37.9%
	VT (parental consent): 34 (68%)			Purging type: IT 6%, VT 15%	HONOSCA: IT-28.1 ± 10.4, VT-18.3 ± 7.2	Readmissions:
				HONOSCA: IT 41.5 ± 4.8, VT 32 ± 5.0	CGAS: IT 47.2 ± 17.0, VT 36.6 ± 15.7	IT 16.7%, VT 34.5%
				Depression: IT 94%, VT 59% CGAS: IT 13 ± 6.5, VT 27 ± 9.0		Deaths: IT =0, VT =2
				Preadmissions: IT 88%, VT 29%		
				Low IQ: IT 19%, VT 3%		
				Abuse: IT 44%, VT 12%		
				Self-harm: IT 75%, VT 12%		
2. Carney et al. [19-21] **Australia** **Naturalistic 5 years inclusion**	Adults and adolescents.	Guardianship or mental health committal. Some tube feeding (46% vs. 16%). Locked ward (42% vs. 1%) Otherwise not defined.	IT: 52 days	BMI: IT 13.2 ± 1.7, VT 14.03 ± 1.8	BMI: IT 14.9 ± 1.4, VT 15.4 ± 2.3	
	Total N = 70		VT: 47 days	Purging type: IT 23%, VT 33%	Weight gain: IT 5.0 ± 6.6, VT 3.7 ± 5.3	
	70 patients with 96 admissions.		Mean: 49 days.	Preadmissions: IT 3.9 ± 3.4, VT 1.7 ± 2.3,		
	IT: 23 (33%)		40% <3 weeks.	Psychiatric comorbidity: IT 2 ± 1.6, VT 1 ± 0.9		
	VT: 47 (67%)					

Table 1 Description and results of studies included in the review *(Continued)*

3. Griffiths et al. [14], Australia Naturalistic,	Age 16–44 years	Guardianship.	IT: 15 weeks	BMI: IT 13.41 ± 1.76, VT 14.3 ± 2.2	BMI: IT 18.05 ± 2.14, VT 17.2 ± 2.9	3 of 15 IT patients reached at follow-up – 1 of 15 died, 4 not located.
IT cases from 4 units compared to VT from one of the units.	Total N = 88	Otherwise not defined.	VT: 9 weeks	Binge/purge type: IT 60%, VT 43%	Weight gain: IT 10 kg, VT 8.7	
	IT: 15 (17%)			Residence - metropolitan: IT 67%, VT 50%	Reached target weight: IT 26.7%, VT 42%	
	VT: 73 (83%)			SES: IT 40%, VT 11%		
4. Kondo et al. [22] Japan	Age 12–44 years	Involuntary admission for treatment and protection.	IT: 216 days	BMI: IT 15.3 ± 5.1,	Good outcome BMI:	
Naturalistic	Total N = 70		VT: 70 days	VT 14.6 ± 8.0	IT 75%, VT 55%	
	IT: 8 (13%)					
	VT: 62					
5. Laakman et al. [17] Germany Naturalistic, all patients from 1 unit.	Age 16-39	Guardianship, forced feeding by tube until BMI = 17.5	Total 158 days	BMI:	BMI:	
	Total N = 25		IT: 183 days	IT: 11.8	IT: 16.6	
	IT: 11 (44%)		P: 166 days	P: 11.9	P: 16.7	
	Persuaded (P):		PC: 145 days	PC: 14.6	PC: 17.8	
	7 (28%)		VT: 98 days	VT: 12.1	VT: 18.8	
	Parental consent (PC): 2 (8%)					
	VT: 5 (20%)					
6. Ramsay et al. [15] UK	Adults	7/81 involuntary admitted, 30/81	IT: 113 days	BMI: IT 14.2 ± 2.7, VT 14.3 ± 2.4),	BMI: IT 18.7 ± 2.3,	5.7 years follow-up:
Time matched controls	Total N = 162	Detained after voluntary admission, 35/81 detained in other hospital before transfer to unit.	VT: 88 days	Bingeing history: IT 41%, VT 44%	VT 18.5 ± 2.0.	Deaths: IT 12.7% vs. VT 2.6%

Table 1 Description and results of studies included in the review *(Continued)*

	IT: 81 (50%)	No tube-feeding or physical restraint.		Vomiting history: IT 51%, VT 44%	Days to target weight (equal to treatment length:	9 out of 12 death certificates included AN
	VT: 81 (50%)			Laxative history: IT 49%, VT 49%	IT 113 days, VT 88 days	
				Preadmissions: IT 3.3, VT 1.8 Childhood abuse: IT 24%, VT 10%		
				Self-harm: IT 59% vs. VT 33%		
7. Serfaty & McCluskey [23] **UK** **Naturalistic cases** **Patients in IT only**	Adults	Involuntary admitted only	Not specified	Mean BMI: 12.7	Mean BMI: 18.6	Mean Follow-up time 1 year
	Total N = 11	7/11 Nasogastric feeding.		Duration of illness 14.1 year	BMI >17.5 = 27%	Mean BMI: 17.9
	All treated involuntary					BMI >17.5 = 45.5%
8. Watson et al. [16] **USA** **Naturalistic** **7 years inclusion**	Adults	Involuntary admitted.	IT: 58 days	BMI: IT 17.4 ± 4.7, VT 18.4 ± 4.7 Preadmissions: IT 3, VT 1.4	BMI: IT 20.5 ± 3.8, VT 20.7 ± 3.6	
	Total N = 397		VT: 41 days	IQ: IT 91, VT 98	Weight gain: IT 18.8 ± 15.9, VT 13.9 ± 14.5 pounds	
	IT: 66 (17%)			Equal eating disorder symptoms, depression, and substance abuse.	Days to restored weight: IT: 58 days	
	VT: 331 (83%)				VT: 41 days (Equal to treatment length)	

IT = Involuntary Treatment; VT = Voluntary Treatment; BMI = Body Mass Index; HONOSCA = Health of the Nation Outcome Scale for Children and Adolescents; CGAS = Children's Global Assessment Scale: IQ = Intelligence quotient from the WAIS-R; SES = Socioeconomic Status; M-R = Morgan – Russell scale (eating disorder psychopathology).

Table 2 Measures at admission, discharge and follow-up

Study (ref.):	1 [18]	2 [19]	3 [14]	4 [22]	5 [17]	6 [15]	7 [23]	8 [16]
Admission/Discharge/Follow-up:								
BMI	A↑*, D↑	A↓*, D↓,	A↓, D↑	A↑, D↑	A↑, D↓	A↓, D↑	A, D, F	A↓, D↓
Duration of illness	A↑*	A↑			A↑	A↑	A	A↑
Age at onset	↓*							
Purging (bingeing) type		A↓	A↑			A↑ (A↓)		
Menstrual period	D↑*							
M-R	A, D↑							
HONOSCA	A↑*, D↓*							
BDI-2	A↑*							
C-GAS	A↓*, D↑*							
Preadmissions	A↑*	A↑*	A↑		A↓	A↑*		A↑*
Prior involuntary treatment						A↑		
Comorbid psychiatric disorders	A↑*	A↑*				A↑		A↑
IQ	A↓							A↓*
Physical or sexual abuse	A↑					A↑*		
Self-harm	A↑*					A↑*		
Substance abuse								A↑
SES			A↓*					
Treatment:								
Duration of treatment	↑*	↑	↑*	↑*	↑	↑*		↑*
Premature discharge	↓							
Frequency of re-feeding syndrome		↑*						
Frequency of tube feeding	↑*	↑*			↑		?	
Locked vs. open ward		↑*						
Treatment outcome:								
Weight increase			D↑		D↑	D↑		D↑*
Days to restored weight						↑*		↑
Reached target weight			D↓					D↓
Rate of weight restoration lb/week								D↑
Good outcome	F↑*			D↑				
Readmissions	F↓							
Death	F↓					F↑*		

A = Admission; D = Discharge; F = Follow-up; ↑ = higher for the involuntary group; ↓ = lower for the involuntary group; * = significant differences between groups ($p < 0.05$); ? = not specified; BMI = Body Mass Index; M-R = Morgan – Russell scale (eating disorder psychopathology); HONOSCA = Health of the Nation Outcome Scale for Children and Adolescents; BDI-2 = Beck Depression Inventory –2; CGAS = Children's Global Assessment Scale: IQ = Intelligence quotient from the WAIS-R; SES = Socioeconomic Status.

severity and co-morbidity. For example, in the 44% group [17] adults had a mean admission BMI of 11.8, while in a 17% group adults had a mean admission BMI of 17.4 [16]. However, when comparing mean BMI at admission with the percentage of involuntary treatment across all studies the picture is less clear. Due to the controversial nature of forced intervention, cultural, organisational and procedural/legal differences between institutions and countries must also be considered, as decisions regarding treatment may be based more on tradition and local regulations and procedures and less on symptom severity or evidence of treatment efficacy [24,25]. A study examining compulsory admission regulations and procedures across countries in the European Union reported that the differences in regulations and procedures across countries were the most significant source of variance [26]. Also, in addition to patient characteristics, hospital characteristics were shown to be an independent predictor of involuntary treatment in a Swiss population [27].

Table 3 Quality-assessment of study methodology*

Study (ref.):	1 [18]	2 [19]	3 [14]	4 [22]	5 [17]	6 [15]	7 [23]	8 [16]	Mean	Max.**
Reporting	8	7	4	6	5	8	3	9	6.25	11
External validity	1	1	0	1	1	2	0	2	1.00	3
Internal validity - bias	2	3	1	1	1	2	1	2	1.63	7
Internal validity – selection bias	3	3	1	3	1	3	0	3	2.13	6
Total score	14	14	6	11	8	15	4	16	11.0	27

*Sub-scale scores on the *checklist for measuring study quality* by Downs & Black.[27]
Note: Higher scores indicate better methodological quality.
Reporting: degree to which information provided in the study is sufficient to allow an unbiased assessment of the findings (scale 0–11).
External validity: degree to which the findings from the study could be generalised to the population from which the study subjects were derived (scale 0–3).
Internal validity-bias: degree to which the study addressed biases in the measurement of the intervention and the outcome (scale 0–7).
Internal validity - selection bias: degree to which the study addressed bias in the selection of study subjects (scale 0–6).
**The highest possible mean score on the subscale.

Information on the type and process of involuntary treatment was very limited in the studies included for review. Type of involuntary treatment can include, but is not limited to, use of physical restraint (including use of straps), locked wards, forced feeding and forced medication. Four of the studies reviewed reported the use of tube feeding [17-19,23], and one study explicitly reported the non-use of tube feeding and physical restraint [15]. Overall, studies show that there is a higher frequency of tube feeding for involuntary patients, however the notable lack of information on type of involuntary treatment needs to be addressed in future studies.

Effect of involuntary treatment

Treatment under involuntary conditions seems to last longer and include more tube feeding, more re-feeding syndrome and use of locked wards. Interestingly, the overall effect of involuntary treatment appears to be comparable to voluntary treatment. When comparing group differences in BMI at discharge across studies the results are inconclusive with any variance in treatment outcome probably masked by treatment continuing until target-weight was reached [14-18]. Weight increase was shown to be significantly higher [16] and time taken to restore weight significantly longer for involuntary patients [15]. The follow-up data on treatment effect is sparse and results are mixed making any conclusions on the long-term effect of involuntary versus voluntary treatment difficult. The higher mortality rate observed in the Ramsey et al. [15] study compared to the Ayton et al. [18] study for involuntary patients is likely due to the difference in mean age across samples. Studies evaluating the long-term effect of voluntary versus involuntary treatment should control for age as outcome measures may differ between adolescent and older-adult populations.

The effect of different types of involuntary treatment is also unclear. To the best of our knowledge there is only one randomised controlled trial in which the efficacy of an "involuntary-type" treatment modality was examined (the study was not included in the review as the treatment was not reported as involuntary). Rigaud et al. [28] randomly assigned inpatients to either combined tube-feeding and normal meals or normal meals only. The combined tube feeding and normal meals group were found to gain more weight, display fewer bingeing episodes and have longer relapse-free periods compared to the normal meals only group [28].

Determinants of involuntary treatment/patient characteristics

When looking at severity in eating disorder symptoms at admission across studies the results are mixed with more similarities than differences observed between involuntary and voluntary groups. Duration of illness was a significant predictor of involuntary treatment for adolescent patients in the Ayton et al. [18] study, with four other studies finding duration of illness to be higher for involuntary patients – although not reaching significance [15-17,19]. Longer duration of illness, together with findings of higher psychiatric co-morbidity, more preadmissions, and more incidences of self-harm for involuntary patient groups, suggest that involuntary treatment is not a reaction to the severity of eating disorder symptoms alone, but is most likely a response to the complexity of the patient's situation as a whole. BMI at admission was expected to partly determine treatment choice, however, this was not clearly shown in the present review. Involuntary treatment is initiated on the basis of either the dangerousness criterion or the need-for-treatment criterion indicating a more severe status. If, as the current review suggests, involuntary treated patients are not predominantly more somatically threatened by eating disorder pathology than voluntary patients, then what other factors are being taken into consideration when prescribing this forced intervention? Somatic problems such as cardiac arrhythmia or severe electrolyte imbalance, or threat due to suicidal thoughts/ideation could all be reasons for involuntary treatment, however, none of these problems are reported in any of the studies reviewed.

Study limitations and concluding remarks

Due to the relatively small number of studies evaluating involuntary treatment in anorexia nervosa it is difficult to know if the results reported in the present review are representative of involuntary treatment in general. The majority of studies included compulsory admission and involuntary treatment cohorts. Information on treatment admission was limited in two of the studies [14,23] making it unclear as to whether treatment admission was involuntary for all patients or whether some patients were admitted on a voluntary basis and then treated involuntary. In two of the studies [14,18] it was noted that is was possible for voluntary treatment to precede involuntary treatment, but further information was not made available. Also, the studies reviewed provide sparse information on the involuntary treatment applied. In general the methodological quality of the studies was low. This was due in part to the reliance on retrospective data collection (from medical journals) and naturalistic research designs. Table 3 shows an assessment of the methodological quality of each study (measured using the *checklist for measuring study quality* by Downs and Black [29]) with overall scores indicating issues with external validity, internal validity, and selection bias. Moreover, with the exception of the studies by Ramsey et al. [15] and Watson et al. [16], studies included in the review lacked sufficient statistical power to detect medium (clinically relevant) effect sizes due to limited sample sizes in the involuntary treatment groups. The overall low level of methodological quality in the studies included in the review is a limitation and must be taken into consideration when interpreting the present findings.

The present findings reflect the complexity of the situation that people with severe anorexia nervosa find themselves in. There is a clear need for large, well designed studies reporting the frequency, type and effect of involuntary treatment in relation to voluntary treatment, as well as the characteristics of patients admitted to involuntary treatment. A better understanding of the determining conditions and effect of involuntary treatment may aid in developing clearer guidelines in the use of this forced intervention.

While this article was under review a comparable article was published [30]. The comparable article includes a more recent search, and uses different inclusion criteria than the present study with less focus on predictors and the effect of involuntary treatment, and more focus on clinical analysis. Despite these differences, the overall results and conclusions are similar across studies.

Competing interests

The authors declare that they have no competing interests.

Author's contributions

Both authors have contributed mutually to the completion of the article. LC was responsible for the conception of the study, the acquisition of data, and the preparation of the first draft of the article. AJ gave intellectual and critical input to all aspects of the article and contributed to several draft revisions. Both authors read and approved the final draft of the article.

Author details

[1]Centre of Child- and Adolescent Psychiatry, Aarhus University Hospital, Skovagervej 2, DK-8240 Risskov, Denmark. [2]Institute of Psychology, University of Southern Denmark, Campusvej 55, DK-5230 Odense M, Denmark.

References

1. Arcelus J, Mitchell AJ, Wales J, Nielsen S: **Mortality rates in patients with anorexia nervosa and other eating disorders. A meta-analysis of 36 studies.** *Arch Gen Psychiatry* 2011, **68**:724–731.
2. Berkman ND, Bulik CM, Brownley KA, Lohr KN, Sedway JA, Rooks A, Gartlehner G: **Management of eating disorders.** *Evid Rep Technol Assess (Full Rep)* 2006, **135**:1–166.
3. Brown TA, Keel PK: **Current and emerging directions in the treatment of eating disorders.** *Subst Abuse* 2012, **6**:33–61.
4. Holm JS, Brixen K, Andries A, Horder K, Stoving RK: **Reflections on involuntary treatment in the prevention of fatal anorexia nervosa: a review of five cases.** *Int J Eat Disord* 2012, **45**:93–100.
5. Nielsen J, Jeppesen NE, Brixen KT, Horder K, Stoving RK: **Severe anorexia nervosa: five fatal cases.** *Ugeskr Laeger* 2008, **170**:1158.
6. Campbell AT, Aulisio MP: **The stigma of "mental" illness: end stage anorexia and treatment refusal.** *Int J Eat Disord* 2012, **45**:627–634.
7. Mishra R: **The case: Starving for perfection.** *Camb Q Healthc Ethics* 2012, **21**:396–397.
8. Guarda AS, Pinto AM, Coughlin JW, Hussain S, Haug NA, Heinberg LJ: **Perceived coercion and change in perceived need for admission in patients hospitalized for eating disorders.** *Am J Psychiatry* 2007, **164**:108–114.
9. Tan JO, Hope T, Stewart A, Fitzpatrick R: **Control and compulsory treatment in anorexia nervosa: the views of patients and parents.** *Int J Law Psychiatry* 2003, **26**:627–645.
10. Tan JOA, Stewart A, Fitzpatrick R, Hope T: **Attitudes of patients with anorexia nervosa to compulsory treatment and coercion.** *Int J Law Psychiatry* 2010, **33**:13–19.
11. Thiel A, Paul T: **Compulsory treatment in anorexia nervosa.** *Psychother Psychosom Med Psychol* 2007, **57**:128–135.
12. Thiels C: **Forced treatment of patients with anorexia.** *Curr Opin Psychiatry* 2008, **21**:495–498.
13. Russell GFM: **Involuntary treatment in anorexia nervosa.** *Psychiatr Clin North Am* 2001, **24**:337–349.
14. Griffiths RA, Beumont PJ, Russell J, Touyz SW, Moore G: **The use of guardianship legislation for anorexia nervosa: a report of 15 cases.** *Aust N Z J Psychiatry* 1997, **31**:525–531.
15. Ramsay R, Ward A, Treasure J, Russell GF: **Compulsory treatment in anorexia nervosa. Short-term benefits and long-term mortality.** *Br J Psychiatry* 1999, **175**:147–153.
16. Watson TL, Bowers WA, Andersen AE: **Involuntary treatment of eating disorders.** *Am J Psychiatry* 2000, **157**:1806–1810.
17. Laakmann G, Ortner M, Kamleiter M, Ufer S, Frodl T, Goldstein-Muller B, Jäger M, Padberg F, Sadowsky N, Tischinger M, Stec I: **Treatment of vitally endangered anorexia nervosa patients based on guardianship laws.** *Nervenarzt* 2006, **77**:35–40.
18. Ayton A, Keen C, Lask B: **Pros and cons of using the mental health act for severe eating disorders in adolescents.** *Eur Eat Disorders Rev* 2009, **17**:14–23.
19. Carney T, Wakefield A, Tait D, Touyz S: **Reflections on coercion in the treatment of severe anorexia nervosa.** *Isr J Psychiatry Relat Sci* 2006, **43**:159–165.
20. Carney T, Tait D, Touyz S: **Coercion is coercion? Reflections on trends in the use of compulsion in treating anorexia nervosa.** *Aust Psychiatry* 2007, **15**:390–395.
21. Carney T, Tait D, Richardson A, Touyz S: **Why (and when) clinicians compel treatment of anorexia nervosa patients.** *Eur Eat Disord Rev* 2008, **16**:199–206.
22. Kondo T, Takaoka K, Ikawa N, Niwa N: **Law relating to compulsory treatment of patients with anorexia nervosa.** *Int Med J* 2004, **11**:281–284.

23. Serfaty M, McCluskey S: **Compulsory treatment of anorexia nervosa and the moribund patient.** *Eur Eat Disorders Rev* 1998, **6**:27–37.
24. Jacobsen TB: **Involuntary treatment in Europe: different countries, different practices.** *Curr Opin Psychiatry* 2012, **25**:307–310.
25. Touyz SW, Carney T: *Compulsory (involuntary) treatment for anorexia nervosa.* New York: The Guilford Press; 2010.
26. Salize HJ, Dressing H, Peitz M: *Compulsory admission and involuntary treatment of mental ill patients - Legislation and practice in EU-member states.* Mannheim Germany: Central Insitute of Mental Health; 2002.
27. Lay B, Nordt C, Rossler W: **Variation in use of coercive measures in psychiatric hospitals.** *Eur Psychiatry* 2011, **26**:244–251.
28. Rigaud D, Brondel L, Poupard AT, Talonneau I, Brun JM: **A randomized trial on the efficacy of a 2-month tube feeding regimen in anorexia nervosa: A 1-year follow-up study.** *Clin Nutr* 2007, **26**:421–429.
29. Downs SH, Black N: **The feasibility of creating a checklist for the assessment of the methodological quality both of randomised and non-randomised studies of health care interventions.** *J Epidemiol Community Health* 1998, **52**:377–384.
30. Elzakkers I, Danner U, Hoek H, Schmidt U, Elburg A: **Compulsory treatment in anorexia norvosa: a review.** *Int J Eat Disord* 2014, **00**:000-000. doi:10.1002/eat.22330.

Psychosocial outcomes of a non-dieting based positive body image community program for overweight adults: a pilot study

Lisa Bloom[1], Beth Shelton[2,3], Melissa Bengough[3] and Leah Brennan[4*]

Abstract

Background: The limited success of traditional diet focused obesity interventions has led to the development of alternative non-dieting approaches. The current study evaluated the impact of a community based non-dieting positive body image program for overweight/obese people on a range of psychosocial outcomes. The characteristics of this real-world sample presenting for a non-dieting weight management intervention are also described.

Method: Overweight and obese participants enrolled in the eight week 'No More Diets' (NMD) group program completed self-report questionnaires assessing disordered eating thoughts and behaviours, body image, motivation for exercise and psychopathology pre- and post-treatment.

Results: Participants (n = 17; 16 female) were aged between 19 and 78 years, with a BMI ranging from 25.2 kg/m^2 (Overweight) to 55.9 kg/m^2 (Severely Obese). They reported elevated levels of eating disorder pathology, body shape preoccupation, depression, anxiety and stress compared to community norms ($p < .05$). Following treatment there were significant improvements in reported body shape preoccupation, shape concern and eating attitudes ($p < .05$), and clinically significant changes (small to medium effect sizes; 0.3-0.35) for improvements in reported weight concern, eating competence, stress and health evaluation. There were no changes in reported dietary restraint, emotional eating and uncontrolled eating, or eating concern ($p > .05$).

Conclusion: Individuals presenting for the NMD program demonstrated increased eating disorder pathology and more generalised psychopathology compared to community norms. The NMD program was particularly beneficial for body image and shape concern. Addressing these body image factors may help to address some of the perpetuating factors of obesity and disordered eating, which are often not addressed in the traditional diet-based weight loss interventions.

Keywords: Obesity, Non-dieting, Community, Body image, Intervention, Disordered eating

Background

Eating disorders, obesity and unhealthy dieting practices share common psychopathology, and can have serious adverse effects on psychological and physical health [1-3], For example, there is evidence that obesity can eventuate in people with bulimic eating disorders and Binge Eating Disorder [4] and levels of body dissatisfaction can be higher in obese populations compared to populations with Anorexia Nervosa [5,6]. Regardless of the method, the goal of traditional obesity interventions, including diet, exercise, behavioural, pharmacological and surgical weight loss, is a reduction in excess body fat, and these approaches often fail to address the perpetuating factors common to both obesity and eating disorders. This emphasis on weight loss is driven by beliefs that excess weight increases morbidity and mortality, sustainable weight loss is possible, and the risks associated with obesity will decrease when weight is lost [7].

The link between obesity and mortality and morbidity is generally accepted [8], however, recent research suggests that this relationship may not be as strong as once thought in the mild to moderately obese [9]. It has also been proposed that some obesity related co-morbidities may be the result of ineffective dieting rather than excess weight [10]. High levels of dietary restraint have been linked to weight

* Correspondence: leah.brennan@acu.edu.au
[4]School of Psychology, Australian Catholic University, Melbourne, Australia
Full list of author information is available at the end of the article

gain [11] and to weight cycling [12]. Weight cycling (the repeated gains and losses of weight over time) has been shown to increase risk for cardiovascular disease, depression, and mortality [13-15].

Dietary restraint has also been associated with psychological distress, including anxiety, food and weight preoccupation, disordered eating and eating disorders, particularly binge eating [16-18]. It is believed that dieting creates a vulnerability to binge eating and problems with eating regulation [19]. Research is not clear about what comes first, dieting or binge-eating in obese individuals [20]. Despite this, levels of binge eating and dietary restraint are positively correlated [21] and binge eating, not overall weight, has been found to be a predictor of psychopathology amongst obese treatment-seeking individuals [22]. Additionally, levels of dietary restraint have been found to be comparable between populations with obesity and populations with Anorexia Nervosa [5,19].

Failure to achieve desired weight loss may also lead to further psychological distress [17,18]. Most people enrolling in a weight loss interventions expect to lose up to 30% of their body weight, however short-term weight loss goals of 5-10% are more commonly achieved [21]. A 5-10% weight loss is considered to be clinically significant and is recommended by most expert bodies [23-25]. There are few studies available examining the impact of long-term weight loss on obesity related risk. Those that are available indicate that long-term maintenance of weight loss is rare [26,27] and that the majority of participants are likely to have returned to baseline weight or higher at 2–5 year follow-up [28,29]. There is also increasing evidence that health improvements can occur without significant weight loss in mild to moderately overweight individuals. For example, cardiovascular fitness, blood pressure improvement and reduction in medical symptoms have been shown to occur in response to health behaviour change independently of weight loss [7,30]. Individuals can also improve a number of health outcomes (e.g., recommended physical activity levels, healthy blood pressure, reduced mortality and morbidity rates), whilst still being classified as overweight or obese [31].

Considering that the prevalence of obesity is rising [32], weight loss is difficult to maintain long-term [26,27], and health outcomes can improve in some individuals without weight loss [7,30], alternatives to the traditional obesity treatment paradigm are being explored. Such alternatives include non-dieting programs. Non dieting approaches view weight management from a health-centred approach, with health outcomes as goals rather than weight loss per se. This philosophy is based on the belief that biopsychosocial outcomes can improve without significant weight loss [33,34]. Healthy eating patterns in response to internal satiety and hunger cues, physical activity for the purpose of pleasure and health acceptance of bodies at different shapes and sizes are encouraged [35].

Efficacy studies of non-dieting interventions have demonstrated improvements in eating behaviours and attitudes, including decreases in dietary restraint, disinhibition, overall eating disorder risk, and binge eating, and greater awareness of hunger and satiety cues [5,36-41]. They have also shown physiological changes, including improvements in metabolic fitness (e.g., pulse reading, blood pressure, cholesterol) without significant weight loss [5,36-40]. In a recent review, in four of seven studies, these improvements in the non-dieting group were significantly better than traditional weight control groups [42]. These studies have all examined the efficacy of non-dieting interventions, in controlled efficacy studies [42]. Effectiveness trials (interventions implemented in real-world clinical and community settings) of non-dieting approaches are still required.

The 'No More Diets' (NMD) program is an example of a non-dieting community intervention. The program targets those experiencing weight cycling and disordered eating patterns with the goal of achieving a range of health improvements. It targets health behaviours such as; healthy normalised eating patterns based on cues of hunger and satiety, positive body image, and maintained physical movement that is practical, sustainable and enjoyable. The current pilot study will provide an opportunity to examine the effectiveness of the NMD program delivered to overweight and obese adults in a community setting. The current study aimed to examine (1) the psychosocial characteristics of NMD participants, (2) differences in pre-treatment characteristics of participants who did and did not complete the program, and (3) the impact of NMD on psychosocial outcomes of participants.

Method

Participants

Participants were recruited to the NMD program via advertisements distributed by MonashLink Community Health Centre, an article in the local newspaper, or through referral from participants' current health professional at MonashLink. There were no formal exclusion criteria.

Materials

Participants completed a number of self-report questionnaires:

Demographic Questionnaire This questionnaire was developed for the purpose of the NMD program. It includes information about height and weight, family structure, educational level, employment status, eating and activity history.

Eating Disorder Examination - Questionnaire (EDE-Q) [43]. This 28-item questionnaire measures four aspects of the psychopathology of eating disorders. The items are rated on a 6-point scale with higher scores reflecting greater severity of psychopathology. The four subscales are Restraint (e.g., avoidance of food, dietary rules), Eating Concern (e.g., food preoccupation), Weight Concern and Shape Concern (e.g., preoccupation and dissatisfaction with weight and shape). It has adequate internal consistency (α = .70, .73, .72 and .83 respectively) and convergent and discriminant validity (r = .79-.81 and .78-.85) [43,44].

Three Factor Eating Questionnaire - Revised 21 Items (TFEQ-21) [45]. This revised version of the Three Factor Eating Questionnaire measures eating behaviour in three domains [46]. Twenty-one items comprise the revised scale; Cognitive Restraint (restricting food intake in order to influence weight), Emotional Eating (eating in response to negative mood states) and Uncontrolled Eating (overeating behaviours). Items are rated on a 4-point scale. The scales have adequate internal consistency (α = .76, .83 and .85 respectively) and convergent and discriminant validity [45].

ecSatter Inventory [47]. This 16-item scale measures eating competence. Items are rated on a 5-point Likert scale. The four subscales are Contextual Skills (measuring skills relate to selecting, preparing and planning meals), Eating Attitude (measuring levels of comfort associated with food and eating), Food Acceptance (openness to a wide range of foods) and Internal Regulation (eating behaviours in response to internal satiety cues), and a total Eating Competence score. It has adequate construct validity and internal consistency (α = .79, .82, .70, .71 and .85 respectively) [47,48].

Multidimensional Body Self-Relations Questionnaire (MBSRQ) [49]. This 69-item questionnaire measures body image and attitudes towards the self. The Appearance Evaluation (measuring self-ratings and attitudes towards one's appearance), Fitness Evaluation (self-ratings and attitudes towards fitness levels) and Health Evaluation (self-ratings of feelings of healthiness) subscales were used for the current study. Items are rated on a 5-point scale ranging from 'definitely disagree' to 'definitely agree'. The scales have adequate internal consistency (α = .88, .77 and .83 respectively) [49].

Body Shape Questionnaire (BSQ) [50]. This 36-item scale measures body shape preoccupations and levels of body dissatisfaction and associated distress over a 4 week period. Items are rated on a 6-point Likert scale ranging from 'Never' to 'Always'. It has adequate reliability (α = .88) and good concurrent validity for clinical and non-clinical samples [51].

Depression, Stress and Anxiety Scale (DASS) [52]. This 42-item questionnaire measures symptoms of depression, anxiety and stress. The three subscales (Depression, Anxiety and Stress) are answered on a 4-point severity/frequency scale of symptoms over the last week. It has adequate internal consistency (α = .81, .73 and .81 respectively) [42] and convergent and discriminant validity [53].

Exercise Motivations Inventory - version 2 (EMI-2) [54]. This 51-item questionnaire measures reasons for exercise. The subscales used in the current study were Enjoyment and Weight Management (e.g., Personally I exercise, or might exercise to stay slim). Items are rated on a 5-point scale. It has adequate reliability (α = .89 and .91) and convergent and discriminant validity for both exercisers and non-exercisers [54].

Procedure

This study was approved by the Monash University Human Research Ethics Committee and the RMIT University Human Research Ethics committee prior to commencement. The program was delivered at MonashLink Community Health Service, a non-profit organization funded by a variety of government programs, providing a range of health and well-being services to people living and working within the City of Monash, Melbourne, Victoria, Australia. Participants approached the community centre for the purposes of attending the NMD program.

A psychologist (BS) and a dietician (MB) from MonashLink Community Health's Disordered Eating Service adapted the NMD program from the Set Your Body Free programs of Paxton and colleagues [55-57]. The program consisted of 8 weekly 2 hour sessions; session content is outlined in Table 1. The program ran twice over a 6 month period. The first program was facilitated by a psychologist and dietician, and the second by a dietician and mental health counsellor. The initial group had 12 participants; the second group had 9 participants.

In the first week of the program, participants completed the questionnaire booklet as part of the program evaluation. A plain language statement and consent form invited the participants to allow the data in the questionnaires to be used in the current study. During the final session, all participants were given the questionnaire booklet to complete after the program and post back to the NMD facilitators. Missing data was collected via telephone contact with participants following the return of their questionnaires. The researcher was provided with the data of those participants who had consented for their data to be used in research.

Statistical analyses

All statistical analyses were completed using the software package Statistical Package for Social Sciences (SPSS; Version 20). Data screening, missing data analysis and assumption testing were conducted prior to commencement of data analysis. There was no missing data. As this was a study of a 'real-world' intervention taking place in the community, power analysis was not completed. Similarly, as this was an exploratory study alpha levels were not adjusted to account for inflation in Type 1 error due to multiple comparisons. Given the small sample size and the

Table 1 NMD weekly session outline

Week	Food & eating topics	Body image topics	Movement activity
1	Why diets do not work	Looking at spine and identifying basic spinal movements to music	
2	Regular eating pattern	Exploration of pros and cons of body acceptance and body dissatisfaction	Introduction to image-based movement improvisation
3	Hunger Scale	Introduction of concept of overvaluation of shape & weight	Integration of a learnt sequence in pairs and improvisation
4	Hungry eating vs non-hungry eating	Introduction of concepts of extreme &/or unhelpful cognitions regarding body image	Continued integration of learnt sequences and reflection of effects of movement
5	How to reduce non-hungry eating	Coping with extreme &/or unhelpful cognitions regarding body image	Movement composition to music
6	Eating with awareness	Review of concepts & effects of overvaluation of shape & weight, avoidance & body checking	Movement sequences and improvisation with reflection
7	Fine tuning nutritional knowledge	Linking movement with community options: guest instructor to demonstrate available exercise programs	
8	Overview and reflection		

Note: Each session ran for 2 hours.

exploratory nature of this study both statistically significant and clinically significant results are discussed. Effect sizes are also presented using the following range: $r = .2$ small, $r = .5$ medium, and $r = .8$ large effect size [58]. Non-parametric tests were used due to the small sample size. In line with the requirements of non-parametric tests, medians are reported instead of means for analyses where appropriate.

The psychosocial characteristics of the sample were described by comparing scores on the measures to published norms from normal and clinical samples using a Wilcoxon Signed Rank test. Normative comparative samples were selected on the basis that they used the appropriate measures, and participant characteristics (e.g., sex) could be matched where possible. The EDE-Q normal sample consisted of females aged over 16 years [59]. The TFEQ sample consisted of middle-aged females [60]. The EcSatter sample consisted of overweight and physically active adults [47]. The MBSRQ sample consisted of females aged over 18 years [49]. The BSQ normal sample consisted of female university students [50] and the DASS 21 normal sample consisted of males and females aged over 17 years [52]. For clinical samples, a diagnosis of an eating disorder and the relevant measure was required, as well as matching characteristics where possible. The EDE-Q clinical sample consisted of females with Anorexia Nervosa [59]. The BSQ sample consisted of females with Bulimia Nervosa [50]. The DASS 21 sample consisted of adolescents and adults with Anorexia Nervosa [61]. The sample was also compared to clinical cut-offs where available. Participants who completed the program were compared with data from participants who dropped out using a Mann–Whitney test. Pre- and post-scores on the outcome measures were compared using related samples Wilcoxon Signed Rank tests.

Results

Of the 21 participants who enrolled in the NMD program, 17 (81%) consented to participate in the study, as outlined in Figure 1. The participants (16 females, 1 male) were aged between 19 and 78 years ($M = 56.45$, $SD = 16.19$). The majority were born in Australia (71%) and 82% identified Australian as their ethnicity. Thirty-five per cent

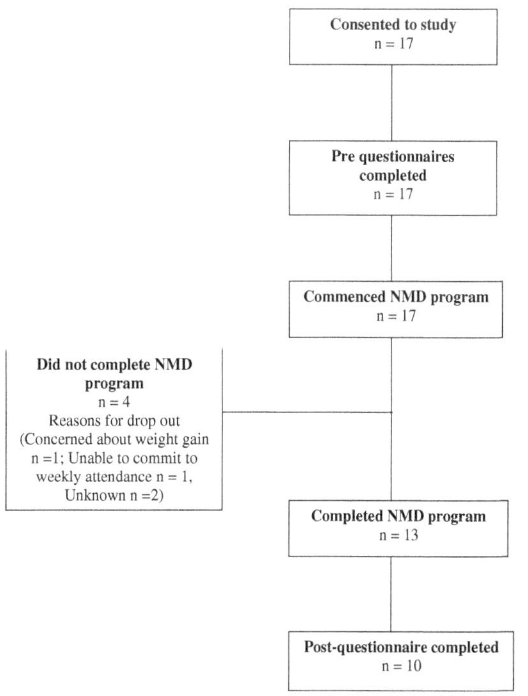

Figure 1 Data collection process from consent stage to return of post-questionnaire.

were married, 6% defacto, 18% divorced or separated, 18% never married, and 23% widowers. Almost half (47.1%) had trade or tertiary qualifications. Twenty-four percent were employed (12% part-time; 12% full-time), 35% were retired and 41% were either unemployed, unable to work, or not working due to caring/parenting commitments. Participants' self-reported weight ranged between 69.8 to 156.0 kg ($M = 92.69$, $SD = 20.88$) and their body mass index (BMI; kg/m^2), calculated based on self-reported height and weight, ranged between 25.2 (Overweight) to 55.9 (Severely Obese) ($M = 34.17$, $SD = 8.57$).

Table 2 illustrates the means and standard deviations for each variable, and clinical-cut offs where appropriate. Over a third (35.4%) of participants scored within the clinical range for concerns about weight. More than half (59%) the participants scored within the clinical range on levels of depression, while almost half scored within the clinical range on levels of stress (41%) and anxiety (47%). Participants reported that binge eating episodes occurred on a mean of 4.65 days ($SD = 6.23$) in the past 28 days.

Scale scores obtained from the study sample were compared to the most appropriate community and clinical samples (Table 3). Severity of eating disorder pathology was compared to a normal [43] and a clinical eating disorder female sample [59]. Participants reported significantly higher scores compared to the community sample on levels of eating concern, shape concern and weight concern. Participants obtained lower scores compared to a sample of females with Anorexia Nervosa on levels of restraint, eating concern, and weight concern.

Level of preoccupations and concerns about body image were also compared to a community sample of women and a clinical sample of women with Bulimia Nervosa [50]. Participants scored significantly higher on the BSQ than the community sample, and lower than the clinical sample. Compared to a normal sample of adult females [52], participants scored significantly higher on measures of depression, anxiety and stress. Participants scored significantly lower compared to an Australian sample of females with Anorexia Nervosa [61].

Eating behaviour was compared to a normal sample of middle-aged adults [60]. Participants obtained significantly higher scores compared to the normal sample on levels of eating restraint, emotional eating, and uncontrolled eating. Attitudes towards the self and body image scales were compared to a normal sample of female adults aged over 18 years [49]. Participants obtained significantly lower scores on the Appearance Evaluation subscale (feelings of attractiveness) and the Health Evaluation subscale (feelings of health).

Table 4 illustrates the results examining predictive characteristics of treatment retention and outcome. At pre-intervention, the level of endorsement of weight management as a motivator for exercise was the only statistically significant difference between NMD completers and non-completers. Completers endorsed weight management for exercise significantly more than non-completers. Small to medium effect sizes were observed for differences between completers and non-completers on shape concern, cognitive restraint and health evaluation; completers scoring higher than non-completers on these subscales.

Table 5 illustrates results of statistical testing for differences between pre- and post-intervention variables. There were statistically significant improvements in scores on shape concern and attitudes towards eating. Concerns and preoccupation with the body image also significantly decreased from pre- to post-intervention. Small to moderate effect sizes were observed for improvements in levels of restraint, weight concern, stress, food acceptance, and the health evaluation and fitness evaluation subscales.

Discussion

The study aimed to describe the characteristics of participants in the community attending the NMD program and to investigate characteristics that were predictors of treatment retention. The primary aim of the current study was to evaluate the NMD program on a range of health outcomes in an uncontrolled pilot study.

Compared to community samples, participants enrolled in the NMD reported elevated levels on all eating behaviour and psychosocial outcomes, except for subscales of the ecSatter Inventory, the restraint scale from the EDE-Q, and subjective feelings of fitness (Fitness Evaluation subscale), although a medium to large effect size for this difference ($r = -.47$) was observed. These findings are consistent with previous research that has indicated that although obese individuals do not exhibit a greater level of psychopathology than the normal population, treatment-seeking individuals are more likely to exhibit a greater level of psychological disturbance and disordered eating patterns [8,62,63]. Compared to clinical eating disorder samples, participants scored lower on eating disorder pathology (restraint, weight and eating concern), depression, anxiety, stress and body preoccupation. NMD participants had similar levels of shape concern to the clinical sample, highlighting the need for obesity treatment to tackle body image problems.

Pre-treatment characteristics were generally not predictive of treatment retention or treatment outcomes. The exception was reasons for exercise; completers endorsed weight management as a motivator for exercise significantly more than non-completers. There were small to medium effect sizes for differences between completers and non-completers on levels of shape concern, cognitive restraint and health evaluation, with a trend for completers to have greater shape concern, higher cognitive restraint and higher ratings of feelings of healthiness. These findings are

Table 2 Descriptive statistics and clinical cut-offs for all variables

Variable	*M*	*SD*	Range	Clinical cut-off score	% in clinical range
Self-report weight (kg)	92.69	20.88	69.8 – 156.0	N/A	N/A
Body Mass Index	34.17	8.57	25.2 - 55.9	Above 25 = Overweight, Above 30 = Obese	29.470.6
Eating Disorders Examination - Questionnaire					
Binge Eating Frequency (per 28 days)	4.65	6.24	0- 23		
Restraint	1.51	0.94	0 - 6	≥ 4	0
Eating Concern	1.71	1.44	0 - 6	≥ 4	11.8
Shape Concern	3.67	1.63	0 - 6	≥ 4	59.0
Weight Concern	3.24	1.50	0 - 6	≥ 4	35.4
Three Factor Eating Questionnaire - Revised					
Cognitive Restraint	2.50	0.68	0 - 4	N/A. Higher scores indicate higher cognitive restraint.	N/A
Emotional Eating	2.76	0.89	0 - 4	N/A. Higher scores indicate higher levels of emotional eating.	N/A
Uncontrolled Eating	2.56	0.52	0 - 4	N/A. Higher scores indicate higher levels of uncontrolled eating and impulsivity.	N/A
ecSatter Inventory					
Eating Attitudes	8.94	3.88	0 - 15	N/A. Higher scores indicate more relaxed and open attitudes to eating	N/A
Food Acceptance	4.71	2.37	0 - 9	N/A. Higher scores indicate higher levels of cognitive and behavioural food acceptance.	N/A
Internal Regulation	6.47	2.79	0 - 9	N/A. Higher scores indicate stronger endorsement of the experiential processes of hunger, appetite and satiety.	N/A
Contextual Eating Skills	8.35	3.71	0 - 15	N/A. Higher scores indicate more behaviours related to managing the patterns and opportunities for eating and planning meals.	N/A
Eating Competence	28.47	10.94	0 - 48	≥ 32 = Eating competent	47.1
Multidimensional Body Self-Relations Questionnaire					
Appearance Evaluation	2.18	0.98	0 - 5	N/A. High scores indicate more positive feelings about appearance.	N/A
Fitness Evaluation	2.94	0.95	0 - 5	N/A. Higher scores indicate greater feelings of fitness.	N/A
Health Evaluation	3.14	0.84	0 - 5	N/A. Higher scores indicate greater feelings of being in good health.	N/A
Body Shape Questionnaire	106.29	33.20	34 - 204	N/A. Higher scores indicate greater concern and preoccupation with appearance and shape.	N/A
DASS-21					
Depression	14.47	10.04	0 - 42	N/A. Moderate, Severe and Extremely Severe range.	59.0
Anxiety	9.41	6.24	0 - 42	N/A. Moderate, Severe and Extremely Severe range.	47.1
Stress	17.06	10.47	0 - 42	N/A. Moderate, Severe and Extremely Severe range.	41.3
Exercise Motivations Inventory - 2					
Reasons for exercise: Enjoyment	2.01	1.82	0 - 5	N/A. Higher scores indicate more endorsement of enjoyment as a motivator for exercise.	N/A
Reasons for exercise: Weight management	3.69	1.21	0 - 5	N/A. Higher scores indicate more endorsement of weight management as a motivator for exercise.	N/A

Note: The clinical range for the DASS-21 consists of scores in the Moderate range and above.

consistent with a recent review of predictors of attrition in obesity interventions, which found that while there were no consistent predictors of treatment attrition, there were several factors associated with attrition, including greater body dissatisfaction, more dieting attempts and poor mental health [64]. Lack of significant predictors is likely due, at least in part, to the small sample size.

Following the completion of the NMD program, there were improvements on several biopsychosocial health outcomes. There was a significant increase in positive attitudes

Table 3 Results of Wilcoxon Signed Rank test comparing the pre-test study sample to normal and clinical samples

Variable	Study sample (n = 17)	Normal sample		Clinical sample	
	Mdn (Interquartile range; IQR)	*M (SD)*	Wilcoxin *T* & effect size (*r*)	*M (SD)*	Wilcoxin *T* & effect size (*r*)
Eating Disorders Examination - Questionnaire		(n = 243)[a]		(n = 60)[b]	
Restraint	1.2 (1.4)	1.3 (1.3)	$T = 93, p = .434, r = .19$	4.7 (1.6)	$T < .01, p < .001, r = -.88$
Eating Concern	1.4 (2.1)	0.6 (0.9)	$T = 130, p = .011, r = .61$	4 (1.3)	$T = 2, p < .001, r = -.83$
Shape Concern	4.4 (3.0)	2.2 (1.6)	$T = 138, p = ,004, r = .71$	4.6 (1.4)	$T = 39, p = .076, r = .78$
Weight Concern	3.4 (2.8)	1.6 (1.4)	$T = 141, p = .002, r = .74$	4.8 (1.2)	$T = 9, p = .001, r = -.78$
Three Factor Eating Questionnaire - Revised		(n = 284)[c]			
Cognitive Restraint	2.5 (1.2)	1. 6 (0.8)	$T = 150, p < .001, r = .85$	N/A	N/A
Emotional Eating	2.8 (1. 3)	1.7 (1.2)	$T = 146, p = .001, r = .80$	N/A	N/A
Uncontrolled Eating	2.77 (.8)	1.1 (0.8)	$T = 153, p < .001, r = .88$	N/A	N/A
ecSatter Inventory		(n = 832)[d]			
Eating Attitudes	9.0 (4.0)	11.1 (3.0)	$T = 45, p = .135, r = -.36$	N/A	N/A
Food Acceptance	6.0 (3.5)	4.9 (2.2)	$T = 73, p = .868, r = -.04$	N/A	N/A
Internal Regulation	7.0 (3.5)	6.7 (1.8)	$T = 85, p = .686, r = .01$	N/A	N/A
Contextual Eating Skills	9.0 (4.5)	8.5 (3.3)	$T = 76, p = .981, r = -.01$	N/A	N/A
Eating Competence	29.0 (13.5)	31.1 (7.5)	$T = 59, p = .407, r = -.20$	N/A	N/A
Multidimensional Body Self-Relations Questionnaire		(n = 1070)[e]			
Appearance Evaluation	2.0 (1.1)	3.4 (0.9)	$T = 7, p = .001, r = -.80$	N/A	N/A
Fitness Evaluation	2. 7 (1. 7)	3.5 (1.0)	$T = 36, p = .055, r = -.47$	N/A	N/A
Health Evaluation	3.7 (1.2)	3.9 (0.8)	$T = 15, p = .004, r = -.71$	N/A	N/A
		(n = 535)[f]		(n = 38)[g]	
Body Shape Questionnaire	112.0 (57.5)	81.5 (28.4)	$T = 128, p = .015, r = .59$	136.9 (22.5)	$T = 17, p = .005, r = -.68$
DASS-21		(n = 592)[h]		(n = 27)[i]	
Depression	14.0 (18.0)	6.3 (7.0)	$T = 132, p = .009, r = .64$	21.6 (10.7)	$T = 28, p = .022, r = -.58$
Anxiety	18.0 (10.0)	4.7 (4.9)	$T = 131, p = .010, r = .63$	16.2 (9.1)	$T = 8, p = .001, r = -.79$
Stress	16.0 (17.0)	10.1 (7.9)	$T = 122, p = .031, r = .52$	24.8 (9.3)	$T = 26, p = .017, r = -.58$

Note: *N/A*: analysis not completed as no appropriate comparable sample available.
[a]females over 16 years [59]. [b]females with Anorexia Nervosa [59].[c]middle-aged females [60]. [d]overweight and physically active adults [47]. [e]females over 18 years [49]. [f]female university students and family planning clinic attendees [50]. [g]females with Bulimia Nervosa [50]. [h]males and females, aged over 17 years, in the community [52]. [i]adolescents and adults with Anorexia Nervosa [61].

towards food and eating, and a decrease in body shape preoccupation, dissatisfaction and shape concern. This finding is consistent with previous research [5,6,38,65-67]. For example, Tanco and colleagues found that a non-dieting intervention resulted in improvements in eating related psychopathology compared to a dieting intervention despite similar weight loss. Non-dieting interventions, such as NMD may be particularly beneficial for treating the psychological correlates of obesity including body image dissatisfaction.

The results for improvements in restraint, weight concern, stress, food acceptance, and the health evaluation and fitness evaluation subscales were not statistically significant, however small to medium effect sizes were observed. These results suggest there have been clinically significant improvements which were not statistically significant as a result of the small sample size. There was also a small to medium effect for improvements in overall eating competence (which incorporates the factors of eating attitudes, food acceptance, internal regulation and contextual eating skills), which suggest there may have been some clinically meaningful change in eating attitudes. Descriptively, the pre-treatment median (29) falls outside of the Eating Competent range, whereas the post-treatment median (36.5) falls within the Eating Competent range, suggesting a trend for a meaningful improvement in eating competence.

Despite changes in these eating and body image factors, there were no differences post-intervention on levels of dietary restraint, emotional eating and uncontrolled eating,

Table 4 Results of Mann–Whitney tests domparing completers and non-completers for all variables

Variable	Completion n = 13 *Mdn (IQR)*	Non-completion n = 4 *Mdn (IQR)*	Mann–Whitney *U* & effect size (*r*)
Self - reported weight (kg)	91 (28.3)	85 (56.5)	$U = 27, p = 1.00, r = -.03$
Body Mass Index	32 (8.7)	31.55 (23.6)	$U = 26, p = 1.00, r < .01$
Eating Disorders Examination - Questionnaire			
Restraint	1.4 (1.5)	1.1 (1.4)	$U = 21.5, p = .624, r = -0.12$
Eating Concern	1.4 (2.7)	1.2 (2.0)	$U = 18, p = .412, r = -0.22$
Shape Concern	4.4 (2.1)	2.4 (3.4)	$U = 12, p = .130, r = -0.39$
Weight Concern	3.4 (1.9)	2.4 (3.4)	$U = 17.5, p = .350, r = -0.23$
Three Factor Eating Questionnaire - Revised			
Cognitive Restraint	2.9 (1.2)	2.2 (1.0)	$U = 14.5, p = .201, r = -0.32$
Emotional Eating	2.8 (1.6)	2.4 (1.2)	$U = 20.5, p = .549, r = -0.15$
Uncontrolled Eating	2.33 (0.9)	2.8 (0.9)	$U = 18.5, p = .412, r = -0.21$
ecSatter Inventory			
Eating Attitudes	9 (5.0)	10 (8.8)	$U = 25, p = 1.00, r = -0.03$
Food Acceptance	6 (4.5)	4 (2.5)	$U = 20, p = .549, r = -0.17$
Internal Regulation	7 (3.5)	7 (6.8)	$U = 23, p = .785, r = -0.08$
Contextual Eating Skills	9 (5.0)	7 (5.5)	$U = 17, p = .350, r = -0.25$
Eating Competence	29 (18.0)	28.5 (22.5)	$U = 21, p = .624, r = -0.14$
Multidimensional Body Self-Relations Questionnaire			
Appearance Evaluation	2.0 (0.71)	2.6 (2.0)	$U = 22.5, p = .703, r = -0.1$
Fitness Evaluation	2. 7 (1.8)	2.67 (1.4)	$U = 19, p = .477, r = -0.19$
Health Evaluation	3.1 (1.4)	2.8 (1.1)	$U = 14, p = .202, r -0.33$
Body Shape Questionnaire	112.0 (42.0)	104.0 (92.5)	$U = 25.5, p = .956, r = -0.01$
DASS - 21			
Depression	14 (17.0)	9 (24.5)	$U = 20, p = .549, r = -0.17$
Anxiety	8 (10.0)	10 (18.5)	$U = 23.5, p = .785, r = -0.07$
Stress	16 (15.0)	20 (27)	$U = 20.5, p = .549, r = -0.15$
Exercise Motivations Inventory - 2			
Reasons for exercise: Enjoyment	1.5 (3.6)	1.1 (2. 6)	$U = 18.5, p = .412, r = -0.21$
Reasons for exercise: Weight management	4.5 (1.4)	2.8 (2.4)	$U = 5.5, p = .015, r = -0.57$

or eating concern [43]. Given that non-dieting approaches encourage intuitive eating and normalised eating as a sustainable approach to healthy eating, rather than a short-term weight loss solution [10], and that level of restraint was elevated in the current sample, it would be expected there would be improvements in measures of eating behaviours and attitudes in the current NMD intervention. Studies have shown improvements in disordered eating post-intervention [5,6,37-39]. The programs from these studies ranged in length from 10 to 24 sessions, with an average length of 14 sessions. The current NMD program ran for 8 weeks, and it may be that eating behaviours (restraint, uncontrolled eating and emotional eating) are more resistant to change, and therefore require a longer time period (more sessions) or more targeted intervention for changes to achieve significant improvements in eating behaviours. The degree of endorsement of weight management and enjoyment as motivators for exercise also did not change following the intervention. As people who seek treatment are likely to be more motivated than non-treatment seekers, this may account for why the NMD participants' positive endorsement of exercise did not change post-intervention.

Small (non significant) effects were observed for changes in levels of depression and anxiety, suggesting there was little improvement following the intervention. As the NMD program had no exclusion criteria, it is possible that some participants were experiencing co-morbid disorders. The baseline characteristics are consistent with this explanation, with more 50% of participants scoring within

Table 5 Results of related samples Wilcoxon Signed Ranks test for differences between pre- and post-intervention for all variables

Variables	Pre *Mdn* (*IQR*)	Post *Mdn* (*IQR*)	Wilcoxon T and effect size (*r*)
Self - reported weight (kg)	90.5 (23.3)	90.0 (25.7)	$T = 21$, $p = .507$, $r = -.16$
Body Mass Index	31.2 (8.6)	31.8 (7.2)	$T = 23$, $p = .646$, $r = -.11$
Eating Disorders Examination - Questionnaire			
Binge Eating Frequency (per 28 days)	2.0 (6.2)	0.0 (3.6)	$T = 15$, $p = .176$, $r = -.33$
Restraint	1.2 (1.4)	0.6 (2.3)	$T = 15$, $p = .202$, $r = -.31$
Eating Concern	1.4 (2.1)	0.5 (2)	$T = 10.5$, $p = .153$, $r = -.35$
Shape Concern	4.4 (3)	2.3 (2.8)	$T = 0$, $p = .005$, $r = -.68$
Weight Concern	3.4 (2.8)	2.8 (3.2)	$T = 9.5$, $p = .066$, $r = -.44$
Three Factor Eating Questionnaire - Revised			
Cognitive Restraint	2.5 (1.2)	2.5 (0.6)	$T = 16$, $p = .439$, $r = -.19$
Emotional Eating	2.8 (1.3)	2.5 (2.0)	$T = 23$, $p = .646$, $r = -.11$
Uncontrolled Eating	2.7 (0.8)	2.4 (1.5)	$T = 29.5$, $p = .838$, $r = -.05$
ecSatter Inventory			
Eating Attitudes	9.0 (4)	11.5 (6)	$T = 33.5$, $p = .028$, $r = -.53$
Food Acceptance	6.0 (3.5)	7.0 (2)	$T = 13$, $p = .131$, $r = -.37$
Internal Regulation	7.0 (3.5)	7.0 (3)	$T = 11$, $p = .334$, $r = -.23$
Contextual Eating Skills	9.0 (4.5)	9.5 (6.3)	$T = 20.5$, $p = .725$, $r = -.09$
Eating Competence	29.0 (13.5)	36.5 (19.3)	$T = 36$, $p = .108$, $r = -.39$
Multidimensional Body Self-Relations Questionnaire			
Appearance Evaluation	2.0 (1.1)	2.4 (1.3)	$T = 39.5$, $p = .220$, $r = -.30$
Fitness Evaluation	2.7 (1.7)	4.2 (1.6)	$T = 22$, $p = .161$, $r = -.34$
Health Evaluation	3.0 (1.2)	3.5 (1.5)	$T = 36.5$, $p = .095$, $r = -.40$
Body Shape Questionnaire	112.0 (57.5)	89.0 (73.5)	$T = 1$, $p = .007$, $r = -.66$
DASS-21			
Depression	14 (18.0)	5 (15.0)	$T = 15.5$, $p = .398$, $r = -.20$
Anxiety	8 (10.0)	3 (8.5)	$T = 13.5$, $p = .284$, $r = -.26$
Stress	16 (17.0)	10 (14.5)	$T = 7$, $p = .121$, $r = -.38$
Exercise Motivations Inventory - 2			
Reasons for exercise: Enjoyment	1.5 (3.4)	3.4 (4.4)	$T = 18$, $p = .490$, $r = -.17$
Reasons for exercise: Weight management	4 (1.4)	3.9 (2.3)	$T = 6$, $p = .172$, $r = -.33$

the clinical range of depression, and over 40% within the clinical range for anxiety and stress. This is consistent with previous research indicating elevated levels of depression and anxiety in obese treatment seekers. The presence of co-morbid mood disorders and mood regulation difficulties was not a target of treatment. These would be common phenomena in real-world obesity interventions that may not be reflected in efficacy studies, as participants with co-morbid disorders are typically excluded from such studies.

Weight and BMI was maintained post-intervention. This was expected as weight loss was not a goal of the current intervention. The non-dieting approach posits that weight loss is not required for health improvements (unless at extreme ends of the spectrum) and this weight maintenance is similar to previous findings in non-dieting interventions [36,38,39,66]. Some healthcare professionals fear that this approach will lead to weight gain [38], however, the current results add to previous research demonstrating an absence of significant weight gain following non-dieting interventions [10]. The frequency of binge episodes did not decrease significantly, but there was a trend for a reduction in the frequency post-intervention. Bacon and Aphramor's review evaluates the evidence and rationale for a shift from the traditional weight-focused treatment paradigm, which induces only short-term weight loss, and little benefits of improved morbidity and mortality. Together, the results of the current study add further support for a paradigm shift in the treatment of overweight and obesity [10].

This study has a number of strengths. The major strength is that it is an effectiveness study with high external validity. These participants are representative of treatment-seeking individuals from the community, accepted without exclusion criteria unlike some other studies of non-dieting interventions. In comparison, with the goal of achieving high internal validity, efficacy trials typically require participants to meet strict inclusion criteria, often excluding those with common mental health conditions and/or or medical complications. In comparison to some other non-dieting interventions, the NMD program also has a large focus on movement that is practised in session. This movement does not require specialist skills, as opposed to exercise or moderate physical activity promoted in other studies. The movements were demonstrated in session, and were aimed at people of all ages, all sizes, and those with limited mobility. Furthermore, much of the previous research into obesity treatment focuses on medical and surgical interventions or traditional diet-based weight loss programs; this is one of few evaluations of non-dieting approaches. This study examines an intervention that is easily accessible, easily delivered within the community, and may potentially be suited to a wider range of treatment-seekers.

A number of limitations should be considered when interpreting the results of the current study. Firstly, as this is an effectiveness study without a control group, internal validity is limited. In addition, as the sample size is small the conclusions drawn from the statistical analyses should be interpreted with caution, as a larger sample size is required to confirm results, and determine if results are able to be generalised to the population. Additionally, the impact of self-selection bias cannot be ruled out. Participants that selected into the study may be different to participants who completed the NMD program but did not elect to take part in the current study, and this needs to be considered when interpreting the results.

A significant limitation which is common to other studies of non-dieting interventions is that physiological health indicators (e.g., cholesterol, blood pressure, metabolic rates) were not included in the outcome measures. Evidence of changes in physiological outcomes are important in order to understand the role of physiological health improvements independent of significant weight loss and should be assessed in future non-dieting interventions.

The limitations could be addressed in future research by conducting larger-scale studies with larger sample sizes within the community. Follow-up data would also provide useful information. In addition, as obesity is associated with a number of physical, psychological and behavioural profiles, in order to understand the effectiveness and sustainability of alternative obesity treatments evaluations of future interventions should incorporate physiological, psychological and behavioural (including eating and exercise behaviours) outcome measures. This will add to the current understanding of obesity and associated characteristics, and how to best target these factors in treatment.

Conclusion

The current study provides preliminary evidence of the effectiveness of the NMD program for improvements in body shape preoccupation and dissatisfaction and attitudes towards eating. The study has also highlighted the physical, psychosocial and behavioural characteristics of a treatment-seeking overweight/obese sample in a non-dieting based community program. As obesity has been associated with several disordered eating maintaining factors (binge eating, emotional eating, body image dissatisfaction, weight cycling, disordered eating [10]), these factors need to be incorporated as part of treatment. They are not addressed entirely through weight loss focused interventions, and alternative approaches, such as the NMD program, may be a viable alternative treatment paradigm which focus on health outcomes, including normalised eating, body self-acceptance and sustainable and realistic physical activity.

Competing interests

The authors declare that they have no competing interests.

Authors' contributions

LB, a research student, contributed to the design of the study, was responsible for data collection, analysis and interpretation and lead the manuscript development. BS and MB adapted and delivered the intervention and provided feedback on study design, measure selection and manuscript development. LB supervised LB and was responsible for the design of the study, measure selection, planning of statistical analyses, and overseeing manuscript development. All authors read and approved the final manuscript.

Author details

[1]School of Health Sciences, RMIT University, Melbourne, Australia. [2]MonashLink Community Health Service, Melbourne, Australia. [3]Southern Health Wellness Recovery Adult Outpatient Eating Disorder Service, Melbourne, Australia. [4]School of Psychology, Australian Catholic University, Melbourne, Australia.

References

1. Fairburn CG: *Cognitive Behavior Therapy and Eating Disorders.* New York: The Guilford Press; 2008.
2. Neumark-Sztainer D, Wall M, Guo J, Story M, Haines J, Eisenberg M: **Obesity, disordered eating, and eating disorders in a longitudinal study of adolescents: How do dieters fare 5 years later?** *J Am Diet Assoc* 2006, **106**(4):559–568.
3. Fairburn CG, Brownell KD: *Eating Disorders and Obesity.* 2nd edition. New York: The Guilford Press; 2002.
4. Fairburn C, Cooper Z, Doll H: PN, O'Connor M: **The natural course of bulimia nervosa and binge eating disorder in young women.** *Arch Gen Psychiatry* 2000, **57**(7):659–665.
5. Ciliska D: **Evaluation of two nondieting interventions for obese women.** *West J Nurs Res* 1998, **20**(1):119–135.
6. Polivy J, Herman CP: **Undieting: A program to help people stop dieting.** *Int J Eat Disord* 1992, **11**(3):261–268.
7. Ernsberger P, Koletsky RJ: **Biomedical rationale for a wellness approach to obesity: An alternative to a focus on weight loss.** *J Soc Issues* 1999, **55**(2):221–260.
8. Wilfley DE, Vannucci A, White EK: **Early intervention of eating- and weight-related problems.** *J Clin Psychol Med Settings* 2010, **17**(4):285–300.

9. Flegal KM, Graubard BI, Williamson DF, Gail MH: **Excess deaths associated with underweight, overweight, and obesity.** *JAMA* 2005, **293**(15):1861–1867.
10. Bacon L, Aphramor L: **Weight science: Evaluating the evidence for a paradigm shift.** *Nutr J* 2011, **10**(9):2–13.
11. Drapeau V, Provencher V, Lemieux S, Després JP, Bouchard C, Tremblay A: **Do 6-y changes in eating behaviors predict changes in body weight? Results from the Quebec Family Study.** *Int J Obes (Lond)* 2003, **27**(7):808–814.
12. Marchesini G, Cuzzolaro M, Mannuci E, Dalle Grave R, Gennaro M, Tomasi F, Barantani EG, Melchionda N: **Weight cycling in treatment-seeking obese persons: data from the QUOVADIS study.** *Int J Obes (Lond)* 2004, **28**(11):1456–1462.
13. Diaz CA, Mainous AG III, Everett CJ: **The association between weight fluctuation and mortality: Results from a population-based cohort study.** *J Community Health* 2005, **30**(3):153–165.
14. Lissner L, Odell PM, D'Agostino RB, Stokes J III, Kreger BE, Belanger AJ, Brownell KD: **Variability of body weight and health outcomes in the Framingham population.** *N Engl J Med* 1991, **324**(26):1839–1844.
15. Petroni ML, Vilanova N, Aragnina S, Fusco MAGF, Compare A, Marchesini G: **Psychological distress in morbid obesity in relation to weight history.** *Obes Surg* 2007, **17**(3):391–399.
16. Carrier K, Steinhardt M, Bowman S: **Rethinking traditional weight management programs: A 3 year follow-up evaluation of a new approach.** *J Psychol* 1994, **128**(5):517.
17. McFarlane T, Polivy J, McCabe RE: **Help, not harm: Psychological foundation for a non dieting approach toward health.** *J Soc Issues* 1999, **55**(2):261–276.
18. Stice E: **A prospective test of the dual-pathway model of bulimic pathology: Mediating effects of dieting and negative affect.** *J Abnorm Psychol* 2001, **110**(1):124–135.
19. Polivy J: **Psychological consequences of food restriction.** *J Am Diet Assoc* 1996, **96**(6):589–592.
20. Yanovski SZ, Billington CJ, Epstein LH, Goodwin NJ, Hill JO, Pi-Sunyer FX, Rolls BJ, Stern JS, Wadden TA, Weinsier RL, Wilson GT, Wing RR, Van Hubbard S, Hoofnagle JH, Everhard J, Harrison B: **Dieting and the development of eating disorders in overweight and obese adults.** *Arch Intern Med* 2000, **160**(17):2581–2589.
21. Leon GR, Fulkerson JA, Perry CL, Cudeck R: **Personality and behavioral vulnerabilities associated with risk status for eating disorders in adolescent girls.** *J Abnorm Psychol* 1993, **102**(3):438–444.
22. Telch CF, Agras WS: **Obesity, binge eating and psychopathology. Are they related?** *Int J Eat Disord* 1994, **15**(1):53–61.
23. Foster G, Wadden T, Vogt R, Brewer G: **What is a reasonable weight loss? Patient's expectations and evaluations of obesity treatment outcomes.** *J Consult Clin Psychol* 1997, **65**:79–85.
24. Dalle Grave R, Calugi S, Molinari E, Petroni ML, Bondi M, Compare A, Marchesini G, Group QS: **Weight loss expectations in obese patients and treatment attrition: an observational multicenter study.** *Obes Res* 2005, **13**(11):1961–1969.
25. National Health and Medical Research Council: *Clinical practice guidelines for the management of overweight and obesity in adults.* Melbourne, VIC: National Health and Medical Research Council; 2003.
26. Miller WC: **How effective are traditional dietary and exercise interventions for weight loss?** *Med Sci Sports Exerc* 1999, **31**(8):1129–1134.
27. Wadden TA, Crerand CE, Brock JB: **Behavioral Treatment of Obesity.** *Psychiatr Clin N Am* 2005, **28**:151–170.
28. Reinehr T, Widhalm K, L'Allemand D, Wiegand S, Wabitsch M, Holl RW: **Two-year follow-up in 21,784 overweight children and adolescents with lifestyle intervention.** *Obesity* 2009, **17**(6):1196–1199.
29. Wadden TA, Sternberg JA, Letizia KA: **Treatment of obesity by very low calorie diet, behavior therapy, and their combination. A five-year perspective.** *Int J Obes (Lond)* 1989, **51**:167–172.
30. Guagnano MT VP-P, Carrans C, Merlittli D, Sensi S: **Weight fluctuations could increase blood pressure in android obese women.** *Clin Sci* 1999, **96**:677–680.
31. Harrington M, Gibson S, Cottrell RC: **A review and meta-analysis of the effect of weight loss on all-cause mortality risk.** *Nutr Res Rev* 2009, **22**(1):93–108.
32. Pal S, Egger G, Wright G: **Dealing with obesity: An Australian perspective.** *Asia Pac J Public Health* 2003, **15**:33–36.
33. Miller WC: **The weight-loss-at-any-cost environment: How to thrive with a health-centred focus.** *J Nutr Educ Behav* 2005, **37**(SUPPL. 2):s89–s93.
34. Provencher V, Begin C, Tremblay A, Mongeau L, Boivin S, Lemieux S: **Short-term effects of a "health at every size" approach on eating behaviors and appetite ratings.** *Obesity* 2007, **15**(4):957–966.
35. Robison J: **Weight, health and culture: Shifting the paradigm for alternative health care.** *Complement Health Pract Rev* 1999, **5**(1):45–69.
36. Hawley G, Horwath C, Gray A, Bradshaw A, Katzer L, Joyce J, O'Brien S: **Sustainability of health and lifestyle improvements following a non-dieting randomised trial in overweight women.** *Prev Med* 2008, **47**(6):593–599.
37. Provencher V, Begin C, Tremblay A, Mongeau L, Corneau L, Dodin S, Boivin S, Lemieux S: **Health-at-every-size and eating behaviors: 1-year follow-up results of a size acceptance intervention.** *Am Diet Assoc* 2009, **109**:1854–1861.
38. Bacon L, Stern JS, Van Loan MD, Keim NL: **Size acceptance and intuitive eating improve health for obese, female chronic dieters.** *J Am Diet Assoc* 2005, **105**(6):929–936.
39. Rapaport L, Clark M, Wardle J: **Evaluation of a modified cognitive-behavioural programme for weight management.** *Int J Obes (Lond)* 2000, **24**(12):1726–1737.
40. Goodrick GK, Poston WSC II, Kimball KT, Reeves RS, Foreyt JP: **Nondieting versus dieting treatment for overweight binge-eating women.** *J Consult Clin Psychol* 1998, **66**(2):363–368.
41. Tanco S, Linden W, Earle T: **Well-being and morbid obesity in women: a controlled therapy evaluation.** *Int J Eat Disord* 1998, **23**(3):325–339.
42. Clarke GN: **Improving the transition from basic efficacy research to effectiveness studies: Methodological issues and procedures.** *J Consult Clin Psychol* 1995, **63**(5):718–725.
43. Fairburn CG, Beglin SJ: **Assessment of eating disorders: Interview of self-report questionnaire?** *Int J Eat Disord* 1994, **16**(4):363–370.
44. Peterson CB, Crosby RD, Wonderlich SA, Joiner T, Crow SJ, Mitchell JE, Bardone-Cone AM, Klein M, Le Grange D: **Psychometric properties of the eating disorder examination-questionnaire: Factor structure and internal consistency.** *Int J Eat Disord* 2007, **40**(4):386–389.
45. Karlsson J, Persson LO, Sjostrom K, Sullivan M: **Psychometric properties and factor structure of the Three-Factor Eating Questionnaire (TFEQ) in obese men and women. Results from the Swedish Obese Subjects (SOS) study.** *Int J Obes (Lond)* 2000, **24**(12):1715–1725.
46. Stunkard AJ, Messick S: **The three-factor eating questionnaire to measure dietary restraint, disinhibition and hunger.** *J Psychosom Res* 1985, **29**(1):71–83.
47. Lohse B, Satter E, Horacek T, Gebereslassi T, Oakland MJ: **Measuring Eating Competence: Psychometric Properties and Validity of the ecScatter Inventory.** *J Nutr Educ Behav* 2007, **39**(5):141–198.
48. Stotts JL, Lohse B: **Reliability of the ecSatter Inventory as a tool to measure eating competence.** *J Nutr Educ Behav* 2007, **39**(5 SUPPL):s167–s170.
49. Cash TF: *MBSRQ User's Manual.* 3rd edition. Norfolk, VA: Old Dominion Univer. Press; 2000.
50. Cooper PJ, Tayor MJ, Cooper Z, Fairburn CG: **The development and validation of the Body Shape Questionnaire.** *Int J Eat Disord* 1987, **6**(4):485–494.
51. Rosen JC, Jones A, Ramirez E, Waxman S: **Body Shape Questionnaire: Studies of validity and reliability.** *Int J Eat Disord* 1996, **20**(3):315–319.
52. Lovibond PF, Lovibond SH: *Manual for the depression, anxiety, and stress scales.* Sydney: Psychology Foundation; 1995.
53. Crawford JR, Henry JD: **The Depression Anxiety Stress Scale (DASS): Normative data and latent structure in a large non-clinical sample.** *Br J Clin Psychol* 2003, **42**:111–131.
54. Markland DA, Ingledew DK: **The measurement of exercise motives: Factorial validity and invariance across gender of a revised Exercise Motivations Inventory.** *Br J Health Psychol* 1997, **2**(4):361–376.
55. Gollings EK, Paxton SJ: **Comparison of internet and face-to-face delivery of a group body image and disordered eating intervention for women: A pilot study.** *Eat Disord: J Treat Prev* 2006, **14**:1–15.
56. Paxton SJ, McLean SA, Gollings EK, Faulkner C, Wertheim EH: **Comparison of face-to-face and internet interventions for body image and eating problems in adult women: an RCT.** *Int J Eat Disord* 2007, **40**:692–704.
57. McLean SA, Paxton SJ, Wertheim EH: **A body image and disordered eating intervention for midlife women: A randomised controlled trial.** *J Consult Clin Psychol* 2011, **79**(6):751–758.
58. Cohen JW: *Statistical power analysis for the behavioral sciences 2nd ed.* Hillsdale, NJ: Lawrence Erlbaum Associates; 1988.
59. Wolk SL, Loeb KL, Walsh BT: **Assessment of patients with anorexia nervosa: Interview versus self-report.** *Int J Eat Disord* 2005, **37**:92–99.

60. de Lauzon B, Romon M, Deschamps V, Lafay L, Borys J, Karlsson J, Ducimetiere P, Charles MA, Group FLVSS: **The three-factor eating questionnaire-R18 is able to distinguish among different eating patterns in a general population.** *J Nutr* 2004, **134**:2372–2380.
61. Moor S, Vartanian LR, Touyz SW, Beuamont PJV: **Psychopathology of EDNOS patients: To whom do they compare?** *Clin Psychol* 2004, **8**(2):70–75.
62. Friedman MA, Brownell KD: **Psychological Correlates of Obesity: Moving to the next research generation.** *Psychol Bull* 1995, **117**(1):3–20.
63. Hrabosky JI, Thomas JJ: **Elucidating the relationship between obesity and depression: Recommendations for future research.** *Clin Psychol Sci Pract* 2008, **15**(1):28–34.
64. Moroshko I, Brennan L, O'Brien P: **Predictors of dropout in weight loss interventions: a systematic review of the literature.** *Obes Rev* 2011, **12**:912–934.
65. Nauta H, Hospers H, Jansen A: **One-year follow-up effects of two obesity treatments on psychological well-being and weight.** *Br J Health Psychol* 2001, **6**(3):271–284.
66. Crerand CE, Ta W, Foster GD, Sarwer DB, Paster LM, Berkowitz RI: **Changes in obesity-related attitudes in women seeking weight reduction.** *Obesity* 2007, **15**:740–747.
67. Jackson EG: **Eating Order: A 13-Week Trust Model Class for Dieting Casualties.** *J Nutr Educ Behav* 2008, **40**(1):43–48.

4

Measuring eating disorder attitudes and behaviors

David H Gleaves[1*], Crystal A Pearson[2], Suman Ambwani[3] and Leslie C Morey[2]

Abstract

Background: Although score reliability is a sample-dependent characteristic, researchers often only report reliability estimates from previous studies as justification for employing particular questionnaires in their research. The present study followed reliability generalization procedures to determine the mean score reliability of the Eating Disorder Inventory and its most commonly employed subscales (Drive for Thinness, Bulimia, and Body Dissatisfaction) and the Eating Attitudes Test as a way to better identify those characteristics that might impact score reliability.

Methods: Published studies that used these measures were coded based on their reporting of reliability information and additional study characteristics that might influence score reliability.

Results: Score reliability estimates were included in 26.15% of studies using the EDI and 36.28% of studies using the EAT. Mean Cronbach's alphas for the EDI (total score = .91; subscales = .75 to .89), EAT-40 (total score = .81) and EAT-26 (total score = .86; subscales = .56 to .80) suggested variability in estimated internal consistency. Whereas some EDI subscales exhibited higher score reliability in clinical eating disorder samples than in nonclinical samples, other subscales did not exhibit these differences. Score reliability information for the EAT was primarily reported for nonclinical samples, making it difficult to characterize the effect of type of sample on these measures. However, there was a tendency for mean score reliability to be higher in the adult (vs. adolescent) samples and in female (vs. male) samples.

Conclusions: Overall, this study highlights the importance of assessing and reporting internal consistency during every test administration because reliability is affected by characteristics of the participants being examined.

Keywords: Eating disorders, Assessment, Psychometric properties, Reliability generalization, Eating disorder inventory, Eating attitudes test

Background

Although estimates for anorexia nervosa and bulimia nervosa approximate .3% and 1% respectively when using strict diagnostic criteria [1], disturbances in eating behavior and body image affect large numbers of individuals [2,3] and recent evidence suggests increases in the annual incidence of EDs in the U.K. [4] and a substantial rise in the point prevalence of ED behaviors in Australia [5]. Several measures are available for the assessment of ED symptomatology, but researchers or clinicians may falsely assume that these tools retain adequate psychometric properties such as internal consistency across all circumstances [6]. For instance, while reporting research results, authors frequently refer to the "reliability of a test", a shorthand phrase that contributes to the misunderstanding by many researchers and students that tests, rather than scores, may be reliable [7]. This distinction between the reliability of test scores during a particular administration versus test reliability is significant; as emphasized by Wilkinson and the APA Task Force on Statistical Inference [8], "It is important to remember that a test is not reliable or unreliable. Reliability is a property of the scores on a test for a particular population of examinees" (p. 596) and thus reliability coefficients may vary depending on characteristics of the sample.

There are several reasons why it is important to examine and report reliability of test scores every time a measure is used. First, if score reliability is poor, the ability to measure the intended construct may be compromised,

* Correspondence: David.Gleaves@unisa.edu.au
[1]School of Psychology, Social Work and Social Policy, University of South Australia, Magill Campus, GPO Box 2471, Adelaide, SA 5001, Australia
Full list of author information is available at the end of the article

leading to a potential problem with validity of the data [9]; reliability of test scores is viewed theoretically as a necessary condition to establish validity, as "unreliable scores measure nothing" ([9], p. 6). Second, poor score reliability may hinder the ability to find statistically, clinically, or practically significant effects [9]. When interpreting effect sizes, score reliability is an important factor to consider because measurement error impacts effect size [10-13], as a larger standard error contributes to a less precise effect size value [14]. Measurement errors cause observed effects to fluctuate across studies and may lead to underestimation of true effects [10]. This has led to recommendations for correcting effect size estimates for unreliable scores [15]. Third, total score variance affects reliability of the data set, and total score variance is impacted by characteristics of the participants [6,7]. Because score variability is a property of the data, reliability estimates will not remain constant across studies and should therefore be evaluated and reported as part of the process of describing the data.

Given the importance of test score reliability to scientific research, it is surprising that the editorial policies of journals often do not require this information to be reported and many authors do not report reliability estimates for their data [13,16]. Studies examining reporting rates for score reliability have estimates ranging from 7.5% for the Beck Depression Inventory [6] to 15.2% for the NEO Five-Factor Inventory [17], and Henson and Thompson [18] suggested that reporting rates are unlikely to exceed 40% for any test. Although reliability generalization studies have been conducted for self-report measures assessing various aspects of psychopathology, such as autism [19], substance abuse [20], depression [21], obsessive-compulsive symptoms [22] and general psychopathology [23], no published studies to date have evaluated the same for eating disorder symptoms.

Given the significance of accurately assessing test reliability, the present study employed reliability generalization (RG) procedures to report the mean score reliability for common measures of eating disorder symptoms and to examine variability in these estimates across sample characteristics. RG, a type of meta-analysis, characterizes the typical (i.e., mean) reliability of scores across studies, the amount of variability in reliability coefficients, and the sources of variability in reliability coefficients [16]. RG is consistent with previous work on validity generalization [24], in which researchers conduct analyses to determine if the validity of scores on a test was generalizable to different samples [12]. As with other types of meta-analysis, RG allows researchers to understand a large body of literature which may be producing inconsistent findings, in this case helping to understand differences in score reliability across multiple studies [6].

Two commonly used self-report measures of eating disordered attitudes and behaviors are the Eating Disorder Inventory (EDI; [25]) and the Eating Attitudes Test (EAT; [26]), both of which are available in revised forms (EDI-2; [27]; EAT-26; [28]). Research suggests that the EDI can distinguish individuals with AN [25] and BN [29] from nonclinical respondents. Conversely, the Eating Attitudes Test (EAT; [26]) assesses thoughts and behaviors related to anorexia nervosa and may be administered in the original 40-item version or a 26-item short form (EAT-26; [28]), both of which are typically highly correlated ($r = .98$; [30]). The EAT has also been shown to discriminate individuals with bulimia nervosa from control participants [29], eating disordered patients and controls, and binge eating patients from those with anorexia nervosa and bulimia nervosa [31].

An examination of the factors that influence reliability in eating disorder assessment can facilitate an understanding of how sample characteristics may contribute to variability in score quality. For example, other factors being equal, a heterogeneous set of participants will produce higher score reliability than a more homogenous group of participants [6]. Participant characteristics such as the type of sample, age and gender should be considered in evaluating score reliability. Other study factors potentially impacting test score reliability are sample size, type of reliability, culture/ethnicity, test format, test length, and test language. By identifying the conditions under which a test's scores display higher or lower reliability, researchers will be able to tailor future studies about eating disordered attitudes and behaviors to conditions that will maximize score reliability and thereby yield additional control over one factor that influences effect sizes. Thus, in the present study we used RG procedures to study the mean score reliability for different versions of the EDI and the EAT to explore how score reliability of these eating disorder measures varies across studies, and explore the study characteristics that account for this variation.

Methods

Procedure

The present study followed five steps for designing an RG study as recommended by Henson and Thompson [18]: selecting the measures to be analyzed, developing a coding sheet, collecting data, identifying potential dependent variables, and conducting analyses. For test selection, studies that utilized various forms of the EDI or the EAT were selected due to their common use as measures of eating disorder symptomatology in clinical and research settings. For developing a coding form and data collection, relevant reports were gathered through database searches of PsycINFO using the terms Eating Disorder Inventory and Eating Attitudes Test. The search period was from when the tests were first published (1979 for the EAT and 1983 for the EDI) through to the end of 2005, so approximately 27 years and 23 years of research publications for the EAT and EDI, respectively. The searches resulted in 873 references for the EDI and 601 for the EAT during that time period. Included references were published empirical journal articles; books/book chapters, theoretical articles, review articles, case studies, dissertations, and meta-analyses, articles not published in English were excluded from this study. Based on these criteria, 283 studies of the EDI and 215 studies of the EAT were reviewed and coded (see Figure 1 for a flow chart). The data coding sheet included codes for whether or not reliability information for the sample was reported and what type of reliability information was provided (i.e., internal consistency or stability). Additional study factors were also coded, including type of reliability coefficient reported, type of sample (clinical–eating disorder, clinical–general psychiatric, nonclinical, or mixed sample), type of study (treatment or other), age of participants, gender of participants, test language, test form, test length, and sample size. A single coder was used to code all studies because, unlike in more traditional meta-analyses, this study did not require any calculations to be made. Separate analyses were conducted using internal consistency and test-retest coefficients as dependent variables.

When using reliability estimates, some researchers combine Cronbach's alpha [32] estimates with test-retest reliability estimates as a single dependent variable, but Dimitrov [33] cautioned against combining these estimates as they are not equivalent, and combining them together could lead to "mixing apples and oranges" ([33],

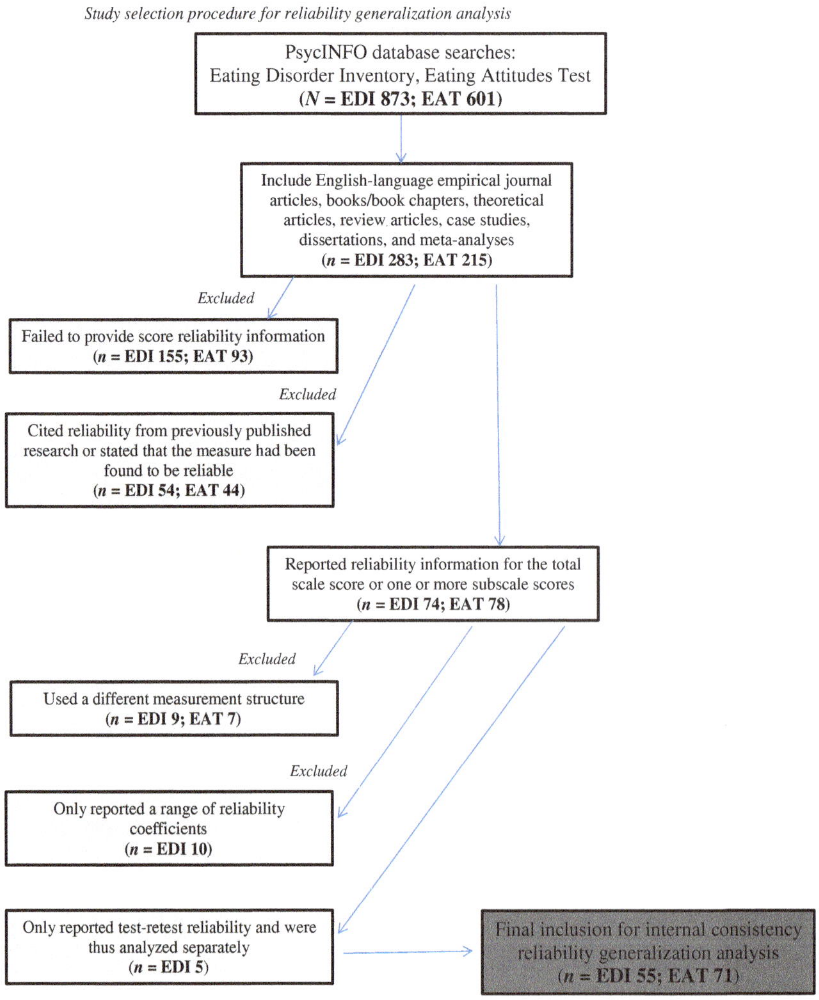

Figure 1 Study selection procedure for reliability generalization analysis.

p. 792). Thus, after coding all the studies, we determined which study features were used in the analyses as independent variables based on whether enough data were available using that feature.

Data analyses

SAS 8.2 software was used for all analyses, and published guidelines for conducting a reliability generalization study [18] and for conducting a meta-analysis [34] were followed. Overall mean reliability coefficients weighted by sample size were calculated for each measure, and sample-weighted mean reliability estimates broken down by predictor variables were also calculated. Sample size is one source of sampling error, with larger sample sizes providing more stable estimates of the population parameter because they are less susceptible to sampling error than smaller samples. Therefore, sample weighted means were used to reduce the effects of sampling error from smaller samples. If data were available, mean reliability coefficients are reported for the subscales of the measures. Additionally, the 95% confidence interval and percent of variance accounted for by sampling error were also calculated.

Results

Eating disorder inventory

In 155 (54.77%) out of 283 studies that used the EDI or EDI-2, the researchers did not provide any score reliability information (see Figure 1). In 54 (19.08%) studies, the researchers cited reliability estimates of scores from previously published studies or stated that the measure had been found to be reliable. The researchers reported reliability information for either the total scale score or one or more subscale scores for their sample in 74 (26.15%) studies; however, 10 of these studies were excluded from the analyses because the authors only reported a range of reliability coefficients for the subscale scores, and 9 studies were excluded for using a different measurement structure (see [25,27,29,31,35-87] for included studies). Five studies included only test-retest reliability and were analyzed separately. In some studies, researchers reported reliability information for more than one group of participants (e.g., control group and clinical group), resulting in more reliability coefficients for that scale than there were studies reporting score reliability information for that scale.

Table 1 presents the mean estimates of internal consistency for the EDI and its subscales and the means broken down by gender and age of participants, as well as type of sample and test language. All of the coded study factors could not be analyzed due to low variability or insufficient reporting of the characteristic. Only one of the articles reporting score reliability information was a treatment study, and the majority of authors did not provide sufficient information regarding participant ethnicity to allow for further analysis. Mean estimates of internal consistency for scores on the subscales ranged from .75 to .89 and for scores on the EDI, the mean estimate was .90. No studies reported estimates of internal consistency for the total score on the EDI-2. The Bulimia subscale had higher score reliability in clinical eating disorder samples than in nonclinical samples, whereas the Drive for Thinness and Body Dissatisfaction subscales did not display this difference. Mean estimates of score reliability also tended to be higher in the adult samples compared to the adolescent samples, as well as the female samples compared to the male samples.

An examination of moderators of score reliability suggested that for the total EDI, there were some differences across adult vs. adolescent samples and clinical vs. nonclinical samples (see Table 1 for confidence intervals). For the most commonly employed EDI subscales (Body Dissatisfaction, Drive for Thinness, and Bulimia), mean estimates for internal consistency were .89, .85, and .75, respectively. For the Body Dissatisfaction subscale, the mean score reliability was higher in the female and mixed gender samples than in the male samples, and the adult samples had greater reliability than the adolescent samples. For the Drive for Thinness subscale, reliability was highest in the mixed gender samples followed by the female and male samples. For the other study characteristics, the adult and clinical samples displayed score reliability similar to their comparison samples, and the English language samples displayed greater reliability in their scores than the non-English test language samples. For the Bulimia subscale, the female and mixed gender samples displayed greater reliability than the male samples with the confidence interval for the male samples not including the means of the other two categories. The adult estimate was also greater than the score reliability estimate for the adolescent samples and the clinical eating disorder samples were greater than the nonclinical samples (see Table 1).

The percent of variance explained by sampling error varied widely for the EDI and its subscales, ranging from 1.65% to 100%. Generally, analyses conducted with a smaller number of data points frequently had a greater percentage of variance accounted for by sampling error. A smaller percentage of variance accounted for by sampling error suggests a greater percentage of variance is accounted for by true score variance across the observed studies.

Eating attitudes test

Reliability information was not provided in 93 (43.26%) of 215 studies utilizing the EAT, and in 44 (20.47%) studies, the researchers made some reference to score

Table 1 Mean internal consistency estimates for the eating disorders inventory (EDI)

Study characteristics		# of data points K	Total sample size N	Sample-weighted mean alpha (SD)	95% CI	PVA_{SE}
		Reliability				
EDI total		**6**	**3269**	**.91 (.06)**	**.86 - .95**	**1.65%**
Gender:	Female	6	3269	.91 (.06)	.86 - .95	1.65%
Age:	Adult	4	995	.85 (.08)	.77 - .93	4.35%
	Adolescent	2	1137	.93 (<.01)	.93 - .93	100.00%
Type of sample:	Nonclinical	4	2989	.90 (.06)	.84 - .96	1.24%
	Clinical: Eating disorder	2	280	.95 (.01)	.93 - .96	99.32%
Test language:	English	4	995	.85 (.08)	.77 - .93	4.35%
	Non-English	2	2274	.93 (<.01)	.93 - .93	100.00%
EDI body dissatisfaction subscale		**55**	**22120**	**.89 (.04)**	**.88 - .90**	**6.51%**
Gender:	Female	44	17240	.90 (.03)	.89 - .91	9.82%
	Male	5	2443	.81 (.03)	.79 - .84	26.56%
	Mixed gender	6	2437	.90 (.03)	.88 - .92	11.02%
Age:	Adult	35	8311	.91 (.03)	.90 - .92	17.16%
	Adolescent	20	13809	.88 (.04)	.86 - .90	3.92%
Type of Sample:	Nonclinical	43	19844	.89 (.04)	.87 - .90	5.63%
	Clinical: Eating Disorder	11	2156	.90 (.03)	.89 - .92	19.05%
Test Language:	English	42	13557	.89 (.03)	.88 - .90	10.70%
	Non-English	13	8563	.88 (.05)	.85 - .91	3.17%
EDI drive for thinness subscale		**49**	**22335**	**.85 (.05)**	**.83 - .86**	**6.24%**
Gender:	Female	37	15831	.84 (.05)	.83 - .86	6.56%
	Male	4	2277	.79 (.03)	.77 - .82	37.17%
	Mixed gender	8	4227	.89 (.02)	.87 - .90	27.54%
Age:	Adult	32	7784	.86 (.04)	.85 - .88	15.07%
	Adolescent	17	14551	.84 (.06)	.81 - .86	3.29%
Type of sample:	Nonclinical	36	19788	.85 (.05)	.83 - .87	4.78%
	Clinical: Eating disorder	12	2427	.83 (.04)	.80 - .85	37.93%
Test language:	English	37	13943	.86 (.05)	.84 - .87	8.58%
	Non-English	12	8392	.83 (.06)	.80 - .86	4.17%
EDI bulimia subscale		**47**	**21875**	**.75 (.07)**	**.73 - .77**	**9.47%**
Gender:	Female	37	15905	.77 (.07)	.74 - .79	9.18%
	Male	3	2081	.67 (.02)	.65 - .69	100.00%
	Mixed gender	7	3889	.74 (.04)	.71 - .77	20.89%
Age:	Adult	31	7437	.81 (.07)	.79 - .83	11.55%
	Adolescent	16	14438	.72 (.04)	.70 - .74	14.17%
Type of sample:	Nonclinical	35	19861	.74 (.06)	.72 - .76	9.98%
	Clinical: Eating disorder	11	1894	.84 (.07)	.79 - .88	10.76%
Test language:	English	35	13483	.76 (.07)	.74 - .78	10.71%
	Non-English	12	8392	.74 (.06)	.70 - .77	7.57%

Note. CI = Confidence Interval. PVA_{SE} = Percent of variance accounted for by sampling error.

reliability from previously published studies (see Figure 1 for a flow chart). Reliability information for either the total EAT score or one or more factor scores for their sample was reported in 78 (36.28%) studies. Seven of these studies were excluded from further analysis because the authors modified the measure or used different factors based on their own factor analysis of the EAT (see [26,28-30,69-135] for included studies). Results indicate that the sample-weighted mean estimates of internal consistency were .81 for the EAT-40 and .86 for the EAT-26. The mean estimates of internal consistency for scores on the EAT-26 factors were .80 for the Dieting factor, .67 for the Bulimia and Food Preoccupation factor, and .56 for the Oral Control factor. Table 2 presents the sample-weighted mean estimates of internal consistency for the EAT, as well as the means broken down by gender, age, type of sample, and test language.

An examination of prospective moderators suggested that for the EAT-40, the female samples had higher reliability than the male and mixed gender samples, and the mixed gender group displayed higher reliability than the male group. However, with a small number of data points for analyses, it is important to interpret these comparisons with caution. The adult and clinical eating disorder samples displayed greater reliability than their respective comparison samples. For the EAT-26, the reliability was similar among the gender and age categories. The clinical eating disorder samples displayed greater reliability than the nonclinical samples, with the mixed clinical and nonclinical samples also displaying greater reliability than the nonclinical samples. The English-speaking samples also had a higher mean estimate of internal consistency than the non-English samples. Regarding subscale scores, female and male samples also displayed similar score reliability on the EAT-26 Dieting Factor. The adult samples had greater reliability than the adolescent samples, and the English test language samples had a higher mean estimate of reliability than the non-English samples. For the Bulimia and Food Preoccupation subscale, the mean estimate of reliability for the adult samples had higher reliability than the adolescent samples. For the Oral Control factor, the score reliability for the male samples was greater than the female samples, and the adolescent samples had a similar mean estimate of internal consistency as compared to the adult samples. The non-English language test samples had higher reliability than the English samples. Overall, for the EAT, the percentage of variance explained by sampling error ranged widely from approximately 5% to 100%. For the majority of the analyses, these values were less than 20%.

Test-retest reliability analyses

Table 3 presents sample-weighted mean estimates of test-retest reliability for the EDI and EAT-26. For the EDI, the mean test-retest score reliability was .81, and for the EDI subscales, mean test-retest reliability estimates ranged from .42 to .77. The lowest mean test-retest reliability estimates were for the Drive for Thinness [60] and Bulimia [64] subscales. For the EAT-26, the mean test-retest reliability estimate was .87. However, due to the low number of data points available for each scale or subscale, these results should be interpreted with caution.

Discussion

This study used reliability generalization procedures to find the mean score reliability for different versions of the EDI and the EAT and to examine study characteristics (i.e., moderators) that might explain the variation in score reliability across studies. The reporting rate of score reliability information for the measures was higher (26.15% - 41.46%) than the reporting rate for other RG studies, such as the BDI (7.5%) [6] and the NEO (15.2%) [17]. However, given that score reliability information should be reported every time a measure is used, it is disappointing that such a large proportion of the studies using the EDI and the EAT failed to provide such information.

Overall, mean reliability estimates for the measures were acceptable, with only the Oral Control factor on the EAT-26 exhibiting questionable mean internal consistency [56]. For the EDI, the Bulimia subscale, which was designed to measure specific eating disorder attitudes and behaviors, displayed higher score reliability in clinical eating disorder samples than in nonclinical samples. Conversely, the Drive for Thinness and Body Dissatisfaction subscales exhibited similar score reliability in clinical and nonclinical groups. One potential explanation for this discrepancy is that the attitudes measured by the Body Dissatisfaction and Drive for Thinness subscales are common in both nonclinical and eating disorder samples, contributing to more reliable measurement of these attitudes across sample type. It is more difficult to characterize the effect of sample type on the two versions of the EAT because scores on these measures were primarily reported for nonclinical samples.

Regarding participant age and gender, mean score reliability tended to be slightly higher in the adult samples than in adolescent samples for all measures; however, reliability was generally acceptable in both groups. However, the EAT-26 Bulimia and Food Preoccupation subscale scores displayed mean reliability above .70 in the adult group but below .70 in the adolescent group. The higher reliability in the adult group may be expected as the measures were developed in adult samples. For all measures, there was a tendency for score reliability to be slightly higher in female samples than in the male samples, perhaps because eating disorder attitudes and behaviors are more prevalent among women resulting in greater score variability for this subpopulation.

Test-retest reliability analyses indicate that this type of reliability was generally acceptable for both measures, with the lowest estimate found for the EDI Drive for Thinness subscale, followed by the EDI Bulimia subscale. Although the EDI Bulimia scale did exhibit lower internal consistency estimates among certain samples, the

Table 2 Mean internal consistency estimates for the eating attitudes test (EAT)

Study characteristics		*Reliability*				
		# of data points K	**Total sample size N**	**Sample-weighted mean alpha (SD)**	**95% CI**	**PVA_{SE}**
EAT-40		**15**	**3925**	**.81 (.09)**	**.77 - .86**	**5.89%**
Gender:	Female	10	1950	.86 (.04)	.84 - .89	19.54%
	Male	2	492	.68 (.06)	.59 - .77	18.90%
	Mixed gender	3	1483	.79 (.08)	.70 - .88	4.55%
Age:	Adult	11	1855	.87 (.05)	.84 - .90	13.32%
	Adolescent	4	2070	.76 (.08)	.68 - .84	5.07%
Type of sample:	Nonclinical	12	3538	.80 (.08)	.75 - .85	6.45%
	Clinical: Eating disorder	2	193	.90 (.05)	.83 - .97	16.45%
Test language:	English	11	2833	.82 (.08)	.78 - .87	6.47%
	Non-English	4	1092	.78 (.10)	.69 - .88	5.72%
EAT-26		**54**	**11963**	**.86 (.05)**	**.84 - .87**	**11.50%**
Gender:	Female	42	9566	.85 (.05)	.83 - .87	11.06%
	Male	4	488	.85 (.03)	.82 - .88	72.61%
	Mixed gender	8	1909	.87 (.05)	.84 - .90	10.28%
Age:	Adult	42	9049	.86 (.05)	.85 - .88	12.89%
	Adolescent	11	2717	.85 (.05)	.82 - .88	11.94%
Type of sample:	Nonclinical	48	11321	.85 (.05)	.84 - .87	11.08%
	Clinical: Eating disorder	4	423	.90 (.02)	.89 - .92	100.00%
	Mixed clinical and nonclinical	2	219	.88 (.05)	.81 - .95	20.57%
Test language:	English	44	9077	.87 (.05)	.85 - .88	11.30%
	Non-English	10	2886	.81 (.04)	.79 - .84	25.69%
EAT-26 dieting factor		**24**	**10924**	**.80 (.07)**	**.77 - .83**	**5.50%**
Gender:	Female	22	10693	.80 (.07)	.77 - .83	5.06%
	Male	2	231	.81 (.03)	.77 - .85	100.00%
Age:	Adult	17	3870	.87 (.04)	.86 - .89	19.92%
	Adolescent	7	7054	.77 (.05)	.72 - .81	5.74%
Type of sample:	Nonclinical	22	10602	.80 (.07)	.77 - .83	5.27%
Test language:	English	21	10150	.80 (.07)	.77 - .83	5.35%
	Non-English	3	774	.86 (.04)	.81 - .90	17.23%
EAT-26 bulimia and food preoccupation factor		**23**	**10751**	**.67 (.11)**	**.63 - .71**	**5.44%**
Gender:	Female	21	10520	.67 (.11)	.62 - .72	5.12%
	Male	2	231	.71 (.11)	.56 - .87	17.26%
Age:	Adult	17	3870	.79 (.07)	.75 - .82	10.99%
	Adolescent	6	6881	.60 (.06)	.56 - .65	9.70%
Type of sample:	Nonclinical	21	10429	.67 (.11)	.62 - .71	5.29%
Test language:	English	20	9977	.67 (.11)	.62 - .72	4.92%
	Non-English	3	774	.71 (.04)	.67 - .76	60.81%
EAT-26 oral control factor		**18**	**4475**	**.56 (.10)**	**.51 - .60**	**21.02%**
Gender:	Female	16	4244	.56 (.10)	.51 - .61	19.03%
	Male	2	231	.60 (.02)	.57 - .63	100.00%
Age:	Adult	14	3065	.56 (.11)	.50 - .61	19.04%
	Adolescent	4	1410	.57 (.06)	.51 - .63	34.67%

Table 2 Mean internal consistency estimates for the eating attitudes test (EAT) *(Continued)*

Type of sample:	Nonclinical	16	4153	.55 (.08)	.51 - .59	27.63%
Test language:	English	15	3701	.54 (.10)	.50 - .59	21.52%
	Non-English	3	774	.63 (.04)	.59 - .67	100.00%

Note. CI = Confidence Interval. PVA_{SE} = Percent of variance accounted for by sampling error.

EDI Drive for Thinness scale appeared to have similar score reliability across diverse samples; thus, it is somewhat surprising that this scale should exhibit the lowest overall test-retest reliability. One possibility for this might be that the construct assessed by this scale may be more subject to temporal fluctuations than some of the other constructs assessed by the EDI. Alternatively, the EDI Drive for Thinness scale is frequently employed in experimental studies involving brief interventions designed to change participants' attitudes toward thinness (e.g., [136]), suggesting that this tool may be sensitive to fluctuations in drive for thinness. Finally, given the small amount of data available regarding test-retest reliability, these findings may be less statistically meaningful than the findings for internal consistency reliability estimates.

Although mean reliability estimates for scores on the EDI, EAT, and their subscales were generally acceptable, the data indicate that some of the subscales display greater score reliability in female, adult, and clinical (eating disorder) subpopulations, but with some variability across the different subscales. It is important that researchers measure internal consistency for their sample every time a measure is used as characteristics of the sample affect test score reliability. The present study demonstrates that reliability estimates do not remain constant across studies; therefore, researchers should ensure that the scores for their sample are found to be reliable as an initial step in any study. Examining and reporting test score reliability should be included as descriptive information about the data. Additionally, researchers can tailor future studies to maximize score reliability, which is one factor that influences effect sizes.

One limitation of this study is the small number of data points available for some analyses. Although information was reported for analyses where only 2–4 internal consistency estimates were available, these findings are less stable than a mean estimate based on 30–50 data points and therefore should be cautiously interpreted and were presented here only for the sake of completeness. Another potential limitation is having only one coder for the study. This decision was made because, unlike in traditional meta-analysis, the coder did not have to calculate effect sizes or other statistics and was only recording information as reported in articles; however, there is always the possibility that two coders could have disagreed about some of this basic information. In addition to addressing some of these design limitations and conducting a more recent search of the literature, future research could also examine the predictors of reliability estimates for other frequently employed assessment tools for eating symptomatology, such as the Eating Disorder Examination-Questionnaire [137].

Conclusions

Reliability generalization is a valuable method of educating other researchers about reliability issues and emphasizing that reliability is "not an immutable unchanging property of tests" ([18], p. 124). This study indicates that test score reliability for the EDI and EAT is greater for adult and clinical samples than for adolescent and nonclinical samples. Although it is important that disordered eating be reliably measured in an adult, clinical population, these findings are potentially troubling as it is also important that these concepts be reliably measurable in nonclinical adolescents who are at high risk for developing disordered eating attitudes and behaviors. In some cases, the differences in score reliability between adult and adolescent samples were small, and mean score reliability for adolescent samples remained acceptable overall. However, the differences between clinical eating disorder and nonclinical samples were generally larger. Without reliable measurement of these concepts

Table 3 Mean test-retest reliability estimates for the EDI and EAT

			Reliability		
Study characteristics	**# of data points K**	**Total sample size N**	**Sample-weighted mean reliability (SD)**	**95nnnnn CI**	**PVA_{SE}**
EDI total	2	471	.81 (.06)	.72 - .90	12.68%
EDI body dissatisfaction subscale	3	256	.77 (.14)	.62 - .92	10.66%
EDI drive for thinness subscale	4	715	.60 (.15)	.45 - .75	10.07%
EDI bulimia subscale	4	715	.64 (.12)	.53 - .76	14.12%
EAT-26	4	920	.87 (.02)	.85 - .88	100.00%

Note. CI = Confidence Interval. PVA_{SE} = Percent of variance accounted for by sampling error.

in an at-risk adolescent population, researchers will have difficulty determining the true effectiveness of prevention programs designed to avoid or reduce future symptoms of eating disorders. Therefore, it is important for researchers to assess and report test score reliability with the measures they are using to determine the effectiveness of their programs.

Competing interests
The authors declare that they have no competing interests.

Authors' contributions
DG developed the idea for the study, assisted with the research conceptualization and design; statistical analyses, writing and revising of the manuscript. CP obtained and coded articles for reliability generalization analyses, conducted analyses and drafted the manuscript from her doctoral dissertation under the supervision of DG and LM. SA assisted with the research conceptualization, literature research, and revising the manuscript. LM assisted with the design of the study and supervised article coding and statistical analyses. All authors read and approved the final manuscript.

Acknowledgements
The authors wish to thank Ms. Lea Simms for her editorial assistance.

Author details
[1]School of Psychology, Social Work and Social Policy, University of South Australia, Magill Campus, GPO Box 2471, Adelaide, SA 5001, Australia. [2]Texas A&M University, College Station, TX, USA. [3]Dickinson College, Carlisle, PA, USA.

References
1. Hoek HW, Van Hoeken D: **Review of the prevalence and incidence of eating disorders.** *Int J Eat Disorder* 2003, **34**:383–396.
2. Berg KC, Frazier P, Sherr L: **Change in eating disorder attitudes and behavior in college women: prevalence and predictors.** *Eat Behav* 2009, **10**(3):137–142.
3. Touchette E, Henegar A, Godart NT, Pryor L, Falissard B, Tremblay RE, Côté SM: **Subclinical eating disorders and their comorbidity with mood and anxiety disorders in adolescent girls.** *Psychiat Res* 2011, **185**(1–2):185–192.
4. Micali N, Hagberg KW, Petersen I, Treasure JL: **The incidence of eating disorders in the UK in 2000–2009; findings from the General Practice Research Database.** *BMJ Open* 2013, **3**:e002646.
5. Hay PJ, Mond J, Buttner P, Darby A: **Eating disorder behaviors are increasing: findings from two sequential community surveys in South Australia.** *PLoS One* 2008, **3**(2):e1541.
6. Yin P, Fan X: **Assessing the reliability of Beck Depression Inventory scores: reliability generalization across studies.** *Educ Psychol Meas* 2000, **60**:201–223.
7. Thompson B: **Guidelines for authors reporting score reliability estimates.** *Educ Psycho Meas* 1994, **54**:837–847.
8. Wilkinson L, APA Task Force on Statistical Inference: **Statistical methods in psychology journals: guidelines and explanations.** *Am Psychol* 1999, **54**:594–604.
9. Thompson B: **Understanding reliability and coefficient alpha, really.** In *Score reliability: Contemporary thinking on reliability issues.* Edited by Thompson B. Thousand Oaks, CA: Sage Publications; 2003.
10. Baugh F: **Correcting effect sizes for score reliability: a reminder that measurement and substantive issues are linked inextricably.** *Educ Psychol Meas* 2002, **62**:254–263.
11. Thompson B: **Significance, effect sizes, stepwise methods, and other issues: strong arguments move the field.** *J Exp Educ* 2001, **70**:80–93.
12. Vacha-Haase T: **Reliability generalization: exploring variance in measurement error affecting score reliability across studies.** *Educ Psychol Meas* 1998, **58**:6–20.
13. Vacha-Haase T, Henson RK, Caruso JC: **Reliability generalization: moving toward improved understanding and use of score reliability.** *Educ Psychol Meas* 2002, **62**:562–569.
14. Lipsey MW, Wilson DB: *Practical meta-analysis.* Thousand Oaks: Sage Publications; 2001.
15. Hunter JE, Schmidt FL: **Correcting for sources of artificial variation across studies.** In *The Handbook of Research Synthesis.* Edited by Cooper H, Hedge LV. New York: Russell Sage Foundation; 1994:323–336.
16. Meier ST, Davis SR: **Trends in reporting psychometric properties of scales in counseling psychology research.** *J Couns Psychol* 1990, **37**:113–115.
17. Caruso JC: **Reliability generalization of the NEO Personality Scales.** *Educ Psychol Meas* 2000, **60**:236–254.
18. Henson RK, Thompson B: **Characterizing measurement error in scores across studies: Some recommendations for conducting "reliability generalization" studies.** *Meas Eval Couns Dev* 2002, **35**:113–126.
19. Breidbord J, Croudace TJ: **Reliability generalization for childhood autism rating scale.** *J Autism Dev Disord* 2013, **43**:2855–2865.
20. Miller CS, Woodson J, Howell RT, Shields AL: **Assessing the reliability of scores produced by the substance abuse subtle screening inventory.** *Subst Use & Misuse* 2009, **44**:1090–1100.
21. Vassar M, Bradley G: **A reliability generalization meta-analysis of coefficient alpha for the Reynolds Adolescent Depression Scale.** *Clin Child Psychol Psychiat* 2012, **17**:519–527.
22. Meca JS, Lopez-Pina JA, Lopez-Lopez JA, Marin-Martinez F, Rosa-Alcazar AI, Gomez-Conesa AA: **The Maudsley obsessive-compulsive inventory: a reliability generalization meta-analysis.** *Int J Clin Health Psychol* 2011, **11**:473–493.
23. Rouse SV: **Using reliability generalization methods to explore measurement error: an illustration using the MMPI-2 PSY-5 scales.** *J Pers Assess* 2007, **88**:264–275.
24. Hunter JE, Schmidt FL: *Methods of meta-analysis: Correcting error and bias in research findings.* Newbury Park: Sage Publications; 1990.
25. Garner DM, Olmstead MP, Polivy J: **Development and validation of a multidimensional eating disorder inventory for anorexia nervosa and bulimia.** *Int J Eat Disorder* 1983, **2**:15–34.
26. Garner DM, Garfinkel PE: **The Eating Attitudes Test: An index of the symptoms of anorexia nervosa.** *Psychol Med* 1979, **9**:273–279.
27. Garner DM: *Eating Disorder Inventory-2 Professional Manual.* Odessa: Psychological Assessment Resources, Inc; 1991.
28. Garner DM, Olmsted MP, Bohr Y, Garfinkel PE: **The eating attitudes test: psychometric features and clinical correlates.** *Psychol Med* 1982, **12**:871–878.
29. Gross J, Rosen JC, Leitenberg H, Willmuth ME: **Validity of the eating attitudes test and the eating disorders inventory in bulimia nervosa.** *J Consult Clin Psych* 1986, **54**:875–876.
30. Scheinberg Z, Koslowsky M, Bleich A, Mark M, Apter A, Danon Y, Solomon Z, Babur I: **Sensitivity, specificity, and positive predictive value as measures of prediction accuracy: the case of the EAT-26.** *Educ Psychol Meas* 1993, **1993**(53):831–839.
31. Williamson DA, Anderson DA, Gleaves DH: **Anorexia nervosa and bulimia nervosa: structured interview methodologies and psychological assessment.** In *Body image, eating disorders, and obesity: An integrative guide for assessment and treatment.* Edited by Thompson JK. Washington, DC: American Psychological Association; 1996:205–223.
32. Cronbach LJ: **Coefficient alpha and the internal structure of tests.** *Psychometrika* 1951, **16**:197–334.
33. Dimitrov DM: **Reliability: arguments for multiple perspectives and potential problems with generalization across studies.** *Educ Psychol Meas* 2002, **62**:783–801.
34. Arthur W Jr, Bennett W Jr, Huffcutt AI: *Conducting meta-analysis using SAS.* Mahwah: Lawrence Erlbaum Associates; 2001.
35. Adkins EC, Keel PK: **Does "excessive" or "compulsive" best describe exercise as a symptom of bulimia nervosa?** *Int J Eat Disorder* 2005, **38**:24–29.
36. Birkeland R, Thompson JK, Phares V: **Adolescent motherhood and postpartum depression.** *J Clin Child Adol Psychol* 2005, **34**:292–300.
37. Compian L, Gowen LK, Hayward C: **Peripubertal girls' romantic and platonic involvement with boys: associations with body image and depressive symptoms.** *J Res Adolescence* 2004, **14**:23–47.

38. Davies K, Wardle J: Body image and dieting in pregnancy. *J Psychosom Res* 1994, 38:787–799.
39. Eberenz KP, Gleaves DH: An examination of the internal consistency and factor structure of the eating disorder inventory-2 in a clinical sample. *Int J Eat Disorder* 1994, 16:371–379.
40. Espelage DL, Mazzeo SE, Aggen SH, Quittner AL, Sherman R, Thompson R: Examining the construct validity of the eating disorder inventory. *Psychol Assess* 2003, 15:71–80.
41. Fitzgibbon ML, Sánchez-Johnsen LA, Martinovich Z: A test of the continuity perspective across bulimic and binge eating pathology. *Int J Eat Disorder* 2003, 34:83–97.
42. Franko DL, Striegel-Moore RH, Barton BA, Schumann BC, Garner DM, Daniels SR, Schreiber GB, Crawford PB: Measuring eating concerns in black and white adolescent girls. *Int J Eat Disorder* 2004, 35:179–189.
43. Janelle CM, Hausenblas HA, Fallon EA, Gardner RE: A visual search examination of attentional biases among individuals with high and low drive for thinness. *Eat Weight Disord* 2003, 8:138–144.
44. Joiner TE Jr, Heatherton TF, Keel PK: Ten-year stability and predictive validity of five bulimia-related indicators. *Am J Psychiat* 1997, 154:1133–1138.
45. Keery H, Boutelle K, van den Berg P, Thompson JK: The impact of appearance-related teasing by family members. *J Adolescent Health* 2005, 2005(37):120–127.
46. Leung F, Wang J, Tang CW: Psychometric properties and normative data of the eating disorder inventory among 12 to 18 year old Chinese girls in Hong Kong. *J Psychosom Res* 2004, 57:59–66.
47. Martin KA, Hausenblas HA: Psychological commitment to exercise and eating disorder symptomatology among female aerobic instructors. *Sport Psycho* 1998, 12:180–190.
48. Pelletier LG, Dion S, Lévesque C: Can self-determination help protect women against Sociocultural influences about body image and reduce their risk of experiencing bulimic symptoms? *J Soc Clin Psychol* 2004, 23:61–88.
49. Podar I, Hannus A, Allik J: Personality and affectivity characteristics associated with eating disorders: a comparison of eating disordered, weight-preoccupied, and normal samples. *J Pers Assess* 1991, 73:133–147.
50. Rhea DJ: Eating disorder behaviors of ethnically diverse urban female adolescent athletes and non-athletes. *J Adolescence* 1999, 22:379–388.
51. Robinson TN, Killen JD, Litt IF, Hammer LD, Wilson DM, Haydel KF, Hayward C, Taylor CB: Ethnicity and body dissatisfaction: are Hispanic and Asian girls at increased risk for eating disorders? *J Adolescent Health* 1996, 19:384–393.
52. Ryu HR, Lyle RM, Galer-Unti RA, Black DR: Cross-cultural assessment of eating disorders: psychometric characteristics of a Korean version of the Eating Disorder Inventory-2 and the Bulimia Test-Revised. *Eat Disord* 1999, 7:109–122.
53. Shore RA, Porter JE: Normative and reliability data for 11 to 18 year olds on the Eating Disorder Inventory. *Int J Eat Disorder* 1990, 9:201–207.
54. Schoemaker C, van Strien T, van der Staak C: Validation of the eat disord inventory in a nonclinical population using transformed and untransformed responses. *Int J Eat Disorder* 1994, 15:387–393.
55. Tasca GA, Illing V, Lybanon-Daigle V, Bissada H, Balfour L: Psychometric properties of the Eating Disorders Inventory-2 among women seeking treatment for binge eating disorder. *Assessment* 2003, 10:228–236.
56. Thurfjell B, Edlund B, Arinell H, Hägglöf B, Engström I: Psychometric properties of Eating Disorder Inventory for children (EDI-C) in Swedish girls with and without a known eating disorder. *Eat Weight Disord* 2003, 8:296–303.
57. Tiggemann M: Television and adolescent body image: the role of program content and viewing motivation. *J Soc Clin Psychol* 2005, 24:361–381.
58. Tylka TL, Subich LM: A preliminary investigation of the eating disorder continuum with men. *J Couns Psychol* 2002, 49:273–279.
59. van Strien T, Ouwens M: Validation of the Dutch EDI-2 in one clinical and two nonclinical populations. *Eur J Psychol Assess* 2003, 19:66–84.
60. Vincent MA, McCabe MP, Ricciardelli LA: Factorial validity of the Bulimia Test-Revised in adolescent boys and girls. *Behav Res Therapy* 1999, 37:1129–1140.
61. Vohs KD, Bardone AM, Joiner TE Jr, Abramson LY, Heatherton TF: Perfectionism, perceived weight status, and self-esteem interact to predict bulimic symptoms: a model of bulimic symptom development. *J Abnormal Psychol* 1999, 108:695–700.
62. Wassenaar D, le Grange D, Winship J, Lachenicht L: The prevalence of eating disorder pathology in a cross-ethnic population of female students in South Africa. *Eur Eat Disord Rev* 2000, 8:225–236.
63. Wear RW, Pratz O: Test-retest reliability for the eating disorder inventory. *Int J Eat Disorder* 1987, 6:767–769.
64. Welch G, Hall A: The reliability and discriminant validity of three potential measures of bulimic behaviours. *J Psychiat Res* 1987, 23:125–133.
65. Wilhelmsson M, Andersson AL: An attempt at distinguishing subgroups of women with anorexia nervosa and bulimia nervosa by means of the Defense Mechanism Technique modified (DMTm) and the Eating Disorder Inventory (EDI). *Eat Weight Disord* 2005, 10:175–186.
66. Wonderlich AL, Ackard DM, Henderson JB: Childhood beauty pageant contestants: associations with adult disordered eating and mental health. *Eat Disord* 2005, 13:291–301.
67. Zabinski MF, Calfas KJ, Gehrman CA, Wilfley DA, Sallis JF: Effects of a physical activity intervention on body image in university seniors: Project GRAD. *Ann Behav Med* 2001, 23:247–252.
68. Breen HB, Espelage DL: Nutrition expertise in eating disorders. *Eat Weight Disord* 2004, 9:120–125.
69. Brookings JB, Wilson JF: Personality and family-environment predictors of self-reported eating attitudes and behaviors. *J Pers Assess* 1994, 63:313–326.
70. Botta RA: For your health? The relationship between magazine reading and adolescents' body image and eating disturbances. *Sex Roles* 2003, 48:389–399.
71. Joiner GW, Kashubeck S: Acculturation, body image, self-esteem, and eating-disorder symptomatology in adolescent Mexican American women. *Psychol Women Quart* 1996, 20:419–435.
72. Tylka TL, Subich LM: Revisiting the latent structure of eating disorders: Taxometric analyses with nonbehavioral indicators. *J Couns Psychol* 2003, 50:276–286.
73. van den Berg P, Thompson JK, Obremski-Brandon K, Coovert M: The Tripartite Influence model of body image and eating disturbance. A covariance structure modeling investigation testing the mediational role of appearance comparison. *J Psychosom Res* 2002, 53:1007–1020.
74. Vanderheyden DA, Fekken GC, Boland FJ: Critical variables associated with bingeing and bulimia in a university population: A factor analytic study. *Int J Eat Disorder* 1988, 7:321–329.
75. Williams TL, Gleaves DH: Childhood sexual abuse, body image, and disordered eating: a structural modeling analysis. *J Trauma Dissociation* 2003, 4:91–108.
76. Tachikawa H, Yamaguchi N, Haianaka K, Kobayashi J, Sato S, Mizukami K, Asada T, Sugie M: The Eating Disorder Inventory-2 in Japanese clinical and non-clinical samples: Psychometric properties and cross-cultural implications. *Eat Weight Disord* 2004, 9:107–113.
77. Tylka TL: The relation between body dissatisfaction and eating disorder symptomatology: an analysis of moderating variables. *J Couns Psychol* 2004, 51:178–191.
78. Nobakht M, Kezhkam M: An epidemiological study of eating disorders in Iran. *Int J Eat Disorder* 2000, 28:265–271.
79. Sherry SB, Hewitt PL, Besser A, McGee BJ, Flett GL: Self-oriented and socially prescribed perfectionism in the Eating Disorder Inventory Perfectionism subscale. *Int J Eat Disorder* 2004, 35:69–79.
80. Sim L, Zeman J: Emotion awareness and identification skills in adolescent girls with bulimia nervosa. *J Clin Child Adolescent Psychol* 2004, 33:760–771.
81. Hund AR, Espelage DL: Childhood sexual abuse, disordered eating, alexithymia, and general distress: a mediation model. *J Couns Psychol* 2005, 52:559–573.
82. Harrison K: The body electric: thin-ideal media and eating disorders in adolescents. *J Comm* 2000, 50:119–143.
83. Siervo M, Boschi V, Papa A, Bellini O, Falconi C: Application of the SCOFF, Eating Attitude Test 26 (EAT 26) and Eating Inventory (TFEQ) questionnaires in young women seeking diet-therapy. *Eat Weight Disord* 2005, 10:76–82.
84. Raciti MC, Norcross JC: The EAT and EDI: screening, interrelationships, and psychometrics. *Int J Eat Disorder* 1987, 6:579–586.

85. Rizvi SL, Stice E, Agras WS: **Natural history of disordered eating attitudes and behaviors over a 6-year period.** *Int J Eat Disorder* 1999, **26**:406–413.
86. Piran N, Cormier HC: **The social construction of women and disordered eating patterns.** *J Couns Psychol* 2005, **52**:549–558.
87. Spillane NS, Boerner LM, Anderson KG, Smith GT: **Comparability of the Eating Disorder Inventory-2 between women and men.** *Assessment* 2004, **11**:85–93.
88. Aarnio K, Lindeman M: **Magical food and health beliefs: A portrait of believers and functions of the beliefs.** *Appetite* 2004, **43**:65–74.
89. Banasiak SJ, Wertheim EH, Koemer J, Voudouris NJ: **Test-retest reliability and internal consistency of a variety of measures of dietary restraint and body concerns in a sample of adolescent girls.** *Int J Eat Disorder* 2001, **29**:85–89.
90. Baş M, Aşçı H, Karabudak E, Kızıltan G: **Eating attitudes and their psychological correlates among Turkish adolescents.** *Adolescence* 2004, **39**:593–599.
91. Boerner LM, Spillane NS, Anderson KG, Smith GT: **Similarities and differences between women and men on eating disorder risk factors and symptom measures.** *Eat Behav* 2004, **5**:209–222.
92. Bittinger JN, Smith JE: **Mediating and moderating effects of stress perception and situation type on coping responses in women with disordered eating.** *Eat Behav* 2003, **4**:89–106.
93. Cash TF, Hrabosky JI: **The effects of psychoeducation and self-monitoring in a cognitive-behavioral program for body-image improvement.** *Eat Disord* 2003, **11**:255–270.
94. Cash TF, Melnyk SE, Hrabosky JI: **The assessment of body image investment: an extensive revision of the appearance schemas inventory.** *Int J Eat Disorder* 2004, **35**:305–316.
95. Daubenmier JJ: **The relationship of yoga, body awareness, and body responsiveness to self-objectification and disordered eating.** *Psychol Women Quart* 2005, **29**:207–219.
96. Espina Eizaguirre A, de Cabezón AOS, de Alda IO, Olariaga LJ, Juaniz M: **Alexithymia and its relationships with anxiety and depression in eating disorders.** *Pers Indiv Diff* 2004, **36**:321–331.
97. Favaro A, Rodella FC, Santonastaso P: **Binge eating and eating attitudes among Nazi concentration camp survivors.** *Psychol Med* 2000, **30**:463–466.
98. Davison KK, Markey CN, Birch LL: **A longitudinal examination of patterns in girls' weight concerns and body dissatisfaction from ages 5 to 9 years.** *Int J Eat Disorder* 2003, **33**:320–332.
99. Fung MSC, Yuen M: **Body image and eating attitudes among adolescent Chinese girls in Hong Kong.** *Percept Motor Skill* 2003, **96**:57–66.
100. Furnham A, Badmin N, Sneade I: **Body image dissatisfaction: Gender differences in eating attitudes, self-esteem, and reasons for exercise.** *J Psychol* 2002, **136**:581–596.
101. Graber JA, Tyrka AR, Brooks-Gunn J: **How similar are correlates of different subclinical eating problems and bulimia nervosa?** *J Child Psychol Psychiat* 2003, **44**:262–273.
102. Haase AM, Prapavessis H, Owens RG: **Perfectionism, social physique anxiety and disordered eating: A comparison of male and female elite athletes.** *Psychol Sport Exercise* 2002, **3**:209–222.
103. Holt MK, Espelage DL: **Problem-solving skills and relationship attributes among women with eating disorders.** *J Counsel Deve* 2002, **80**:346–354.
104. Francis LA, Birch LL: **Maternal influences on daughters' restrained eating behavior.** *Health Psychol* 2005, **24**:548–554.
105. Humphry TA, Ricciardelli LA: **The development of eating pathology in Chinese-Australian women: Acculturation versus culture clash.** *Int J Eat Disorder* 2004, **35**:579–588.
106. Iyer DS, Haslam N: **Body image and eating disturbance among south Asian-American women: the role of racial teasing.** *Int J Eat Disorder* 2003, **34**:142–147.
107. Jackson T, Weiss KE, Lunquist JJ, Soderlind A: **Sociotropy and perceptions of interpersonal relationships as predictors of eating disturbances among college women: two prospective studies.** *J Genet Psychol* 2005, **166**:346–359.
108. Johnson CE, Petrie TA: **Relationship of gender discrepancy to psychological correlates of disordered eating in female undergraduates.** *J Couns Psychol* 1996, **43**:473–479.
109. Johnson CS, Bedford J: **Eating attitudes across age and gender groups: a Canadian study.** *Eat Weight Disord* 2004, **9**:16–23.
110. Jordan PJ, Redding CA, Troop NA, Treasure J, Serpell L: **Developing a stage of change measure for assessing recovery from anorexia nervosa.** *Eat Behav* 2003, **3**:365–385.
111. Kirk G, Singh K, Getz H: **Risk of eating disorders among female college athletes and nonathletes.** *J Coll Counsel* 2001, **4**:122–132.
112. Koslowsky M, Scheinberg Z, Bleich A, Mark M, Apter A, Danon Y, Solomon Z: **The factor structure and criterion validity of the short form of the Eating Attitudes Test.** *J Pers Assess* 1992, **58**:27–35.
113. Lee S, Kwok K, Liau C, Leung T: **Screening Chinese patients with eating disorders using the Eating Attitudes Test in Hong Kong.** *Int J Eat Disorder* 2002, **32**:91–97.
114. Lee S, Lee AM: **Disordered eating in three communities of China: a comparative study of female high school students in Hong Kong, Shenzhen, and rural Hunan.** *Int J Eat Disorder* 2002, **27**:317–327.
115. Lorenzo CR, Lavori PW, Lock JD: **Eating attitudes in high school students in the Philippines: A preliminary study.** *Eat Weight Disord* 2002, **7**:202–209.
116. Mazzeo SE: **Modification of an existing measure of body image preoccupation and its relationship to disordered eating in female college students.** *J Couns Psychol* 1999, **46**:42–50.
117. McVey GL, Davis R, Tweed S, Shaw BF: **Evaluation of a school-based program designed to improve body image satisfaction, global self-esteem, and eating attitudes and behaviors: A replication study.** *Int J Eat Disorder* 2004, **36**:1–11.
118. McVey GL, Pepler D, Davis R, Flett GL, Abdolell M: **Risk and protective factors associated with disordered eating during early adolescence.** *J Early Adolescence* 2002, **22**:75–95.
119. Miotto P, De Coppi M, Frezza M, Preti A: **The spectrum of eating disorders: Prevalence in an area of Northeast Italy.** *Psychiat Res* 2003, **119**:145–154.
120. Moradi B, Dirks D, Matteson AV: **Roles of sexual objectification experiences and internalization of standards of beauty in eating disorder symptomatology: A test and extension of objectification theory.** *J Couns Psychol* 2005, **52**:420–428.
121. Ohring R, Graber JA, Brooks-Gunn J: **Girls' recurrent and concurrent body dissatisfaction: Correlates and consequences over 8 years.** *Int J Eat Disorder* 2002, **31**:404–415.
122. Prouty AM, Protinsky HO, Canady D: **College women: eating behaviors and help-seeking preferences.** *Adolescence* 2002, **37**:353–363.
123. Russell CJ, Keel PK: **Homosexuality as a specific risk factor for eating disorders in men.** *Int J Eat Disorder* 2002, **31**:300–306.
124. Santonastaso P, Mondini S, Favaro A: **Are fashion models a group at risk for eating disorders and substance abuse?** *Psychother Psychosom* 2002, **71**:168–172.
125. Scheinberg Z, Koslowsky M, Bleich A, Mark M, Apter A, Danon Y, Solomon Z, Babur I: **Sensitivity, specificity, and positive predictive value as measures of prediction accuracy: The case of the EAT-26.** *Educ Psychol Meas* 1993, **53**:831–839.
126. Slater A, Tiggemann M: **A test of objectification theory in adolescent girls.** *Sex Roles* 2002, **46**:343–349.
127. Smith MC, Thelen MH: **Development and validation of a test for bulimia.** *J Consult Clin Psych* 1984, **52**:863–872.
128. Tchanturia K, Katzman M, Troop NA, Treasure J: **An exploration of eating disorders in a Georgian sample.** *Int J Soc Psychiat* 2002, **48**:220–230.
129. Thome J, Espelage DL: **Relations among exercise, coping, disordered eating, and psychological health among college students.** *Eat Behav* 2004, **5**:337–351.
130. Wichstrøm L: **Psychological and behavioral factors unpredictive of disordered eating: A prospective study of the general adolescent population in Norway.** *Int J Eat Disorder* 2000, **28**:33–42.
131. Wood A, Waller G, Miller J, Slade P: **The development of Eating Attitude Test scores in adolescence.** *Int J Eat Disorder* 1992, **11**:279–282.
132. Zmijewski CF, Howard MO: **Exercise dependence and attitudes toward eating among young adults.** *Eat Behav* 2003, **4**:181–195.
133. Wardle J, Watters R: **Sociocultural influences on attitudes to weight and eating: results of a natural experiment.** *Int J Eat Disorder* 2004, **35**:589–596.
134. Vander Wal JS: **Eating and body image concerns among average-weight and obese African American and Hispanic girls.** *Eat Behav* 2004, **5**:181–187.

135. Hopkinson RA, Lock J: **Athletics, perfectionism, and disordered eating.** *Eat Weight Disord* 2004, **9**:99–106.
136. Hausenblas HA, Janelle CM, Gardner RE, Focht BC: **Viewing physique slides: affective responses of women at high and low drive for thinness.** *J Soc Clin Psychol* 2004, **23**:45–60.
137. Fairburn CG, Bèglin SJ: **Assessment of eating disorders: interview or self-report questionnaire?** *Int J Eat Disord* 1994, **16**:363–370.

5

Dysfunctional self-talk associated with eating disorder severity and symptomatology

Ned Scott[1], Tanya L Hanstock[1,2*] and Chris Thornton[3]

Abstract

Background: While self-talk has been argued to play a crucial role in the development and maintenance of eating disorders (EDs), it has received limited research attention. This study aimed to explore the relationship of ED self-talk with ED severity and symptomatology.

Methods: Analysis of the existing literature, supplemented with a small-scale pilot study, identified 24 distinct categories of ED self-talk. The main study involved the completion of on-line questionnaires by 172 women aged 18–49, recruited through clinical services, ED websites, and the general population. Participants were assigned to clinical ($n = 83$) and non-clinical ($n = 89$) samples, using the Eating Disorder Examination Questionnaire to screen for ED psychopathology.

Results: Substantial differences in the levels of ED self-talk were found between the clinical and non-clinical populations. Principal components analysis, conducted within the clinical sample, revealed ED self-talk to have a two-component structure. Self-talk reflecting an 'abusive relationship' between the sufferer and the ED strongly predicted overall severity and several aspects of symptomatology. 'Ascetic attitudes' towards thinness were linked with compulsive exercising and lower BMIs but not with overall severity.

Conclusions: Close examination of the 'abusive relationship' component suggests a need to loosen the connection between negative appraisals of the abused self and the abusive voice of the ED so that the former can fulfil their potential as a force for change. Further, in seeking to counter the impact of the ED voice, it is suggested that the seducer and abuser roles require primary clinical focus.

Keywords: Self-talk, ED severity, ED symptomatology

Background

Eating disorder (ED) self-talk or the 'voice of A/b (anorexia/bulimia)' ([1], p. 21) has been argued to play a crucial role in the development and maintenance of disordered eating behaviour. This voice ensures that weight, shape, and eating issues are never far from one's consciousness [2], that self-worth remains integrally connected with thinness [3], and that the sufferer's original self-identity and values are subjugated, along with thoughts of a healthier/more positive nature [1,4].

Insight into the nature of ED self-talk comes primarily from anecdotal self-reports obtained during the course of clinical treatment e.g., [1] and from first-hand accounts written by past sufferers e.g., [5]. In addition, several exploratory studies have made initial attempts at categorising ED self-talk or cognitions e.g., [2,4,6-8].

An examination of this material reveals the multidimensional nature of ED self-talk. ED sufferers often refer to an ED voice, which, in some instances, speaks to them in the second person and which they perceive as having a different persona, despite it being essentially ego-syntonic and non-psychotic in nature [4]. For example, De Rossi ([5], p. 238) refers to her ED voice as the "drill sergeant". Maisel et al. [1] provide examples of four different roles adopted by the ED voice: the seducer, making promises to remove pain and suffering; the coach, monitoring eating behaviour and providing guidance and exhortation; the mentor or "voice of reason" (p. 22) that helps the

* Correspondence: thansto2@une.edu.au
[1]Clinical Psychology Program, School of Behavioural, Cognitive and Social Sciences, University of New England, Armidale, NSW 2351, Australia
[2]School of Psychology, University of Newcastle, Callaghan, NSW 2308, Australia
Full list of author information is available at the end of the article

sufferer interpret the world through eyes that see thinness and self-discipline/denial as core moral virtues; and the abuser/bully, seizing every opportunity to denigrate the sufferer as unworthy. Tierney and Fox [9] analysing first hand reports by individuals with anorexia nervosa (AN), suggest that the sufferer's relationship with the voice changes markedly over the course of the ED, as the seducer role becomes less prominent and the abuser role more so.

The literature also details a form of self-talk that represents sufferers' appraisals of the ED's impact on their lives. These appraisals reflect the ambivalence felt by many sufferers towards their ED [8]. Hence, on the one hand, there is self-talk that reflects the sufferer's identification with the ED, their pride in what they have achieved as a result, and their sense that their ED is essential to their coping abilities. However, there is also self-talk that reflects the suffering inherent in living with an ED, the weariness resulting from constantly worrying about food, and the sense of loss regarding identity and life ambitions [7].

In this study, we define ED self-talk as including both these aspects: the so-called voice of the ED and the voice of the individual herself. We include all cognitions/inner verbalisations made by the individual that relate to self-worth, eating behaviours, or weight/appearance.

Sufferers' first-hand accounts document the distress they experience as a result of ED self-talk, and also clearly outline the influence they believe the ED voice has in maintaining the ED. Despite this, these accounts also testify to the fear associated with the idea of being separated from that voice e.g., [1,5,9]. Tierney and Fox [9] have linked the power inherent in the ED voice with the high rate of relapse in AN. Maisel et al. [1] argue that treatment efforts have to centre on lessening the hold the "voice of A/b" has on the sufferer. Higbed and Fox [4] suggest that better understanding ED sufferers' beliefs about this voice may be central to reducing its power. Williams and Reid [8] argue that the failure of some health professionals to acknowledge the hold of such pro-cognitions is an important factor in increasing treatment-resistance. Despite this, little attention has been paid to systematically documenting such cognitive styles [2], nor to measuring their change as a result of treatment [10].

Aims

The first objective of this study was to produce a detailed categorisation of ED self-talk so as to better inform clinicians' dealings with such patients. Additionally, the study aimed to investigate the factor structure of such self-talk and the extent to which the factors identified were associated with overall severity and specific forms of ED pathology (e.g., successful dietary restriction versus purging). Specifically, it was hypothesised that:

1. Women with EDs would experience self-talk related to eating, weight, and self-worth that, in its nature and frequency, was qualitatively and quantitatively distinct from that experienced by their same aged peers in the general population.
2. Within the clinical sample, factor components of this self-talk would predict both overall severity and the strength of specific forms of ED pathology: namely, restrictive eating, binge eating, purging, compulsive exercising and body mass index (BMI).

Method

Exclusion criteria

Males were excluded since the vast majority of patients presenting with EDs are female [11]. Additionally, the survey was limited to adult women aged under 50. Females under 18 years of age were excluded, partly due to ethical safety concerns, and also because of the potential additional impact of lifestage on the nature of their self-talk. For the latter reason, women aged 50 and over were also excluded.

Initial pilot study

Analysis of the existing literature produced an initial list of 21 distinct categories of ED self-talk. Based on this review, these different forms of ED self-talk identified were plotted against two dimensions: the ED voice versus the sufferer's voice and whether talk is experienced positively or negatively (see Figure 1).

A small-scale pilot study was conducted to confirm/refine this list of categories and develop first person sample items to represent each category. Participants in the pilot were six women with a history of eating disorders, five of whom had been diagnosed with the restricting form of AN, and one with the purging type of Bulimia Nervosa (BN). At the time of participation, half had current diagnoses of Eating Disorder Not Otherwise Specified (EDNOS) and half were classed as being in remission. Participants were recruited by providing information on the study to clinicians and sufferers, who were encouraged to pass on the material to clients/fellow sufferers. Interested parties then contacted the main researcher (NS) by email. Individuals who were personally known to the researchers were excluded from participation. Methods used to explore self-talk included the keeping of a two-day diary, telephone qualitative interviews, and semi-structured email questionnaires.

Qualitative content analysis [12] was utilised to analyse these pilot interviews. The pilot study served to confirm the presence of all 21 self-talk categories identified in the literary analysis, and also uncovered a further three

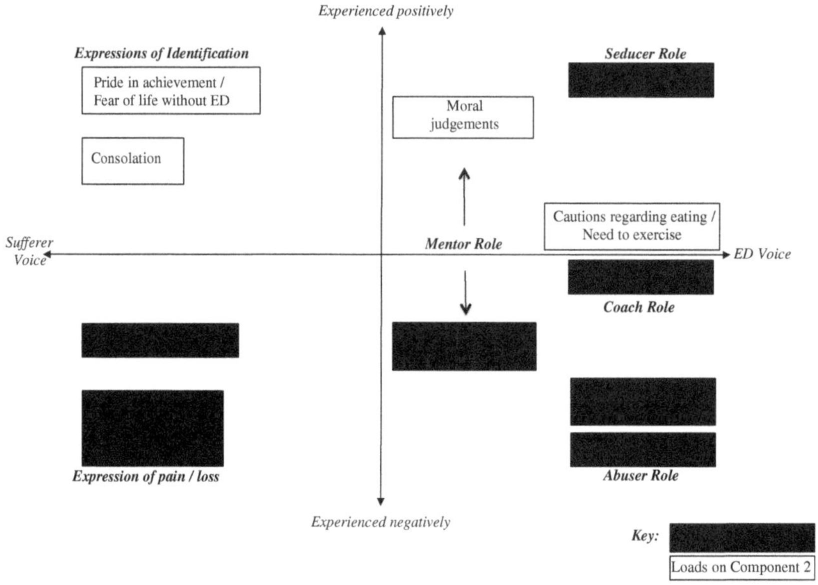

Figure 1 Segmentation of eating disorder (ED) self-talk components based on existing literature.

categories, which were subsequently included in the main study. Content analysis was used to formulate sample first person statements to represent each category as detailed in Table 1.

Main study

Participants included 172 women aged 18 to 49 ($M = 28.86$, $SD = 9.32$). Recruitment involved the use of posters/flyers advertising the study. Two versions were produced, one aimed at women with EDs and the other directed to all women in the study's age range. The former poster/flyer was placed, with clinicians' permission, in a number of private ED in-patient clinics, handed directly to outpatients by treating private clinicians and dietitians, and also placed on a number of ED websites. The latter version was distributed through friends and colleagues. Details of the study were also provided to University of New England (UNE) students enrolled in first year psychology units. Students who chose to participate were awarded one Research Participation (RPO) point upon completion. No other incentives were provided for study participation.

Research design

The study employed a cross-sectional case-control design, using the Eating Disorder Examination Questionnaire EDE-Q [13] to screen for the presence of ED pathology. Screening criteria were based on those recommended by Mond, Hay, Rodgers, Owen, and Beumont [14] who suggest that a positive screen should require both a high score (2.3 or more) on the EDE-Q global scale and the confirmatory presence of some behavioural symptoms. Using the presence of some objective bulimic episodes (OBEs) and/or compulsive exercising for weight/shape reasons at least weekly as confirmatory symptoms, Mond et al. achieved a sensitivity of 0.83, a specificity of 0.96, and a positive predictive value of 0.56. In this study, the presence of some form of purging was also considered as a confirmatory behavioural symptom. On the basis of these amended criteria, 78 participants were assigned to the clinical sample.

Additionally, participants whose reported physical/behavioural symptoms were sufficient to clinically justify an EDNOS diagnosis in their own right were also included in the clinical sample, irrespective of their EDE-Q scale score. Accepted criteria in this respect were the bi-weekly presence of OBEs and/or purging, and/or a BMI of less than 17.5, the accepted criteria for AN [15]. A further 5 participants were added to the clinical sample as a result. In total, 83 women were assigned to the clinical sample (M [age] = 27.01, $SD = 8.32$) and the remainder to the non-clinical sample ($M = 30.58$, $SD = 9.89$). An independent samples t test revealed that this difference in age was significant, $t\ (168.2) = 2.57$, $p = .011$, $d = 0.39$.

Procedure

Ethical approval for the study was granted by UNE's Human Research Ethics Committee. Questionnaires were administered online using Qualtrics. Prospective participants were provided with codes to access the study. Initial screens explained the nature of the research, prior to seeking participants' informed consent and checking their eligibility.

Table 1 Categories of ED self-talk identified

Description	Example selected for inclusion
Promises (of reduced pain)	*If I'm thinner/lose more weight then rejection and criticism won't hurt so much.*
Consolation	*I may not be doing so well in some areas of my life but at least I'm thin.*
Self-congratulations (on eating behaviour etc.)	*I'm doing really well in controlling my eating today.*
Threats	*If I don't keep my eating under control, I'm going to get obese and be rejected by everyone.*
Cautions regarding eating	*That food/eating situation is dangerous. I'm going to have to be really careful about what I eat.*
Need to purge	*I'm worried that I've eaten too much. I need to get rid of it by purging.*
Need to exercise	*I can't afford to just sit around, I have to exercise more.*
Self-disappointment (at ability to meet dietary ideals)	*I'm so disappointed at myself: I've failed to live up to my dietary ideals again.*
Self-abuse	*I am so pathetic and useless. I have no discipline or self-control.*
Self-punishment	*Because I have failed to live up to my dietary ideals I deserve to be punished by denying myself food or exercising harder.*
Self-criticism (lack of self-worth)	*I'm such a failure. I try really hard to do well and make friends but I'm just not the type of person I want to be.*
Comparisons (with others)	*Look at her she's so thin and she does it so easily. Why can't I be like her?*
Reinterpretations	*When they say things like "you're looking well", what they're really meaning is how much weight I've put on.*
Sensory misperceptions	*Just feel that stomach/Look at those thighs (etc.). I feel/look so fat/terrible.*
Denial (of symptoms)	*Feeling tired and/or cold doesn't mean there's anything wrong with me. I just have to be stronger.*
Moral judgements	*Practising self-restraint is an important virtue. I despise people who have no self-control.*
Ruination of life	*My concern about food and weight is threatening the other things I want to achieve/get out of life.*
Weariness (of constantly thinking about food)	*I'm so fed up of constantly thinking about food and what I eat.*
Misery (of living with an ED)	*Life is so miserable/lonely living like this.*
Lost identity	*I feel like I don't really know who I am/what I stand for any more. I've lost touch with the real me.*
Need for secrecy	*People mustn't find out the way I think or behave concerning food.*
Rebellion	*I'm fed up of trying to control what I eat. I'm just going to eat whatever and as much as I want!*
Pride in ED	*When I think about how self-controlled I am around food compared to the average person, I feel quite proud of what I can achieve.*
Fear of life without ED	*If I let go of my strict control and ideals around eating, I'm really quite frightened about what life would be like.*

Questioning in the main study asked participants to first identify which of the 24 categories of self-talk they themselves experienced. For each type mentioned, participants were asked to specify how often they experienced that type of self-talk on an 8-point Likert scale, ranging from 1 (*no longer experienced*) to 8 (*every waking hour*). This was expanded to a 9-point scale by giving those participants who did not specify an item a score of zero.

Additional measures

Severity/Nature of ED pathology

The current level and nature of core ED pathology was assessed using the EDE-Q. The EDE-Q contains three attitudinal subscales covering Eating Concern, Shape Concern, and Weight Concern. A further subscale, entitled Restraint, measures the frequency of attempting to restrict the amount and types of food eaten. All items relate to the preceding 28-day period. The global scale is defined as the mean of these four subscales and is considered to give an overall measure of ED pathology. EDE-Q subscales have been shown to have good internal consistency amongst both community samples of women [16] and women with bulimic symptoms [17]. Cronbach's α's for the current study ranged from .86 for the Restraint subscale to .94 for Shape Concern.

Impact on psychosocial functioning

The overall impact of the ED on psychosocial functioning was assessed using the Clinical Impairment Assessment Questionnaire CIA [18]. The CIA asks the participant to specify to what extent, over the last 28 days, their eating habits, exercising, and feelings about eating, shape, or weight have impacted on particular areas of their life. The CIA has high internal consistency ($\alpha = .97$), acceptable test-retest reliability ($r = .86$), good construct and discriminant validity, and has been demonstrated to be sensitive to change [19]. Cronbach's α for the current study was .98. Fairburn [20] argues that impact on psychosocial functioning is a further valuable indicator of the ED's hold on the individual.

Current and past diagnoses and treatments

Participants were also asked to supply details of any current and past ED diagnoses, perceived periods of remission, and the forms of community or inpatient treatment they had received.

Results

Data cleaning

Of the 216 individuals who consented to participate in the study, 42 dropped out prior to completing the EDE-Q and thus could not be assigned to either the clinical or non-clinical samples. Examination of a further two response sets (revealed by Mahalanobis distance calculations to be extreme multivariate outliers within the clinical sample) suggested these cases were not valid members of the clinical population. Hence they were excluded, leaving a total of 172 participants.

The data set was complete for these participants with the exception of two who did not complete the CIA scale and a further seven who omitted/gave nonsensical values for their weight and/or height, and whose BMI was therefore incalculable. Visual examination of other key variables for these participants revealed no systematic pattern of response; hence in analyses of the variables concerned, cases with missing values were simply excluded.

Outliers and violated assumptions

Independent samples t test comparisons of self-talk and ED severity measures between the clinical and non-clinical samples were complicated by the lack of normality for many of these measures, particularly in the non-clinical sample. Where possible, data was transformed to address this. A transformation was also required when a paired sample t test was used to compare mean frequency scores in the clinical and non-clinical samples across the 24 self-talk items. In all instances, the impact of these transformations on results was inconsequential, so the untransformed data is reported to enhance ease of interpretation. Where the data was too severely non-normal to permit transformation, the non-parametric Mann–Whitney test was substituted. For the independent samples t test used to compare the number of self-talk items experienced, Levene's test revealed the assumption of homogeneity of variance was violated. Hence, the results reported are those for equal variances not assumed. In contrast, few problems were encountered with the assumptions relating to the multiple regression analyses conducted. The data was analysed using IBM SPSS Statistics Version 18.

Participants included in the study

Thirty-six (21%) of the 172 participants reported having a current ED diagnosis, all but two of which (both of whose current diagnosis was AN in remission) satisfied the EDE-Q criteria for inclusion in the clinical sample. The current diagnoses reported were AN by 12 (7%) participants, AN in remission by 11 (6%), BN by 4 (2%), and EDNOS by 9 (5%). A further 20 (12%) participants reported past diagnoses. In total, 35 (20%) of participants had had a diagnosis of AN at some point, 20 (12%) a diagnosis of BN, and 17 (10%) a diagnosis of EDNOS.

In total, 83 (48%) participants satisfied the criteria for the clinical sample. Within this clinical sample, 42 (51%) participants had had a formal diagnosis at some time; 59 (71%) reported OBE's and 33 (40%) reported some form of purging in the last 28 days. Weekly episodes of compulsive exercising for weight/shape reasons were reported by 41 (49%). Mean scores for both samples on scales measuring ED severity and clinical impairment are detailed in Table 2. To ensure differences between the clinical and non-clinical samples held across all these scales, a series of Mann–Whitney tests were conducted. All were significant with $p < .001$. Effect sizes range from $d = 1.90$ to 2.93 (Table 2).

Eating disorder self-talk

On average, participants in the clinical sample identified with 12.02 (50%, $SD = 5.39$) of the 24 categories of self-talk presented. This compared with an average of 4.38 (18%, $SD = 3.51$) self-talk categories in the non-clinical sample. An independent samples t test confirmed this difference was significant, $t\ (139.4) = 10.93$, $p < .001$, $d = 1.68$. Multiple regression analysis confirmed that membership of the clinical sample remained a highly significant predictor, $p < .001$, when age was controlled for.

All categories of self-talk were experienced to some degree across both samples. However, as shown in Table 3, in the clinical sample, a substantial proportion experienced each type of self-talk at least several times per day.

Table 2 Mean scores (S.D.s) on severity measures across clinical and non-clinical samples

Scale	Clinical sample	Non-clinical sample	Effect-size d
EDE-Q			
Global scale	4.09 (1.06)	1.22 (0.89)	2.93***
Restraint subscale	3.56 (1.54)	1.05 (1.06)	1.90***
Eating concern subscale	3.29 (1.54)	0.58 (0.85)	2.20***
Shape concern subscale	4.96 (0.97)	1.79 (1.25)	2.82***
Weight concern subscale	4.53 (1.10)	1.43 (1.18)	2.71***
CIA	28.07 (12.52)	4.80 (6.51)	2.36***

Note: EDE-Q = Eating Disorder Examination Questionnaire; CIA = Clinical Impact Assessment Questionnaire; ***$p < .001$.

Table 3 Percentages of sample experiencing different types of eating disorder (ED) self-talk

	Clinical sample		Non-clinical sample	
Self-talk category	**At least several times per day %**	**Ever experience %**	**At least several times per day %**	**Ever experience %**
Sensory misperceptions	59	93	2	54
Comparisons	33	86	4	53
Threats	30	64	-	11
Need for secrecy	29	53	-	11
Need to exercise	28	55	8	42
Self-disappointment	25	70	2	25
Self-abuse	25	69	2	19
Ruination of life	25	54	-	11
Lost identity	25	52	-	8
Self-criticism	25	41	1	16
Fear of life without ED	22	45	1	8
Self-punishment	22	40	-	7
Weariness	22	55	-	12
Need to purge	19	45	-	9
Misery	19	45	-	7
Cautions re. eating	18	55	1	17
Reinterpretations	14	47	-	7
Promises	12	34	1	13
Consolation	10	35	-	15
Self-congratulations	8	63	-	42
Moral judgements	7	24	1	12
Denial	6	35	-	7
Pride in ED	6	23	1	10
Rebellion	4	35	-	21

In the non-clinical sample, such frequencies were extremely rare.

Additionally, a paired sample t test was used to compare the mean frequencies with which each of the 24 self-talk items was experienced in the two samples. As measured on the 9-point Likert scale, mean frequency scores in the clinical sample ($M = 2.53$, $SD = 1.07$) were significantly greater than in the non-clinical sample ($M = 0.57$, $SD = 0.50$), $t\ (23) = 11.60$, $p < .001$, $d = 2.50$.

Principle components analysis

To explore the factor structure of ED self-talk, the data collected from all clinical sample participants on these 24 items was subjected to Principle components analysis (PCA). Prior to the final analysis, four items (*Self-congratulations*, *Self-disappointment*, *Denial*, and *Rebellion*) were omitted due to low communalities (less than .2), and a further two items (*Self-punishment* and *Reinterpretations*) omitted due to cross-loadings. The Kaiser-Myer-Olkin measure of sampling accuracy was .81, indicating strong linear relationships within the item set. Communalities for the retained items were all above .25, indicating that they all contributed a meaningful amount of shared variance to the data set.

Both Cattell's [21] scree test and Velicer's [22] minimum average partial (MAP) test indicated that two components should be retained. Direct oblimin rotation was used with Δ set to zero to permit correlations between components. Table 4 shows the component loadings after rotation. Component 1 has over four loadings in excess of .6, indicating it is reliable despite the relatively small sample size [23]. Component 2 has only three loadings in excess of .6 and therefore findings in relation to this factor need to be treated with a degree of caution.

Examination of these loadings suggests that component 1 combines both sides of the abusive relationship that characterises much of ED self-talk: self-denigration and self-pity; whereas component 2 is connected with a moral or ascetic attitude to thinness. Together, these components accounted for 45% of the variance in these self-talk items. Individually, component 1 accounted for 31%, component 2 for 19%. The correlation between the two

Table 4 Rotated component loadings and Cronbach's α for eating disorder (ED) self-talk item frequencies

Variable	Component 1 Abusive Relationship (α = .88)	Component 2 Ascetic Attitudes (α = .72)
Threats	.79	
Comparisons	.71	
Self-criticism	.71	
Self-abuse	.69	
Sensory misconceptions	.66	
Need to purge	.65	
Misery	.62	
Lost identity	.55	
Ruination of life	.54	
Weariness	.54	
Promises of reduced pain	.51	
Need to retain secrecy	.51	
Moral judgements		.75
Pride in ED		.73
Fear of life without ED		.60
Consolation		.55
Cautions re. eating		.49
Need to exercise		.44

Note: Rotation employed the direct oblimin approach with Δ = 0. Loadings below .4 are not included. As recommended by Tabachnick and Fidell [24] pattern matrix loadings are reported. These values are partial scale correlations between the scale items and the components after controlling for the variance shared by the other retained components.

components was .27, indicating a moderate relationship between the two factors.

Scale scores were computed by averaging the items that loaded above .4 on each component. Cronbach's α for both scales exceeded .7 reflecting adequate internal consistency. Because scale scores were heavily skewed (particularly in the non-clinical sample), the Mann–Whitney U test was employed to evaluate differences between scale scores for the clinical ($n = 83$) and non-clinical ($n = 89$) samples. For both self-talk components, scores were significantly greater in the clinical sample. For Abusive Relationship, the clinical sample had a mean score of 3.04 ($SD = 1.85$) compared to 0.58 ($SD = 0.61$) for the non-clinical; $U = 483.5$, $p < .001$, $d = 1.81$. For Ascetic Attitudes, the clinical sample had a mean score of 1.92 ($SD = 1.65$) compared to 0.58 ($SD = 0.77$) for the non-clinical; $U = 1640$, $p < .001$, $d = 1.05$.

Relationship between components and eating disorder severity

The two measures of severity, the global EDE-Q and the CIA were found to be highly correlated in the clinical sample, $r\ (81) = .81$, $p < .001$. Accordingly, a measure of overall severity was produced by averaging the standardised scores on these two variables. A multiple regression analysis was then conducted to determine, within the clinical sample, the extent to which ED self-talk predicts ED severity. The two self-talk components identified served as predictors, and overall severity served as the dependent variable. Table 5 presents the results of this analysis. Overall, the two self-talk components predicted 60% of the variance in ED severity. However, only the Abusive Relationship component was a significant individual predictor, accounting for 46% of the variance.

Relationship between components and behavioural/outcome symptoms

Further regression analyses were conducted to assess the extent to which self-talk predicts specific ED symptomatology. Again the two self-talk components served as predictors. Dependent variables were OBE, Purging, Compulsive Exercising, Restricted Eating, and BMI. The first three were measured by the number of reported occasions over the last 28 days. Restricted Eating was represented by the EDE-Q Restraint Subscale score. BMI's were calculated from participants' reported weights and heights.

To determine the p value correction necessary for these analyses, the effective number of independent variables (Veff) represented by these five variables was estimated using a factor analysis as described by Nyholt [25]. Veff was 4.63, meaning for $\alpha = .05$, $p < .011$ was required for significance.

Results of all five analyses are detailed in Table 5. Together, the two self-talk components significantly predicted Restricted Eating, Purging, Compulsive Exercise, and BMI, accounting for 45%, 17%, 21%, and 24% of the variance in these measures respectively. Individually, the Abusive Relationship component was a significant predictor of Restricted Eating (accounting for 24% of the variance) and Purging (13%), whereas the Ascetic Attitudes component

Table 5 Predicting eating disorder severity and symptomatology from self-talk components

Variable	Total variance explained %	Variance explained by individual factors	
		Abusive Relationship %	Ascetic Attitudes %
Overall severity	60***	46***	< 1
Specific symptoms:			
Restraint	46***	23***	< 1
Purging	17**	13**	2
OBE	9	7	6
Compulsive exercising	21***	< 1	12**
BMI†	24***	< 1	16***

Note: OBE = Objective Bulimic Episodes, BMI = Body Mass Index, ***Indicates p < .001, **Indicates p < .01. Analyses conducted on clinical sample only. $n = 83$, except for analysis marked † for which $n = 80$.

was a significant predictor of Compulsive Exercising (12% of variance) and BMI (17%). The result for the regression analysis predicting OBE was not significant when the *p* value correction was applied.

Discussion

The study set out to document the nature of ED self-talk and its relationships with ED severity and symptoms. Comparisons were made between ED self-talk in clinical and non-clinical samples and the factor structure of such self-talk within the clinical sample was investigated. The ability of the factors that emerged to predict ED severity and symptomatology was explored, along with the effectiveness of strategies used to counter this self-talk.

The distinctive nature of eating disorder self-talk

The first hypothesis, that women with EDs (as classified using the EDE-Q) would experience a level of self-talk regarding eating, weight, and self-worth that was qualitatively and quantitatively distinct from their same aged peers in the general population, was strongly supported. Although all self-talk items were found in both samples, women in the clinical sample experienced more items, at greater average frequencies, than those in the non-clinical sample. Further statistical confirmation of this difference was obtained by comparing mean scores on the two self-talk components that emerged from the PCA on item frequency. For each component, those items loading upon it occurred with greater average frequency in the clinical than in the non-clinical sample. Effect sizes for these analyses were all large (greater than 1.0). Visual examination of the data provided an important qualitative distinction. Those with EDs commonly reported experiencing certain items several times each day (or more often). Such frequencies were extremely rare in the non-clinical sample.

Self-talk components

The two components of self-talk that emerged from the PCA, Abusive Relationship and Ascetic Attitudes can be reviewed in the light of the theoretical segmentation of self-talk based on the literature (Figure 1). Both components include items considered to represent both the ED voice and the voice of the sufferer. This helps explain the difficulty individuals with ED have in distinguishing their voice from that of the ED [1]. The main distinction between the two factors is whether items are experienced positively or negatively, with the key exception that *Promises* load on the Abusive Relationship component (see below for further discussion), which otherwise consists primarily of negatively experienced items. The three advice components; *Cautions about eating, Need to exercise,* and *Need to purge*; can be viewed as containing both positive and negative experiential aspects [8]. However, the fact that *Need to purge* loads on the predominantly negative Abusive Relationship component is consistent with the shame that commonly accompanies these actions [3].

Predicting eating disorder severity and symptomatology

Hypothesis 2 concerning the ability of these self-talk components to predict ED severity and specific symptomatology was supported with the sole exception that self-talk was not found to predict the frequency of OBEs. However, the two individual components predicted quite distinct aspects. Greater average frequency scores on the Abusive Relationship component predicted greater frequency of purging, greater attempts to restrict eating (as measured on the EDE-Q restraint subscale), and increases in overall ED severity. In contrast, greater average frequency scores on the Ascetic Attitudes component predicted greater frequency of compulsive exercising and lower BMI's. Scores on this second component did not predict overall severity.

These findings are in contrast to past research asking sufferers' to evaluate the impact (positive and negative) of their eating disorder on their lives. Where such beliefs are concerned, it is the strength of positive rather than negative ED cognitions that predict resistance to treatment [8,26] and lesser motivation to change [27]. At an experiential level, however, it is the strength of predominantly negative self-talk that predicts ED severity. This finding lends support to the contention of Maisel et al. [1] that treatment efforts should focus on lessening the hold the ED voice exerts on sufferers. Although the Abusive Relationship component includes several items representing the sufferer's voice, these recognitions of the negative consequences of the ED would appear to have little impact in reducing the grip of the ED, presumably because they are so strongly linked with the ED voice, in both its abuser and seducer roles. According to Walker's [28] cycle of violence theory, these two roles mirror those adopted by perpetrators of domestic violence, which Walker argues explain the difficulty victims of such violence have in leaving those relationships. In the case of EDs, however, the 'perpetrator' is in the victim's head.

The fact that the two self-talk components predict distinct behavioural and physical symptoms would, at first sight, seem to run counter to Fairburn's [20] contention of a common ED psychopathology. However, comparing the relationships between Ascetic Attitudes and Restraint on the one hand, and BMI on the other, suggests an alternative explanation. The restraint subscale of the EDE-Q assesses not restricted eating per se but rather attempts at restricted eating: four of the five items include the words 'tried', 'trying', or 'desire' [13]. A low BMI, in contrast, is linked to actual restriction of food intake. This suggests the possibility that the Ascetic Attitudes component might be the outcome rather than the driver of success in attempts to restrict eating. This would be consistent with the concept of a common psychopathology that finds different forms of expression [20].

The failure of self-talk to predict OBE's could be a reflection of the limited power of the study, with both components having a relationship approaching significance. However, while there were a number of participants with binge eating disorder (BED) in the main study, neither the literature nor the pilot study from which self-talk items were derived involved such individuals. If (BED) involves distinctive forms of self-talk, the inclusion of participants with this disorder in the study could have diluted the relationship between self-talk and OBE's found in ED sufferers whose psychopathology is not limited to binge eating.

Study limitations

In addition to the above, other limitations of the study should be acknowledged. The pilot study sample of six participants contained only one individual with a history of purging behaviours, with the remainder all having suffered from the restrictive type of AN. The failure (despite substantive efforts) to obtain a broader-based sample for the pilot, leaves open the possibility that important items of self-talk predominantly associated with bulimic behaviours were omitted from the study (in addition to possible items connected with (BED) mentioned above). The recruitment bias towards private sector clients, in both the pilot and main studies, should also be acknowledged.

A further issue concerns the lack of any formal ED diagnosis for 49% of participants assigned to the clinical sample. The positive predictive value reported by Mond et al. [14] for the criteria on which assignment was based was only 0.56, implying that approximately 20% of the clinical sample might not qualify for an ED diagnosis. Nevertheless, the fact that such substantial differences were found between the clinical and non-clinical samples on the CIA and on all subscales of the EDE-Q (Table 2), clearly indicates that the clinical sample represents individuals with extreme positions across the continua of ED psychopathology.

The study is also limited in providing no information as to how the relationship between self-talk and ED severity/psychopathology develops over time, both during the development of the disorder and as a result of successful treatment. The cross-sectional nature of the current study means that the extent to which self-talk remains a force driving the development/maintenance of the disorder, as Maisel et al. [1] would argue, as opposed to a mere symptom, remains open to argument.

Future research

Further research is required to confirm the factor structure of ED self-talk to emerge from this exploratory study. Ideally, this research should be preceded by further small-scale pilot work amongst individuals with BN and (BED) to ensure that forms of self-talk specific to those disorders are not excluded. It should also be noted that the exploratory study intentionally involved a large number of self-talk categories, many of which were closely related (e.g., concerning alternative methods of compensating for food intake, and different forms of self-chastisement) to ensure potential differences were not lost. This initial study provides the basis for substantially reducing the number of items in future work.

Also of importance, as mentioned above, is to examine how the nature of self-talk and its relationship with ED severity/psychopathology develop over the course of the ED and in response to treatment. In this respect, it should be noted that Tierney and Fox [9] have suggested that the ED voice evolves over the development of the disorder, such that *Promises* become less prominent, and the abuser role components such as *Threats* and *Self-abuse* much more so. Confirming the extent of this change and, perhaps even more importantly, the process by which the sufferer's own voice becomes locked (in factorial terms) with that of the ED, offers further considerable insight into the ED experience and as to how EDs can be more effectively treated. Additionally, one would wish to explore how ED self-talk changes over the course of recovery and in response to the differing therapeutic strategies employed to counter it.

Clinical implications

This study serves to further clinical understanding of the self-talk experienced by ED sufferers and provides a basis for the more empathic approach to treatment advocated by Williams and Reid [8] and others. In particular, the fact that the component of self-talk that predicts overall ED severity is so characteristic of an abusive relationship suggests that too domineering an approach (argued by Maisel et al. [1] to be common practice in much ED treatment) risks adding to the client's trauma and loss of sense of self. Rather, treatment needs to focus on empowering the ED sufferer to withstand the abuser that resides in her head. To this end, we note Tierney and Fox's ([9], p. 252) exhortation to therapists to persevere with efforts to "infiltrate the relationship" between the sufferer and the eating disorder voice, and the advice of Vitousek, Watson, and Wilson [29] that therapists should seek to develop a collaborative relationship that employs a "judicious blend of empathy and firmness".

Looking further at the structure of the crucial Abusive Relationship component suggests two areas of focus for clinical efforts. First, there may be value in loosening the connection between the negative appraisals of the abused self and the abusive voice of the ED so that the former can fulfil their potential as a force for change. Externalization offers one method by which this might be achieved. The second key point to emerge is that, in seeking to counter the impact of the ED voice, it is the 'seducer' and 'abuser' roles described by Maisel et al. [1] that would seem to merit primary attention. Fairburn et al. ([3], p. 119) suggests the patient be taught to recognise the "eating disorder mindset". This data suggests that helping the patient identify specific types of the eating disorder mindset (e.g., seducer or abuser) may be helpful. Therapists might also be guided by the relationship between "the abuser" and purging and restrictive behaviour, and between ascetic attitudes and exercising and low weight, to more precisely target the type of mindset at work.

Conclusion

The current study examined the relationship between ED self-talk, specific symptomatology, and overall severity. It identified a two factor component mode of self-talk in adult women; self-talk which reflects the 'abusive relationship' between the sufferer and the ED and 'ascetic attitudes' towards thinness. It supports the idea that self-talk plays an important role in ED maintenance and provides strong indications as to those aspects that most require addressing in therapy. It also brings us closer to understanding the experience of those who live with an ED.

Competing interests

The authors received no financial support for the research, authorship, and/or publication of this article. The authors further declare that there are no potential conflicts of interest with respect to the research, authorship, and/or publication of this article.

Authors' contributions

NS conceived of and designed the study under the supervision of TLH. NS conducted the analysis of the literature and all pilot interviews, and designed the final questionnaire. NS also was responsible for publicising the study and generating the main sample. In this, he was substantially aided by CT. NS conducted the statistical analysis and wrote the first draft of the manuscript. TLH and CT have since contributed substantially to the final manuscript. All three authors have read and approved the final submission.

Acknowledgements

The authors thank the following individuals and organisations for their help in publicising the study: Clinicians at the Redleaf Practice, Helen Storey (Accredited Practicing Dietitian), Chris Basten (Basten & Associates), Hazel Williams (Accredited Practicing Dietitian), Sue Paton (EATFED), Dr. Naresh Mondraty (Wesley Eating Disorder Centre, Ashfield), the Mandometer Clinic in Melbourne, the Northside Clinic in Sydney, the Geelong Clinic, the Butterfly Foundation, the Centre for Eating and Dieting Disorders (CEDD), and Recovery is Possible for Everyone (RIPE). Additionally we thank all participants for their contribution to the pilot and main studies. We would also like to thank Dr. Tony Marks and Dr. Will Coventry at UNE for their advice and support during the study.

Author details

[1]Clinical Psychology Program, School of Behavioural, Cognitive and Social Sciences, University of New England, Armidale, NSW 2351, Australia. [2]School of Psychology, University of Newcastle, Callaghan, NSW 2308, Australia. [3]The Redleaf Practice, Wahroonga, NSW 2076, Australia.

References

1. Maisel R, Epston D, Borden A: *Biting the Hand that Starves you: Inspiring Resistance to Anorexia/Bulimia.* New York: W. W. Norton; 2004.
2. Cooper MJ, Fairburn CG: **Thoughts about eating, weight and shape in anorexia nervosa and bulimia nervosa.** *Behav Res Ther* 1992, **30**:501–511.
3. Fairburn CG, Cooper Z, Shafran R, Bohn K, Hawker DM, Murphy R, Straebler S: **Enhanced cognitive behavior therapy for eating disorders: the core protocol.** In *Cognitive Behavior Therapy and Eating Disorders.* Edited by Fairburn CG. New York: Guilford Press; 2008:47–193.
4. Higbed L, Fox JRE: **Illness perceptions in anorexia nervosa: a qualitative investigation.** *Br J Clin Psychol* 2010, **49**:307–325.
5. De Rossi P: *Unbearable Lightness: A Story of Loss and Gain.* New York: Atria Books; 2010.
6. Cooper MJ, Todd G, Wells A: **Content, origins, and consequences of dysfunctional beliefs in anorexia nervosa and bulimia nervosa.** *J Cogn Psychother* 1998, **12**:213–230.
7. Serpell L, Treasure J, Teasdale J, Sullivan V: **Anorexia nervosa: friend or foe.** *Int J Eat Disord* 1999, **25**:177–186.
8. Williams S, Reid M: **Understanding the experience of ambivalence in anorexia nervosa: the maintainer's perspective.** *Psychol Health* 2010, **25**:551–567.
9. Tierney S, Fox JRE: **Living with the 'anorexic voice': a thematic analysis.** *Psychol Psychother Res Pract* 2010, **83**:243–254.
10. Cooper MJ, Wells A, Todd G: **A cognitive model of bulimia nervosa.** *Br J Clin Psychol* 2004, **43**:1–16.
11. American Psychiatric Association (APA): *Diagnostic and Statistical Manual of Mental Disorders.* 4th edition. Washington D.C: American Psychiatric Pub; 2000.
12. Schilling J: **On the pragmatics of qualitative assessment: designing the process for content analysis.** *Eur J Qual Asses* 2006, **22**:28–37.
13. Fairburn CG, Beglin S: **Eating Disorder Examination Questionnaire (EDE-Q 6.0).** In *Cognitive Behavior Therapy and Eating Disorders.* Edited by Fairburn CG. New York: Guilford Press; 2008:311–313.
14. Mond JM, Hay PJ, Rodgers B, Owen C, Beumont PJV: **Validity of the Eating Disorder Examination Questionnaire (EDE-Q) in screening for eating disorders in community samples.** *Behav Res Ther* 2004, **42**:551–567.
15. Wilson GT, Fairburn CG: **Treatments for eating disorders.** In *A Guide to Treatments That Work.* 3rd edition. Edited by Nathan PE, Gorman JM. New York: Oxford University Press; 2007:579–609.
16. Luce KH, Crowther JH: **The reliability of the eating disorder examination – self-report questionnaire version (EDE-Q).** *Int J Eat Disord* 1999, **25**:349–351.
17. Peterson CB, Crosby RD, Wonderlich SA, Joiner T, Crow SJ, Mitchell JE, Bardone-Cone AM, Klein M, le Grange D: **Psychometric properties of the eating disorder examination questionnaire: factor structure and internal consistency.** *Int J Eat Disord* 2007, **40**:386–389.
18. Bohn K, Fairburn CG: **Clinical Impairment Assessment Questionnaire (CIA 3.0).** In *Cognitive Behavior Therapy and Eating Disorders.* Edited by Fairburn CG. New York: Guilford Press; 2008:315–317.
19. Bohn K, Doll HA, Cooper Z, O'Connor ME, Palmer RL, Fairburn CG: **The measurement of impairment due to eating disorder psychopathology.** *Behav Res Ther* 2008, **46**:1105–1110.
20. Fairburn CG: **Eating disorders: the transdiagnostic view and the cognitive behavioral theory.** In *Cognitive Behavior Therapy and Eating Disorders.* Edited by Fairburn CG. New York: Guilford Press; 2008:7–22.
21. Cattell RB: **The scree test for the number of factors.** *Multivar Behav Res* 1966, **1**:245–276.
22. Velicer WF: **Determining the number of components from the matrix of partial correlations.** *Psychometrika* 1976, **41**:321–327.
23. Guadagnoli E, Velicer WF: **Relation of sample size to the stability of component patterns.** *Psychol Bull* 1998, **103**:265–275.
24. Tabachnick BG, Fidell LS: *Using Multivariate Statistics.* 5th edition. Boston: Allyn & Bacon; 2007.
25. Nyholt DR: **A simple correction for multiple testing for SNPs in linkage disequilibrium with each other.** *Am J Hum Genet* 2004, **74**:765–769.
26. Gale C, Holliday J, Troop NA, Serpell L, Treasure J: **The pros and cons of change in individuals with eating disorders: a broader perspective.** *Int J Eat Disord* 2006, **39**:394–403.
27. Delinsky S, Thomas JJ, St. Germain SA, Craigen KE, Weigel TJ, Levendusky PG, Becker AE: **Motivation to change among residential treatment patients with an eating disorder: assessment of the multidimensionality**

of motivation and its relation to treatment outcome. *Int J Eat Disord* 2011, **44**:340–348.
28. Walker LEA: **The battered woman syndrome as a psychological consequence of abuse.** In *Current Controversies in Family Violence.* Edited by Galles RJ, Loseke DR. Newbury Park: Sage Publications; 1993:133–153.
29. Vitousek K, Watson S, Wilson GT: **Enhancing motivation for change in treatment-resistant eating disorders.** *Clin Psychol Rev* 1998, **18**:391–420.

Thinking about internal states, a qualitative investigation into metacognitions in women with eating disorders

Alix Vann[1], Esben Strodl[1*] and Erin Anderson[2]

Abstract

Background: There is a need for qualitative research to help develop case conceptualisations to guide the development of Metacognitive Therapy interventions for Eating Disorders.

Method: A qualitative study informed by grounded theory methodology was conducted involving open-ended interviews with 27 women aged 18–55 years, who were seeking or receiving treatment for a diagnosed ED.

Results: The categories identified in this study appeared to be consistent with a metacognitive model including constructs of a Cognitive Attentional Syndrome and metacognitive beliefs. These categories appear to be transdiagnostic, and the interaction between the categories is proposed to explain the maintenance of EDs.

Conclusions: The transdiagnostic model proposed may be useful to guide the development of future metacognitive therapy interventions for EDs with the hope that this will lead to improved outcomes for individuals with EDs.

Keywords: Eating disorders, Meta cognitions, Qualitative

Background

Given that eating disorders (EDs) are prevalent among women in western countries [1,2], there is an obvious need to develop effective interventions for eating disorders. Psychological therapies have been recommended as important components of interventions for EDs, with cognitive behaviour therapy (CBT) being a commonly recommended treatment [3,4]. While CBT has been helpful for many people, there are still limitations in its effectiveness. For example, meta-analyses have found that only approximately 41% of individuals with Bulimia Nervosa (BN) completing individual CBT interventions recover and only 29% remain recovered 12 months following CBT [5].

Given the variable and often limited impact of diagnosis-specific treatments for EDs, as well a recognition of additional maintaining mechanisms beyond the common cognitive targets of overvaluation and dieting, an enhanced cognitive behaviour therapy (CBT-E) was developed for EDs by Fairburn and colleagues [6,7]. This enhanced therapy was based on a proposed transdiagnostic cognitive model of EDs as well as the inclusion of four additional maintaining mechanisms: perfectionism, core low self-esteem, mood intolerance, and interpersonal difficulties. While Christopher Fairburn's CBT-E has significantly improved the conceptualisation of eating disorders, trials using CBT-E indicate that there is still a need to further refine the case formulations and interventions for EDs. For example, in a sample of 154 patients with an EDs other than Anorexia Nervosa (AN), after receiving 20 weeks of CBT-E only approximately 50% of the sample had a level of eating disorder features less than one standard deviation above the community mean [7].

While such outcomes are still admirable given the complexity and pathology associated with EDs, these findings have resulted in calls by clinicians and researchers to further develop the cognitive models that underpin interventions for EDs [8,9]. One proposition has been to extend the standard cognitive therapy conceptualisation of focusing on the content of cognitions, or *what* people think, to *how* people think [10,11]. The domain of 'how' thinking occurs comprises the concept of metacognition,

* Correspondence: e.strodl@qut.edu.au
[1]Queensland University of Technology School of Psychology & Counselling, Level 5, O Block, B Wing, QUT Kelvin Grove Campus, Victoria Park Road, Kelvin Grove Queensland 4059, Brisbane, Australia
Full list of author information is available at the end of the article

which refers to the cognitive mechanisms involved in the knowledge, interpretation and regulation of thinking itself [10]. One metacognitive theory has stemmed from the Self-Regulatory Executive Function (S-REF) theory of psychological disorder proposed by Adrian Wells [12]. The S-REF model suggests that beliefs comprise two metacognitive components that guide information processing, interpretations and the control of thoughts. The first is metacognitive knowledge, or the positive and negative beliefs which an individual holds about how to regulate internal states. The second is metacognitive regulation, or the coping strategies and changes in focus of attention that result from the chosen means of internal regulation [12]. S-REF theory suggests that in the case of psychological disorder, this metacognitive system becomes dysfunctional and the metacognitive processes become maladaptive [12], resulting in a Cognitive-Attentional Syndrome (CAS) [11,12]. The CAS involves perseverative thinking and excessive conceptual processing, as well as attentional hypervigilance to threat, which lead to the use of unhelpful coping strategies that ultimately fail [10,12].

Metacognitive theory has previously been applied in the conceptualisation and treatment of anxiety and depression with success [12,13]. However, the application to EDs has been limited thus far, with integrated cognitive and metacognitive therapy used only with BN [8]. This is perhaps due, in part, to the current lack of a sound metacognitive model of EDs that specifies which metacognitions underlie EDs, and are therefore important to target. The limited application of metacognitive theory in EDs may also reflect the reliance on deductive research methodologies by employing quantitative measures of metacognition that were developed for other psychological disorders [14,15]. Further, to date metacognitive research in EDs has focused on a single ED diagnosis [14], which is not consistent with emerging transdiagnostic conceptualisations of EDs [6]. As such, the lack of inductive investigations into metacognition in EDs may have restricted the depth of understanding of these disorders and the development of new metacognitive interventions.

Beginning to address these limitations, Woolrich and colleagues [16] recently investigated metacognition in patients with AN, dieters and non-dieting controls, using a qualitative methodology and found evidence for specific metacognitions associated with AN. Whilst providing a starting point for the current inductive research, the study by Woolrich and colleagues was limited by a number of methodological issues. Woolrich and associates [16] extracted data using a simple thematic analysis rather than any interpretative analysis, which would allow for the development of a model to guide case formulation. Further, the study explored metacognitions in a single diagnostic category (i.e. AN), not allowing for any comparison of metacognitions across ED diagnoses. Thus despite preliminary investigation into the existence of metacognition in EDs, there is still no in-depth qualitative investigation of metacognition in EDs available. Another limitation we see in the research is that some metacognitive theories focus solely on metacognitions about verbal cognitions [10-12]. Recently there has been a call to build upon metacognitive theory by also considering meta-cognitions about emotions [17]. Using Well's metacognitive theory as a basis, Manser, Cooper, and Trefusis developed a questionnaire measuring metacognitions about emotions and found that metacogntions of emotions added to the explanation of emotional dysregulation (as measured by borderline personality disorder symptoms) above that explained by metacognitions about verbal cognitions [17].

The current research therefore aimed to propose a theoretical model to guide the conceptualisation of metacognitions in EDs that might guide the development of future metacognitive interventions for EDs. As such given the presence of existing metacognitive therapy strategies and interventions, based upon Wells' SREF model [11], starting questions for the exploration were based upon Wells' SREF model. In addition the study aimed to expand this model by also exploring metacognitions about emotions as well as metacognitions about verbal thoughts. Finally given the emerging evidence of transdiagnostic conceptualisations of EDs, we were also interested to explore if categories of metacognitions varied across diagnosis or tended to be transdiagnostic. A grounded theory approach [18] was chosen as a basis to provide a rigorous framework that would support not just the extraction of themes but also an interpretative analysis for the development of a model. Due to the higher prevalence of EDs in females and in order to keep the sample relatively homogenous, the current research sampled women only.

Method

Participants

Participants were 27 women between the ages of 18 and 55 years, with the majority of participants 30 years old or younger (mean = 26.22 years, *SD* = 8.11 years). Participants were attending the Eating Disorders Outreach Service (EDOS) at a major metropolitan hospital in Brisbane, Australia, and were seeking or receiving treatment for an ED (AN, BN or EDNOS). Participants satisfied criteria for an ED diagnosis according to the DSM-IV-TR[a] [19] and received a diagnosis from a psychiatrist or a psychiatric registrar as part of the intake process at EDOS, which was confirmed by administering the ED section of the Mini International Neuropsychiatric Interview [M.I.N.I.] 6.0. All patients who engaged with EDOS during the data collection period were considered for participation. EDOS clinicians (clinical psychologists, psychiatrists or psychiatric registrars) individually assessed the suitability of patients to participate based on current mental state and overall functioning. No specific exclusionary criteria were applied.

Setting and procedure

Data collection was approved by the hospital and university Human Research Ethics Committees. Interviews were conducted between April 2011 and May 2012 and were audio recorded. Each individual interview lasted between 20 and 60 minutes. Following the interview, participants were administered sections L. Anorexia Nervosa and M. Bulimia Nervosa of the M.I.N.I. 6.0 by the first author (AV). In addition, AV returned to each section of the M.I.N.I. and asked appropriate questions to ensure the diagnosis was congruent with proposed DSM-V diagnoses. Participants were finally asked to complete a brief demographic questionnaire regarding their age, culture, educational background/qualifications, time since diagnosis, and number of hospitalisations related to the ED.

The initial starting questions were based upon Wells' SREF model i.e. positive and negative metabeliefs, attentional bias and coping strategies i.e.

1 What do you think is good about experiencing strong emotions or thoughts?
2 What do you think is bad about experiencing strong emotions or thoughts?
3 When you feel that urge, what do you do to cope with experiencing strong emotions or thoughts?
4 What do you focus your attention on when you experience strong emotions or thoughts?

In line with grounded theory methodology, questions were modified as categories and a model emerged through the process of open and axial coding [18] with metacognitive profiling questions [10] were drawn upon as necessary to further elucidate the emerging themes.

Data analysis

AV transcribed interviews verbatim. All coding was conducted from transcriptions and was done in line with grounded theory methodology using the ATLAS.ti v6.2 (2010) computer software. Open coding proceeded in a two stage process. The labels associated with the codes and concepts extracted from the transcripts were aligned closely with the words used by the participants. As the authors worked with the data generation, the categories appeared to overlap significantly with the constructs proposed by Adrian Well's metacognitive model. As such words and terms were borrowed from this metacognitive model to more accurately describe the categories. As concepts and categories started to emerge from within the data, axial coding was used to relate concepts and categories to each other, with an emphasis on causal relationships, intervening conditions, action strategies and consequences [18]. In addition to the original interview questions posed, more specific questions were asked in following interviews to confirm, disconfirm and explore the emerging core categories and the proposed model. Finally, selective coding was used to relate all other themes, relationships, conditions and consequences to the core categories identified in the overall model. Once saturation of themes was reached in the data analysis, the concurrent data collection and analysis allowed for the final four interviews to be largely confirmatory/disconfirmatory in nature. In these interviews, participants were presented with an outline of the proposed overall model and asked specific questions to determine whether or not this was in line with their experience.

Theoretical memos were used throughout the data collection and analysis process to track working hypotheses and rationales for the process of coding, and aid the generation of a theory with well-connected concepts. Reflexivity was also employed to ensure that the researcher's personal beliefs and biases, and their potential influence on the analysis, were considered. The first author was a postgraduate student who had been briefly trained in psychodynamic therapies, cognitive behaviour therapy, narrative therapy and family therapy, with cursory prior knowledge of metacognitive therapy. She had no strong allegiance to any particular modality of therapy. The second author is an experienced clinician who works primarily from a cognitive behaviour therapy framework and had a relatively strong prior knowledge of metacognitive therapy principles. The third author is an experienced clinician who works primarily from a cognitive behaviour therapy framework and had no prior knowledge of metacognitive therapy. To further address methodological rigour, the second and third authors reviewed interview transcripts in order to confirm the validity and integrity of coding.

Results

Demographic summary

The breakdown of diagnoses of those interviewed was: nine AN, nine BN, and nine EDNOS. All participants were Australian-Caucasian except for one American-Caucasian and one Asian participant. The mean body mass index (BMI: weight [kg]/height [m^2]) at the time of the interview per diagnostic group was as follows: AN mean = 17.22 (*SD* = 1.22); BN mean = 22.79 (*SD* = 1.84); EDNOS mean = 20.44 (*SD* = 2.68). The length of time since initial diagnosis ranged from four months to 20 years, and 21 of the participants had been diagnosed with an ED for over a year. Eleven participants had been hospitalised at some point since diagnosis, due to the ED.

Overall model summary

The results are presented within the structure of the model that emerged from the ongoing data analysis. Comparison of the themes across diagnostic categories supported a transdiagnostic model of metacognitions in EDs and is displayed in Figure 1 below. Axial coding revealed that the sequence of actions within the model started with specific, but not universal, triggers activating participants' positive metacognitive beliefs about internal states (namely negative thinking and strong negative emotions). Once these beliefs were activated, participants would employ the perseverative negative thinking and specific allocation of attention found to be characteristic of the CAS in EDs. It appeared that the CAS itself resulted in some distress for participants. Once the CAS was active, participants' negative metacognitive beliefs about internal states were then activated, with these beliefs adding to the distress participants experienced. Following this, positive beliefs participants held about their coping strategies arose, which resulted in the implementation of several specific cognitive and behavioural coping strategies. Whilst providing some temporary relief, these strategies ultimately increased the experience of distress. Given that distress in itself is an internal state, the experience of distress then had the potential to re-activate positive beliefs about internal states, thus re-activating the original cycle. These themes and actions are described in more detail below.

Metacognitive model for eating disorders

Trigger

All participants idicated that there was usually an external trigger that began the process of activating their metacognitive beliefs. This was often related to body image, weight, food or eating, or as described below, may also have been related to more general events:

> *"Well it usually starts off with, it usually happens... after I've put on weight or I look in the mirror and I see something that upsets me and then it sort of progresses to... a want to be incredibly skinny again... I mean it could be anything from eating an extra apple to someone making a comment, like, completely*

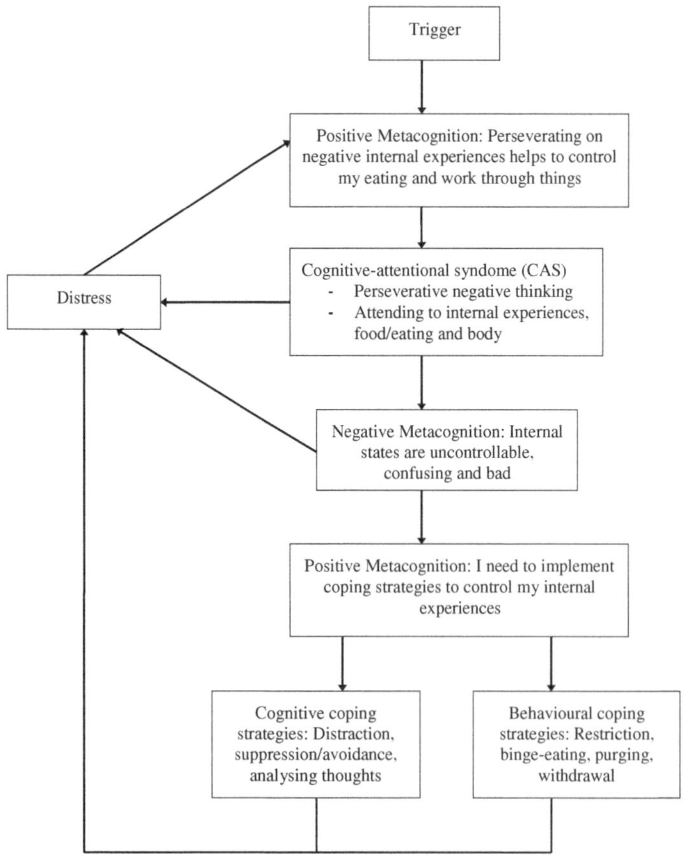

Figure 1 Proposed model of metacognition in EDs.

unrelated to body shape and [the] eating disorder." (Age 18 – BN)

Whilst this trigger was usually external, for the majority of participants it seemed to result in an internal trigger, in the form of either a distressing thought or a strong negative emotion. The internal trigger seemed to lead to the activation of positive beliefs held about certain ways of regulating internal experiences.

Positive metacognitions about internal states

The data revealed three dominant beliefs about positive actions to help regulate the experience of internal states. With the first two metabeliefs below, in both cases the perceived positive action is the same (i.e. engaging in negative perseverative thinking), however in the first case this is due to interpreting emotions as uncontrollable and dangerous, whereas in the second case it is due to interpreting thoughts as uncontrollable and dangerous.

1. Strong negative emotions mean something uncontrollable is happening and therefore I need to focus and perseverate on my negative thoughts to protect me from losing control of my eating, because if I lose control of my eating I will become fat and worthless.

This category was endorsed by most participants. In the quote below, an emotion triggers off the action of perseverative negative thinking as a strategy for protection against losing control of one's eating behaviour.

"[I focus on] not eating. I don't know when that started but when I'm angry, when I'm sad, like I'm a bit sad today, like a bit off, and the next step is [to think] don't go to the fridge, don't you dare go into the kitchen, do not eat, just do not blow it, like you feel shit, there's an opportunity that you'll just lose control, like do not do that." (Age 26 – EDNOS)

2. Negative thoughts mean something uncontrollable is happening and therefore I need to focus and perseverate on my negative thoughts to protect me from losing control of my eating, because if I lose control of my eating I will become fat and worthless.

The quote below illustrates an emergent theme that engaging in negative perseverative thinking was a positive action, in response to experiencing negative thoughts, that resulted in benefits for the person by protecting them from losing control of their eating or protecting them from becoming fat and therefore worthless. The majority of participants endorsed this category.

"If I didn't think those, I suppose if I didn't think that stuff then I might just actually eat all day every day... you know just eat all the time um and then I would become more enormous... Yeah if I beat myself enough with the negative thoughts and stuff somehow that might make me a better person... And certainly, oh I would certainly be a much better person if I were smaller." (Age 55 – EDNOS)

3. Feeling strong negative emotions and thinking negatively is comforting as it is familiar and means that I am working hard at something, therefore it is good for me to focus on my negative internal experiences.

Participants indicated that the experience of strong negative emotions and negative thoughts was often painful, uncomfortable and overwhelming. This category was endorsed by approximately half of the sample. However, paradoxically, the experience of the emotion or thought was still viewed as positive action in regulating their internal state in that it allowed them to feel comforted and reassured by the familiarity of the experiences:

"It gives me something to always think about... because it's become part of me, it's like, if I didn't have it then what's wrong?... What am I supposed to think about all the time?" (Age 29 – AN)

There was also the sense for participants that experiencing perseverative negative thinking allowed them to acknowledge or work through something, so focusing on their negative thoughts may lead to something positive:

"The negative self-talk may have in a way made me go ok you've screwed up, you didn't do that right... Yeah it's good because you feel real and you feel like you're making progress, but it's hard when you're in it." (Age 28 – BN)

Cognitive-Attentional Syndrome (CAS)

In line with previous metacognitive models of psychopathology, it appeared that the majority of women with EDs in the current study had a CAS that was activated at this point. Two aspects of this which appeared to be consistently endorsed by participants included the implementation of perseverative negative thinking and attentional bias.

Perseverative negative thinking

All participants employed perseverative negative thinking in some form. The perseverative thinking described by the participants included worry about the future and rumination about the past, but was predominated by strong themes of repetitive thoughts of food/eating/body image. The quote below is an example of a perseverative negative thinking pattern of one participant.

"I think, no, don't think about that, don't analyse the thoughts just do what you used to do because that made you happy once... and I keep telling myself that

restricting is good and that getting on the scales and weighing less every week is good... but I'll sort of think at the same time that's not good to think that way because is it actually true? Like lately I weigh myself and I don't feel happy anymore and then I think what's wrong with you, you used to love getting on the scales and being so thin. But now I just think, why do you think that... why aren't you happy?" (Age 22 – AN)

Attentional bias

There was a consistent sense for participants that when they were experiencing strong negative emotions or negative thoughts, their attentional focus would become largely internal, such that these experiences caused them to focus on their thoughts (often their negative, ED-related thoughts):

"I should be going out and doing things, well I do go out but then I go out and it's like oh, you're away from the fridge, that's good, that's good, but then [I'm thinking] when you get home don't eat, make sure when you get home you don't eat... so a big focus on thoughts of not eating." (Age 26 – EDNOS)

Participants also reported an increased focus on food and/or eating when they were experiencing a strong negative emotion or negative thoughts:

"I guess [my focus was] on the actual food that I was eating like just, like if I just restricted what I was eating well then I wouldn't have to be worried so much that I was over-eating or that I would gain weight or that kind of thing." (Age 21 – BN)

When in a state of heightened emotion or engaging in negative thinking, it was also common for participants to attend more closely to their bodies, their weight and how they compared to others on these dimensions:

"I think because I was so body focused, mentally as well, I really experienced emotions quite physically and I would, more so than I had in the past like you know feel things here and here [pointing to back and tummy] *and just that drained sadness... I remember being really aware of what was sore and what was, you know like you'd be kind of very body-focused."* (Age 22 – BN)

While most participants endorsed an attentional bias towards thoughts and body image/weight, only some participants reported attentional bias towards food.

Negative metacognitions about internal states

With the CAS activated, all participants described negative metacognitive beliefs related to the regulation of internal states. The negative metacognitive beliefs reported by participants are best represented by the following three categories:

Strong emotions and negative thoughts are uncontrollable and awful

Participants consistently described the sense that their experience of strong negative emotions and negative thoughts was overwhelming and all-consuming, such that they felt powerless to be able to do anything about them or to stop the emotions/thoughts once they had started. This was a category that was endorsed by almost every participant.

"The symptoms of the emotion that I was feeling, like, I had no control of it whatsoever and it was the first time that I ever felt that intensely, like where I couldn't stop crying... I just couldn't turn it off, I didn't know how to turn it off." (Age 28 – EDNOS)

Participants described their strong emotions and negative thoughts as simply awful, and experiencing these internal states as terrible, uncomfortable, painful and exhausting:

"Emotions for me, like feeling emotions means like I'm just hurt, I get hurt, or it's painful... anger for me is, it's just a painful experience, like if you slammed your hand in a car door sort of pain, it just hurts to be angry." (Age 26 – EDNOS)

Strong emotions are confusing – I don't know what I am feeling or what to do about the feeling

Most participants described having difficulty identifying the emotion they were feeling, struggling to label or describe the emotion, and finding it difficult to approach strong negative emotions in a rational sense:

"Yeah I think as well like, with the feeling, a lot of it was suppressed for so long that's why it's really hard to tell, you know, what are you feeling? Cos I'm quite, I'm extremely emotional and I really hate it but... I actually am not really good at picking up, like different types of emotions ... and you know like in one of the therapy sessions she was like 'and how did that make you feel?' and I was just like 'I dunno', like, to label it I find strange." (Age 29 – BN)

From this confusion, these participants also appeared to struggle to know what to do with strong negative emotions, grappling with how strong emotions should be handled and whether there was anything that could be done about them:

> *"I actually had a very strong desire to cut myself um because I was unbelievably angry slash frustrated, I suppose the feeling is anger, and I couldn't think of anything to do and I actually had the conscious thought well what is an appropriate way to react to that?"* (Age 55 – EDNOS)

All negative thoughts are bad, wrong or abnormal and need to be addressed

Approximately half of the participants frequently passed judgements on their thoughts and their thinking, labelling many of their internal experiences as bad, wrong, unjustified or abnormal:

> *"There isn't really anything good about it* [negative thinking]*... it's not something I should feel or think, it's bad, but I do... yeah and then I think that I'm a terrible person because I don't think normally like you know, other normal healthy people do."* (Age 22 – AN)

These participants also appeared to hold strong beliefs about the need to address negative thoughts each time they occurred. It seemed important that they did not simply accept their negative thoughts as they occurred, but that participants worked hard to challenge, control or change their negative thoughts:

> *"If I'm aware of my thoughts and I just challenge them as they come, and if I hear a bad thought, I will tell myself what I need to be thinking to replace that thought."* (Age 23 – BN)

Positive beliefs about coping strategies

Similar to the positive beliefs identified about internal states, more than half of the participants also appeared to hold positive beliefs about the coping strategies they employed to manage their experience of internal states. Such beliefs appeared to be activated after the negative metacognitions and prior to the implementation of their coping strategies. Positive metacognitions about coping strategies were initially explored as they related to managing thoughts and emotions separately, however, as the analysis continued, the data suggested that the types of beliefs held by participants were similar for both of these types of internal experience. As such, the dominant positive belief appeared to be: I need to implement my coping strategies intensely to protect me from being taken over by my internal experiences (e.g., thoughts and emotions) because if I lose control of my internal experiences, I will lose control of my eating and become fat and worthless.

Cognitive coping strategies

Following these beliefs, several cognitive coping strategies were consistently identified by participants as being employed to reduce the distress experienced to this point.

Distraction.

Most participants described using cognitive distraction to ensure that their mind was otherwise engaged or busy. Participants appeared to employ this strategy to escape or manage the experience of strong negative emotions or difficult thoughts:

> *"I'd say even though distracting myself is hard to do, I tend to find that a bit more effective in terms of forgetting about the negative thoughts. Even though it might be hard to actually start a crossword puzzle or to you know make the effort to go and see someone, once I actually do then I tend to you know feel better afterwards, yeah, or less stressed about everything, even though it's harder to actually do."* (Age 22 – AN)

Suppression/avoidance

Most participants also reported trying to mentally block out or avoid some negative thoughts and/or strong emotions completely. For some participants this was done as a way of numbing their minds to avoid reality:

> *"You disconnect from all emotion I think sometimes... and that includes all the positive ones that disconnection, you reject love and things like that as well so you have to, in order to get rid of the bad stuff you have to sacrifice all of the good things, yeah you can't... um block out the sadness and keep the love – either it all goes or it all stays."* (Age 22 – BN)

Analysing/questioning negative thoughts

There also emerged a strong belief amongst participants that it was important to cognitively address their negative thoughts and strong emotions in some way, and that doing so would help them to cope. The data showed that the idea of "thinking things through" was important and this appeared to encompass trying to analyse thoughts and feelings, questioning and challenging negative thoughts, and trying to control negative thinking:

> *"When I was actually out of control was when I was in control, and I think a lot of that would have come from that weighing up and deciding is it good, is it not, should I do it, should I not, and every decision was calculated almost, even if it was subconscious, it was always a calculated thing... it was always controlled."* (Age 22 – EDNOS)

This category was endorsed by approximately half of the sample.

Behavioural coping strategies

Also following from the positive beliefs about coping strategies, several behavioural strategies were employed by participants to cope with their distress.

While there was a general tendency for some diagnostic disorders to use particular behavioural coping strategies more than other diagnoses (e.g., restricting food intake/starvation was typical of participants with AN, while binge-eating was typical of participants with BN), the striking observation was that the underlying purpose for a strategy selection was transdiagnostic.

Restricting food intake/starvation

Participants with AN described using restriction of their food intake as a way of controlling strong negative emotions and perseverative negative thinking. This was often expressed in terms of the "numbing" of the mind that successful restriction allowed, perhaps due to the physiological response of the brain undergoing Starvation Syndrome. In this way, this behavioural coping mechanism may partly have been employed as another way of maintaining cognitive control.

> "*For me it's like a numbing process. Once my brain's starved and I'm fairly numb, you can't think about much at all.*" (Age 24 – AN)

Similarly impacting cognitive functioning, restriction appeared to be employed as a means of consuming the mind with thoughts of food and eating, to avoid thinking about other, more distressing, thoughts:

> "[*I would*] *try to concentrate a lot because you know I'm allowed three milkos* [biscuits] *a day, and you know having five milkos in my bag and then having to concentrate and tell myself even though I'm really really hungry that I can only have three and it's really really hard sometimes to not want to have the fourth so then it takes all my energy and all my focus and all my concentration to be worrying about not having those other two milkos and so then I don't have to think about, you know, my day.*" (Age 39 – AN)

Approximately half of the sample reported using this coping strategy irrespective of the diagnosis.

2. Binge-eating

Across diagnoses, most participants reported binge-eating food as a coping mechanism. Several purposes to this strategy emerged from the data, including using the episode of binge-eating as a distraction or a means of escapism. For some women bingeing appeared to result from building feelings of being out of control. These women initially restricted their food intake in response to feeling out of control, but once the feeling reached a certain threshold, then they felt that they *were* out of control. At this point, feeling like they had to act on their thoughts of being out of control, some women engaged in the disinhibited eating that is characteristic of binge-eating:

> "*I felt really sad and out of control... so I just was like what's the point? I'm just going to give in and have that food suicide... I don't think I really thought past the point I'm just going to eat all this food and become a big slug and I don't know what would happen then I guess I'd be worthless and non-existent and things wouldn't matter and I'd just sort of die.*" (Age 19 – AN)

Binge-eating also seemed to be employed due to the experience of positive cognitive effects during bingeing. Some participants reported that food and eating became their sole focus in this moment, allowing their mind to feel cleared of any thoughts:

> "*And I never realised that until recently but like whenever I would eat, it would be to the extent that I just would, I would zone out, it was just me and my food. And I wouldn't, I just wouldn't think.*" (Age 22 – EDNOS)

Purging

Approximately half of the participants in each diagnostic group reported the use of various purging strategies to cope with strong negative emotions and difficult thoughts. Such strategies included vomiting, exercising, and the use of laxatives and/or diuretics. Purging may have been somewhat of a secondary coping mechanism designed to deal with the added distress caused by the use of the previous two coping strategies. However, purging does appear to act as a form of release to cope with a build up of internal pressure, in particular feelings of guilt:

> "*I end up purging because it's like I need to feel some sense of relief or I need to take the feeling of guilt associated with purging to remove my mind from the intensity of* [*it*]." (Age 28 – EDNOS)

Social withdrawal

Most participants frequently used withdrawal from others as a way of dealing with their strong emotions and/or negative thoughts, regardless of diagnosis. Participants reported that social isolation helped them to control their experiences by allowing them to deal with things alone:

> *"It did take me a few years to kind of get to a place where I was isolated... but when I got there I was like this is my world and like you can come and walk around me and you can say things to me but they're going to bounce straight back off me because I kind of formed like a whole new identity within myself... and like drawing from the eating disorder, that was my only friend I guess, that was the only thing that I would let in my life and so once I got to that place I was like 'Hi, I'm great, life is great, because you're not in it!'"* (Age 27 – BN)

Discussion

Grounded theory guided the combined inductive/deductive interpretative analysis to produce a metacognitive model which may guide the future development of metacognitive interventions for EDs. We found evidence that women with EDs do experience a Cognitive-Attentional Syndrome (CAS) that involves perseverative thinking and attentional bias about food/body image/weight. Consistent with metacognitive model proposed by Adrian Wells [12], we found evidence that women with EDs do have positive and negative metacognitions surrounding the CAS that appear to drive both the experience of the CAS and the selection of unhelpful coping strategies to manage the CAS. While the experiencec of the CAS and coping strategies help to define the manifestation of the ED, the associated metacognitions and attentional bias are proposed also to be causal factors in this presentation and should be considered targets for interventions. The model proposed was transdiagnostic in nature, as the qualitative analysis suggested no clear differences between diagnoses in the existence, or degree of endorsement, of the core categories.

The overarching categories are in line with previous models of metacognition in psychopathology. Similar models have been proposed for generalised anxiety disorder (GAD) [20], obsessive-compulsive disorder [21], post-traumatic stress disorder (PTSD) [22], and depression [23]. In the current study, some of the beliefs identified about negative thinking are similar to the beliefs about worry proposed as important in GAD (e.g., my worries are uncontrollable) and to the beliefs about rumination suggested to be key in understanding depression (e.g., thinking about the causes of depression will help me to prevent it). The results of the present research thus support the application of metacognitive theory to EDs, and suggest that there is some overlap between important metacognitive constructs in EDs and other forms of psychopathology that may help explain the high levels of comorbidity seen in these presentations.

Metacognition about emotions

In line with recent suggestions about the importance of metacognitions about emotions [12], we found support for the role of metacognitions of emotions in EDs. In particular we found themes of beliefs that emotions can be uncontrollable or dangerous, or interestingly also confusing. The concern that emotions can be uncontrollable or dangerous is consistent with Wells' identification of metacognitions that verbal thoughts can be uncontrollable or dangerous [12]. The theme of emotions being confusing is consistent with findings of higher levels of alexithymia in those with EDs [24-27].

Within the construct of alexithymia, the affective elements (e.g., problems identifying and expressing emotional states) has been suggested as more relevant to women with EDs than the cognitive elements (e.g., poor externally oriented thinking) [24]. The current study supports this literature by suggesting that one of the reasons for employing ED behaviours may be to manage the distress associated with feeling confused by strong negative emotions.

Transdiagnostic considerations

An important consideration in this research was the suitability of adopting a transdiagnostic perspective of EDs. The issue of whether metacognitive beliefs and related constructs were transdiagnostic was considered throughout the qualitative analysis process, particularly when undertaking axial and selective coding to relate themes to each other. In line with recent developments [5], the current research supports the view of EDs as transdiagnostic when considered within a metacognitive framework. There did not appear to be meaningful qualitative differences between the metacognitive beliefs, the CAS or the cognitive coping strategies employed by participants with AN, BN and EDNOS. While there were some broad differences in the selection of behavioural coping strategies, the underlying purpose for the implementation of these strategies appeared common across diagnostic groups. Further investigation into the transdiagnostic nature of metacognitions in EDs is recommended.

Treatment implications

Given the variable impact of currently available treatments of EDs on recovery, there is a need to continue to explore new conceptualisations of EDs to develop interventions with improved outcomes. One option is to explore the impact of metacognitive therapy for the treatment of EDs. There is emerging evidence from other diagnostic categories such as PTSD [22], GAD [20,28] and depression [23,29] that metacognitive therapy may be a promising development over traditional CBT. The themes and model identified in this study may guide case formulation required to implement metacognitive therapy for eating disorders and spur further research in this area.

In particular, it is suggested that interventions should target the main themes extracted from this study. That is, clinicians and researchers should target positive metacognitions that motivate the use of perseverative negative thinking about eating, body image, weight etc. In addition, they should target the negative metacognitions that emotions and thoughts are dangerous or uncontrollable and that an individual needs to use a coping strategy to manage their emotions and thoughts when they experience them. We also feel that clinicians and researchers should use metacognitive strategies to address the attentional bias toward internal cues as well as towards cues of food, weight or body image. Moreover, standard metacognitive therapy strategies could be used to help clients or participants change their use of the unhelpful cognitive and behavioural coping strategies identified in this study. However in addition to using standard metacognitive therapy strategies for areas identified in this study, we believe that individuals with EDs would also benefit from further strategies aimed at helping them better understand their emotions. A common theme was that emotions were confusing with the implication that the participants therefore needed to use an unhelpful coping strategy to manage these confusing emotions. The addition of psychoeducation in affect regulation to treatment as usual (CBT) has been shown to improve the skill of down-regulating negative affect in patients with AN and BN, and to also reduce dietary restraint [30]. This suggests that educating individuals with EDs about emotions can improve their ability to handle emotions and impact their ED symptomatology. Other researchers who view EDs as an emotion regulation strategy have administered dialectical behaviour therapy (DBT) [31] to women with EDs. Modified DBT for EDs has been shown to be effective in addressing both ED behaviours and more general forms of psychopathology (e.g., mood disorders, anxiety) in ED samples [311]. However, the effect of DBT for EDs on the core element the treatment theoretically targets – affect tolerance and regulation – is less clear [32]. As such, it is possible that even treatments with a specific distress-tolerance component such as DBT are not directly impacting this ability in women with EDs. Thus, it is important to continue considering methods to directly target the affective difficulties connected with EDs. The current model provides another way of thinking about core emotional difficulties in EDs and may eventually be used to inform other potential treatment modalities, such as detached mindfulness as part of MCT.

Limitations

All participants were recruited via their engagement with a specialist ED treatment service (EDOS) where they were offered or already engaged in CBT treatment. Engagement in structured CBT interventions may have impacted the metacognitions elicited during interviews and may be a limitation in the current study. This impact is particularly relevant to beliefs about the need to challenge/analyse thoughts, as this concept is fundamental to CBT treatment approaches. However, the idea of needing to be aware of, monitor and analyse one's thoughts has been identified as a common cognitive coping strategy in other presentations of psychopathology [33]. It is therefore possible that the identification of the negative metacognitive belief that negative thoughts must be addressed and analysed may be a true metacognitive belief in women with EDs, rather than a belief shaped by treatment experiences. To confirm this aspect of the proposed model, future research should consider samples of women with EDs who have not yet undergone psychological treatment.

The current model does not clearly specify which strong negative emotions are implicated in metacognitive processes, or why ED symptoms are chosen as emotion regulation strategies instead of other behaviours. Such limitations have been previously criticised in cognitive-affective models proposed to understand EDs [34]. It was clear that participants held beliefs about negative, and not positive, strong emotions, and while they referred to a variety of strong negative emotions (including sadness, anger, guilt and fear) these were not specifically accounted for in the current model. The lack of specificity in exploration of emotions was due to the fact that no clear pattern emerged early on, and given the scope of the investigation, it was decided to keep this as a broad category to aid with conceptualisation. Future research should investigate whether particular strong negative emotions are implicated in a metacognitive model of EDs.

Conclusion

To date, interventions targeting EDs have tended to only produce modest effects. It is possible that this may be due to a need for more novel conceptualisations of key psychological processes driving ED presentations. The findings from this study suggest that women with EDs do possess important metacognitions that may explain the psychopathology associated with EDs. In particular, we propose that the positive and negative metacognitions surrounding the CAS identified in this study are important targets for interventions. If the results of this qualitative study are replicated through deductive studies that confirm the generalisability of these findings, the themes identified in this study may provide important constructs to help develop case conceptualisations that guide future metacognitive therapy interventions for EDs.

Endnotes

[a]Proposed DSM-5 criteria (as at April 2011, when data collection began) were also considered, and this altered the diagnostic breakdown accordingly: 10 AN, 8 BN, 1 Binge-eating Disorder, 3 Feeding and Eating Condition Not Elsewhere Classified (FECNEC) – atypical AN, 4 FECNEC – sub-threshold BN, and 1 FECNEC - other. However, this did not meaningfully impact the analysis and so DSM-IV-TR criteria were used for this study.

Competing interests

The authors declare that they have no competing interests.

Authors' contributions

AV conducted the data collection and performed the transcribing of the interviews. AV also contributed to the study design, data coding, the data interpretation, as well as the writing of the manuscript. ES contributed to the study design, data interpretation, as well as the writing of the manuscript. EA contributed to the study design, data interpretation, as well as the writing of the manuscript. All authors read and approved the final manuscript.

Author details

[1]Queensland University of Technology School of Psychology & Counselling, Level 5, O Block, B Wing, QUT Kelvin Grove Campus, Victoria Park Road, Kelvin Grove Queensland 4059, Brisbane, Australia. [2]Eating Disorders Outreach Service, 14 Cartwright Street, Herston Queensland 4029, Brisbane, Australia.

References

1. Wade T, Bergin J, Tiggemann M, Bulik C, Fairburn C: **Prevalence and long-term course of lifetime eating disorders in an adult Australian twin cohort.** *Aust NZ J Psychiat* 2006, **40**:121–128.
2. Hudson JI, Hiripi E, Pope HG, Kessler RC: **The prevalence and correlates of eating disorders in the National Comorbidity Survey Replication.** *Biol Psychiat* 2007, **61**:348–358.
3. Royal Australian and New Zealand College of Psychiatrists Clinical Practice Guidelines Team for Anorexia Nervosa: **Australian and New Zealand clinical practice guidelines for the treatment of anorexia nervosa.** *Aust NZ J Psychiat* 2004, **38**:659–670.
4. National Institute of Clinical Excellence: *Eating Disorders: Core interventions in the treatment and management of anorexia nervosa, bulimia nervosa and related eating disorders.* Leicester, UK: The British Psychological Society; 2004. www.nice.org.uk.
5. Fairburn CG, Cooper Z, Shafran R: **Cognitive behaviour therapy for eating disorders: a "transdiagnostic" theory and treatment.** *Behav Res Ther* 2003, **41**:509–528.
6. Fairburn CG: *Cognitive behavior therapy and eating disorders.* New York, NY: Guilford Press; 2008.
7. Fairburn CG, Cooper Z, Doll H, O'Connor ME, Bohn K, Hawker DM, *et al*: **Transdiagnostic cognitive-behavioral therapy for patients with eating disorders: A two-site trial with 60-week follow-up.** *Am J Psychiatry* 2009, **166**:311–319.
8. Cooper MJ, Todd G, Wells A: *Treating bulimia nervosa and binge eating: An integrated metacognitive and cognitive therapy manual.* East Sussex, London: Routledge; 2009.
9. Wilson GT, Grilo CM, Vitousek KM: **Psychological treatment of eating disorders.** *Am Psychol* 2007, **62**:199–216.
10. Wells A: *Emotional disorders and metacognition: Innovative cognitive therapy.* Chichester: Wiley; 2000.
11. Wells A, Matthews G: **Modelling cognition in emotional disorder: the S-REF model.** *Behav Res Ther* 1996, **34**:881–888.
12. Wells A: *Metacognitive therapy for anxiety and depression.* London: The Guilford Press; 2009.
13. Wells A, King P: **Metacognitive therapy for generalized anxiety disorder: an open trial.** *J Behav Ther Exp Psy* 2006, **37**:206–212.
14. Cooper MJ, Grocutt E, Deepak K, Bailey E: **Metacognition in anorexia nervosa, dieting and non-dieting controls: a preliminary investigation.** *Br J Clin Psychol* 2007, **46**:113–117.
15. Konstantellou A, Reynolds M: **Intolerance of uncertainty and metacognitions in a non-clinical sample with problematic and normal eating attitudes.** *Eat Behav* 2010, **11**:193–196.
16. Woolrich RA, Cooper MJ, Turner HM: **Metacognition in patients with anorexia nervosa, dieting and non-dieting women: a preliminary study.** *Eur Eat Disord Rev* 2008, **16**:11–20.
17. Manser R, Cooper M, Trefusis J: **Beliefs about emotions as a metacognitive construct: initial development of a self report questionnaire measure and preliminary investigation in relation to emotion regulation.** *Clin Psychol Psychot* 2012, **19**:235–246.
18. Strauss A, Corbin J: *Basics of qualitative research: Grounded theory procedures and techniques.* London: Sage; 1990.
19. American Psychiatric Association: *Diagnostic and statistical manual.* 4th edition. Washington, DC; 2004.
20. Wells A: **Meta-cognition and worry: a cognitive model of generalised anxiety disorder.** *Behav Cogn Psychoth* 1995, **23**:301–320.
21. Fisher P, Wells A: **Experimental modification of beliefs in obsessive-compulsive disorder: A test of the metacognitive model.** *Behav Res Ther* 2005, **43**:821–829.
22. Wells A, Colbear JS: **Treating posttraumatic stress disorder with metacognitive therapy: a preliminary controlled trial.** *J Clin Psychol* 2012, **68**:373–381.
23. Wells A, Papageorgiou C: **Metacognitive therapy for depressive rumination.** In *Depressive rumination: Nature, theory and treatment.* Edited by Wells CPA. Chichester: Wiley; 2004.
24. Lawson R, Emanuelli F, Sines J, Waller G: **Emotional awareness and core beliefs among women with eating disorders.** *Eur Eat Disord Rev* 2008, **16**:155–159.
25. Karukivi M, Hautala L, Korpelainen J, Haapasalo-Pesu KM, Liuksila PR, Joukamaa M, Saarijärvi S: **Alexithymia and eating disorder symptoms in adolescents.** *Eat Disord* 2010, **18**:226–238.
26. Schmidt U, Jiwany A, Treasure J: **A controlled study of alexithymia in eating disorders.** *Compr Psychiat* 2009, **34**:54–58.
27. Wheeler K, Greiner P, Boulton M: **Exploring alexithymia, depression, and binge eating in self-reported eating disorders in women.** *Perspect Psychiatr Care* 2005, **41**:114–123.
28. Wells A, Welford M, King P, Papageorgiou C, Wisely J, Mendel E: **A pilot randomized trial of metacognitive therapy vs applied relaxation in the treatment of adults with generalized anxiety disorder.** *Beh Res Ther* 2010, **48**:429–434.
29. Wells A, Fisher P, Myers S, Wheatley J, Patel T, Brewin CR: **Metacognitive therapy in recurrent and persistent depression: a multiple-baseline study of a new treatment.** *Cog Ther Res* 2009, **33**:291–300.
30. Storch M, Keller F, Weber J, Spindler A, Milos G: **Psychoeducation in affect regulation for patients with eating disorders: a randomized controlled feasability study.** *Am J Psychother* 2011, **65**:81–93.
31. Bankhoff SM, Karpel MG, Forbes HE, Pantalone DW: **A systematic review of dialectical behavior therapy for the treatment of eating disorders.** *Eat Disord: J Treat Prevent* 2012, **20**:196–215.
32. Iancu I, Cohen E, Yehuda YB, Kotler M: **Treatment of eating disorders improves eating symptoms but not alexithymia and dissociation proneness.** *Compr Psychiat* 2006, **47**:189–193.
33. Wells A, Davies MI: **The thought control questionnaire: a measure of individual differences in the control of unwanted thoughts.** *Beh Res Ther* 1994, **1994**(32):871–878.
34. Fox JRE, Power MJ: **Eating disorders and multi-level models of emotion: an integrated model.** *Clin Psychol Psychot* 2009, **16**:240–267.

A decade of data from a specialist statewide child and adolescent eating disorder service: does local service access correspond with the severity of medical and eating disorder symptoms at presentation?

Jeremy Alman[1,2], Kimberley J Holles[1,2], Hunna J Watson[1,2,3,4,5*], Sarah J Egan[2], Matthew Hamilton[1,2], Julie McCormack[1], Julie Potts[1], David A Forbes[1,3] and Chloe Shu[1,2]

Abstract

Background: Eating disorders affect up to 3% of children and adolescents, with recovery often requiring specialist treatment. A substantial literature has accrued suggesting that lower access to health care services, experienced by rural populations, has a staggering effect on health-related morbidity and mortality. The aim of this study was to evaluate whether lower service access foreshadowed a more severe medical and symptom presentation among children and adolescents presenting to a specialist eating disorders program.

Method: The data source was the Helping to Outline Paediatric Eating Disorders (HOPE) Project registry (N ~1000), a prospective ongoing registry study comprising consecutive paediatric tertiary eating disorder referrals. The sample consisted of 399 children and adolescents aged 8 to 16 years (M =14.49, 92% female) meeting criteria for a DSM-5 eating disorder.

Results: Consistent with the hypotheses, lower service access was associated with a lower body mass index z-score and a higher likelihood of medical complications at intake assessment. Contrary to our hypothesis, eating pathology assessed at intake was associated with higher service access. No relationship was observed between service access and duration of illness or percentage of body weight lost.

Conclusions: Lower service access is associated with more severe malnutrition and medical complications at referral to a specialist eating disorder program. These findings have implications for service planning and provision for rural communities to equalize health outcomes.

Keywords: Adolescent, Child, Eating disorders, HOPE Project, Medical complications, Rural

Background

Eating disorders, including anorexia nervosa (AN), bulimia nervosa (BN), and other types of eating disorders are estimated to affect between 0.5% to 3% of children and adolescents [1-3]. There are serious consequences of eating disorders in this age group, including risks to growth and brain development and life-threatening medical complications [1,4]. Mortality rates of individuals with eating disorders are amongst the highest of all psychiatric disorders, particularly for AN, due to medical complications and suicide [5-8]. Eating disorders may require intensive treatment programs to facilitate recovery [9]. This is a concern in the context of rural areas where physical, cultural, and systemic barriers to accessing health services may contribute to increased medical compromise [10]. Very little research has investigated impact of service access or differences between rural and metropolitan

* Correspondence: hunna_watson@med.unc.edu
[1]Eating Disorders Program, Child and Adolescent Mental Health Service, Child and Adolescent Health Service, Roberts Road, Subiaco, Western Australia, Australia
[2]School of Psychology and Speech Pathology, Division of Health Sciences, Curtin University, Kent St, Bentley, Western Australia, Australia
Full list of author information is available at the end of the article

populations with eating disorders in their clinical and medical presentation [11,12].

The nature of rural–urban health differential remains unclear with factors such as socioeconomic status, ethnicity, geographical location and access to health services likely contenders to health disadvantage in rural areas, when it is observed [10]. Distance from services may make health care more difficult to access, although in smaller countries this issue is less apparent, suggesting that a critical distance is required before the disadvantage becomes measurable in health behavior or outcomes. In Australia, the standardised mortality ratio for Australian children and adolescents in inner regional areas is 1.26, increasing to 3.44 in very remote areas [13]. Service access may impact capacity for prevention, early identification, and treatment. For example lower levels of screening may occur, therefore reducing detection rates and delaying diagnosis, and treatment may be delayed or inadequate due to reduced service capacity and limits in expertise.

General practitioners and nurses are often the only health service providers available in rural areas; 90% of psychiatric staff are located in major cities, this can lead to care ratios of up to 6000:1 for mental health professionals in rural settings [14]. As such, people in rural areas seeking mental health care are often transferred to the nearest metropolitan city, suggesting specialist psychological care in rural areas is inadequate [15]. This is undesirable for the treatment of child and adolescent eating disorders, as relocation away from home can be a stressor, and treatment is typically long-term and ideally involves the entire family and collaboration of a primary care physician, nutritionist, and therapist [9]. Obtaining appropriate treatment for paediatric eating disorders can be difficult without relocating to a metropolitan city or without an effectively resourced "hub-and-spoke" model. In the hub-and-spoke model, a specialist tertiary service ("hub") provides training, education, and consultation and liaison services to health professionals operating in rural settings ("spoke") [16].

Until present, there has been little research on service access in the context of children and adolescents with eating disorders, with only a few studies exploring differences in rural versus metropolitan areas. Van Son and colleagues [12] investigated incidence rates of eating disorders in children, adolescents, and adults in the Netherlands across three categories of urbanisation: rural, urbanised and large cities. BN incidence was 2.5 times higher in urban areas and 5 times higher in large cities compared to rural areas, with no differences in AN. In a Japanese study, clinical presentations of AN occurred primarily in patients from urban areas [17]. In an Italian adolescent sample, contrasting results were found [11]; more people with symptoms lived in rural areas when using dimensional criteria, but this trend was reversed when using categorical criteria, with more people in urban areas scoring above clinical cut-offs. An Italian study compared urban and suburban populations, and found a higher incidence of all eating disorder diagnoses with urbanisation [18]. Neither of these studies focused on service access, therefore little is known about how service access relates to clinical presentation when people with eating disorders present for specialist care, particularly whether low services access is related to higher morbidity.

The present study

The aim of this study is to explore the association between service access and clinical presentation in treatment-seeking children and adolescents with eating disorders. Scientific literature indicating that people from rural communities often have poorer general physical and mental health outcomes than their metropolitan counterparts informs our predictions, as evidence pertaining specifically to eating disorders is lacking. We predict that children and adolescents with eating disorders who present for specialist care will have poorer physical health and more severe eating pathology as service access decreases. Specifically, we predict they will show higher duration of illness, loss of body weight, eating pathology, and medical complications, and lower body mass index (BMI) z-score.

Methods

Participants and procedure

The study is part of a larger study called the Helping to Outline Paediatric Eating Disorders (HOPE) Project, an ongoing prospective clinical cohort registry study, with 1024 participants at the time of the present study. The participation rate in the HOPE Project is approximately 97% [19]. Ethical approval for this study was obtained from the Princess Margaret Hospital for Children and Curtin University Human Research Ethics Committees.

Western Australia covers an area of 2 532 400 km^2, which is approximately 10 times the size of the United Kingdom. The state consists of 2 430 300 people, of which 621 800 are children or adolescents [20]. Approximately 262 742 (11%) of Western Australians live in outer regional or remote areas, that is, areas that are from 3 hours to 3 days drive from the major city Perth which has the only public specialist paediatric eating disorders service in the state. The HOPE Project registry consists of children and adolescents that consecutively presented to this specialist service, Child and Adolescent Health Service Eating Disorder Program (CAHS EDP) (formerly Princess Margaret Hospital for Children Eating Disorders Program) between 1996 and 2013. All children and adolescents and their families presenting to CAHS EDP undertake routine intake assessment spanning two half-days to determine whether they have an eating disorder diagnosis according to the fifth edition of the Diagnostic and Statistical Manual (DSM-5) [21] and to evaluate mental and physical health status.

Participants were included in the study if they met DSM-5 criteria for an eating disorder and were referred from 2001, so a service access score could be assigned. DSM-5 eating disorder diagnosis was assigned retrospectively based on prospectively collected child and parent eating disorder interviews adapted from Fairburn and Coopers Eating Disorder Examination (EDE) [22] and medical records [19], and prospectively after publication of DSM-5. Participants who attended boarding school in Perth but whose family residence was outside Perth, causing ambiguity to their status, were excluded (n =7) as well as participants who had a postal code for which an access score could not be assigned (n =2). The final sample comprised 399 participants aged 8 to 16 years (M =14.49, 92% female).

Measures

The Access/Remoteness Index for Australia Plus (ARIA+) measured service access and is a relatively stable measure of remoteness and access to services developed by the National Key Centre for Social Applications of Geographic Information Systems for the Department of Health and Aged Care [23]. The ARIA + is a continuous variable (between 0–15) with higher scores reflecting poorer service access - the following categories have been offered to describe accessibility; highly accessible (0–0.19), accessible (0.2 - 2.39) moderately accessible (2.4 - 5.92), remote (5.93 – 10.53), and very remote ([10.54 – 15] [23].

The *Socio-Economic Indexes for Areas (SEIFA)* Index of Economic Resources is a continuous measure of relative socio-economic advantage and disadvantage or a region; with higher scores indicating greater access to resources [24,25]. The SEIFA was used as a covariate as per previous research to adjust for socioeconomic differences across postcodes [13,25].

Duration of illness (months) was the self-reported length of time the patient had been experiencing eating disorder symptoms prior to assessment and was collected in the medical review with the family and child in attendance. *BMI z-score* assessed nutritional status and was calculated with Epi Info 7 [26], entering the patient's height and weight collected at the medical initial assessment, sex, and age into the program. *Z*-scores are age- and sex-adjusted based on the Centres for Disease Control and Prevention [27] growth charts. *Eating pathology* was assessed with the adapted child version of the EDE [22]. The EDE has four subscales – restraint, eating concern, shape concern, and weight concern – that aggregate to a global score. Internal reliability is acceptable and all but three items have been found to have inter-rater reliability coefficients > .9 [28]. *Percentage of body weight lost* was calculated by subtracting the participant's weight at the initial intake assessment from the maximum ever self-reported weight, dividing by maximum ever weight, then converting to a percentage. This is an imperfect method, since (unmeasured) linear growth occurs over the average 8 months illness duration, but is a sufficient proxy. *Potentially life-threatening medical complications* was a categorical variable defined by the presence of at least one medical indicator (1 = yes, 0 = no), specifically bradycardia, hypothermia, hypotension, and poor peripheral perfusion. The medical indicators were defined based on age-appropriate cut-offs [4].

Statistical analysis

General linear and generalized linear modelling (GLM) approaches were used. The predictor for all models was ARIA + and analyses were adjusted for the confounding effects of age, sex, presence of AN, and SEIFA. Presence of AN was added as a covariate because a higher proportion of participants in lower services access presented with AN, and we wanted to be able to tease apart medical and psychological differences attributable to service access, ruling out diagnostic differences. The dependent variables of BMI *z*-score, duration of illness, percentage of body weight lost, and global EDE were modelled with GLMs. The binary dependent variables, medical complications, were modelled with a binomial distribution and a logit link function. Statistical significance was observed at the conventional alpha level of .05.

Prior to analysis, Little's MCAR test was used to assess the pattern of missing data. All variables had less than 5% missing data, except for percentage of weight lost (15%). Missing data were assessed as missing completely at random, χ^2 (93) = 70.44, $p = .96$, and were imputed via SPSS MVA expectation maximization.

Results

Sample characteristics

Although a continuous measure of service access was used in the analyses, sample characteristics (see Table 1) were categorised descriptively by accessibility classification; highly accessible, accessible, and moderately accessible, remote, and very remote. Approximately 11% of referrals were from moderate to low service access areas, which is proportional to the general population distribution. The mean age of the sample was 14.49 (SD = 1.54) years and the predominant diagnosis was AN (39.3%) followed by other specified feeding or eating disorder (28.8%), unspecified feeding or eating disorder (24.1%), BN (7.5%), and binge eating disorder (0.3%).

Table 1 Descriptive and clinical characteristics of children/adolescents with eating disorders for all potential outcomes by accessibility classification

	Highly accessible (*N* = 295)	Accessible (*N* = 61)	Moderately accessible, remote and very remote (*N* = 43)	Total (*N* = 399)
Age (yrs), *M* (*SD*)	14.47 (1.57)	14.70 (1.42)	14.32 (1.46)	14.49 (1.54)
Female, *n*	277 (93.8%)	52 (85.2%)	39 (90.7%)	368 (92.2%)
DSM −5 diagnosis				
Anorexia nervosa	109 (36.9%)	23 (37.7%)	25 (58.1%)	157 (39.3%)
Other specified feeding or eating disorder	94 (31.8%)	15 (24.6%)	6 (14.0%)	115 (28.8%)
Unspecified feeding or eating disorder	70 (23.6%)	15 (24.6%)	11 (25.6%)	96 (24.1%)
Bulimia nervosa	21 (7.1%)	8 (13.1%)	1 (2.3%)	30 (7.5%)
Binge eating disorder	1 (0.3%)	0	0	1 (0.3%)
Age of onset (yrs), *M* (*SD*)	13.61 (1.67)	13.72 (1.56)	13.52 (1.65)	13.62 (1.65)
Illness duration (mths), median ± IQR [range]	8.00 ± 5-12 [1, 48]	9.00 ± 6-18 [1,36]	6.00 ± 4-9 [2,78]	8.00 ± 5-12 [1,78]
BMI *z*-score, *M* (*SD*)	−1.38 (1.41)	−1.45 (1.59)	−2.29 (1.32)	−1.49 (1.45)
Percentage of body weight lost, *M* (*SD*)	16.35 (10.85)	17.50 (10.89)	19.82 (11.33)	16.90 (10.93)
Medical complications, *n*	101 (34.2%)	23 (37.7%)	25 (58.1%)	149 (37.3%)
Bradycardia	70 (23.7%)	14 (23.0%)	17 (39.5%)	101 (25.3%)
Hypotension	32 (10.8%)	8 (13.1%)	8 (18.6%)	48 (12.0%)
Hypothermia	12 (4.1%)	0	4 (9.3%)	16 (4.0%)
Poor peripheral perfusion	27 (9.2%)	7 (11.5%)	10 (23.3%)	44 (11.0%)
EDE-restraint	3.36 (1.73)	3.51 (1.6)	3.08 (2)	3.35 (1.74)
EDE eating concern	2.52 (1.66)	2.58 (1.68)	1.98 (1.49)	2.47 (1.65)
EDE shape concern	3.45 (1.86)	3.66 (1.72)	3.05 (1.92)	3.44 (1.85)
EDE weight concern	3 (1.86)	2.99 (1.64)	2.58 (1.75)	2.95 (1.82)
EDE global score	3.08 (1.63)	3.19 (1.43)	2.67 (1.66)	3.05 (1.60)

Note: Median +/− IQR [range] were reported when variable skewness (>3) was present in 1 or more group.

Service access, medical and eating disorder characteristics at tertiary presentation

As shown in Table 1, a higher percentage of children and adolescents from lower service access areas had AN, and there was a positive association between ARIA+ scores and AN diagnosis (β = 0.12, 95% CI: 1.04 to 1.23, $p = .01$). Therefore, presence of AN was controlled for in subsequent analyses. As hypothesised, there was a significant negative association between ARIA+ and BMI z-score (β = 0.08, 95% CI: −0.13 to −0.03, p = .004) and medical complications (OR = 1.99, 95% CI: 1.01 to 1.21, p = .03), such that lower service access was related to greater medical compromise. Contrary to our predictions, ARIA+ and global EDE scores were significantly negatively associated (β = 0.08, 95% CI: −0.14 to −0.02, p = .01), such that as distance from specialist service increased, pathology was lower. There was a non-significant relationship between ARIA+ and percentage of body weight lost (β = 0.26, 95%CI: −1.16 to 0.68, p = .22) and duration of illness even when adjusting for covariates (β = −0.04, 95% CI: −0.40 to 0.33, p = .85).

Discussion

To the authors' knowledge, this study is the first to investigate the association between service access and clinical characteristics of children and adolescents presenting for specialist eating disorder treatment. The study discovered that children and adolescents with eating disorders assessed at a specialist treatment setting who were located in areas with lower service access presented to specialist treatment at greater physical risk, with lower BMI z-score and more prevalent medical complications.

An issue to consider in the present study is referral bias, since the study described children who were ultimately referred and then assessed at a specialist service and may have more severe and complex presentations than children with eating disorders in the community who do not get referred for treatment. Generalization of the study findings to youth who are not referred to treatment is not possible, without knowledge of the broader epidemiological features of children with eating disorders in Australia. Population-based research would help to determine if clinic-referred youth are sufficiently similar to non-clinic referred youth.

Amongst the assessed youth, we noted that AN was more prevalent in patients referred from rural areas, which we considered to be an artefact of referral bias rather than a true prevalence difference, given the reproducibility of prevalence estimates of AN generally. Hence we adjusted for AN in the analyses to rule this out as a possible confound explaining differences in physical and medical compromise between rural- and locally-assessed youth.

Our findings, based on over a decade of collected data, indicate that young people presenting from areas with lower access to health services had substantially higher physical and medical morbidity related to their eating disorder. The findings are of serious concern because malnutrition and medical complications of eating disorders may lead to increased mortality [5], stunted vertical growth, cardiac complications, and osteoporosis [7,8]. There may be some parallel with depression and cancer, whilst rural areas do not always have higher prevalence of these disorders, morbidity and mortality can be worse, which may reflect rates of screening, recognition and treatment capacity in more isolated and remote areas [29,30]. An important implication of this study is that young people with eating disorders need to be supported by a health system that is accessible, relevant, and timely, regardless of residential location.

Further studies are needed to understand the role of service access in morbidity, as conceptualised in this study, and how this factor works together with other plausible explanations. It may be that other aspects, such as rural cultural values of self-reliance and survival through independence, and higher stigma or concerns about confidentiality in smaller residential areas, impede access also [10]. There may be relationships between rural status and poverty, which may increase risk for extreme weight status of either underweight through lack of nutrition, or overweight through consumption of nutrient-poor, calorie dense, but more affordable foods [31-33]. Findings from the Australian Institute of Health and Welfare [34] suggest that there is an association between low socioeconomic status and childhood rates of obesity. Such data could shed light on differences in child weight status between geographical regions. Sociocultural mechanisms are known to shape eating disorder presentation and symptomatology; future research could explore whether the clinical characteristics observed in this study are a feature of eating disorders in more remote areas, for example, lower eating pathology may correspond with differences in media and Internet access and use.

In contrast to predictions, an increase in rural status was not associated with an increase in severity of eating disorder pathology, but rather the opposite was observed. Eating pathology may not be as conspicuous as physical deterioration and weight loss, and may be less of a factor associated with the decision to refer for specialist treatment, in particular to tertiary inpatient care which is a common entry point of rural patients to metropolitan services. It may also be that this finding is less related to service access and reflects the phenomenology of eating disorders in more geographically isolated settings. Sociocultural theory proposes that urbanisation is associated with greater exposure to the thin ideal and eating concern [35] and consequently those experiencing eating disorders from rural areas may have less developed weight, shape and eating cognitions and share some similarity with those observed in non-Westernised cultures where rationales for self-starvation are more variable [36,37]. Further, the higher levels of overall BMI in rural communities may both reduce and reflect the social pressure to be thin.

Contrary to our predictions, there was no relationship between an increase in rural status and duration of illness or percentage of body weight lost for tertiary assessed children. It is reassuring that duration of illness is not different by health service access, and while not statistically significant there was a trend for greater percentage of body weight lost with lower service access that may be clinically meaningful, particularly when considered in combination with the statistically significant differences in BMI z-score and general malnourishment observed in this clinical population.

Limitations of the study include the lack of information about individuals with an eating disorder not seen by health care professionals, or seen by primary care professionals in the community without referral to specialist care. As a consequence, many young people would not be included in this study and as a result the sample is biased toward treatment-seeking patients and families. BMI-z score and percent body weight loss do not take into account changes in height from the time of premorbid weight to the time of clinic assessment, so conclusions regarding these findings are limited. Socioeconomic status of regions was controlled for in the current study; however a measure of individual wealth status was not, which could explain the association between rurality and weight status in our cohort independent of eating disorder severity and course. The EDE and other measures of eating pathology have shortcomings when applied to AN, making it difficult to compare rural and metropolitan populations with this diagnosis [38,39]. The EDE was the only measure of psychological symptoms. Future studies could investigate comorbid psychological symptoms to identify if differences exist in variables other than physical health.

Conclusions

In conclusion, our findings suggest that lower access to health services is associated with greater danger of malnutrition and medical complications by the time the young person and their family obtains specialist care. The most important implication of our study is that individuals with low access to health services, such as those residing in rural areas, may require better access to services via telehealth and e-health, transport, accommodation assistance, dedicated outreach or training, and consultation services for families required to travel long distances to access specialist services [16]. Additionally, advocacy and education may assist to reduce the possible stigma of mental illness and help seeking in rural communities. Identifying the specific factors underlying rural–urban health differentials, such as distance from services or social or cultural impediments such as stigma or fear of loss of confidentiality, is important to the development of targeted and effective rural health policies and interventions. Further research and policy are needed to focus on improving hub and spoke models, increase access to appropriate care, and reduce health inequities in rural-dwelling communities and others who reside away from specialist care. Our study is based on data from the past decade, it is up to funders, policy makers, and health service planners and providers to work creatively into the next decade to address the needs of lower access populations.

Abbreviations

AN: Anorexia nervosa; BN: Bulimia nervosa; BMI: Body mass index; HOPE: Helping to Outline Paediatric Eating Disorders; CAHS EDP: Child and Adolescent Health Service Eating Disorders Program; DSM-5: Diagnostic and Statistical Manual Fifth Edition; EDE: Eating Disorder Examination; ARIA+: Access/Remoteness Index for Australia Plus; SEIFA: Socio-Economic Index for Areas; GLM: Generalised linear models.

Competing interests

The authors declare that they have no competing interests.

Authors' contributions

All authors contributed to the design of the study and assisted in preparing the manuscript. KH conducted data analysis and HW and MH assisted in data analysis. All authors read and approved the final manuscript.

Authors' information

JA, BSc(Hons)Psych. School of Psychology and Speech Pathology, Curtin University, Perth, Australia. KH, BSc(Hons)Psych. Research Psychologist at CAHS EDP and PhD Candidate at the School of Psychology and Speech Pathology, Curtin University, Perth, Australia. HW, PhD, MPsych(Clin). Senior Research Psychologist at CAHS EDP, Adjunct Research Fellow at the School of Paediatrics and Child Health, The University of Western Australia, Adjunct Lecturer at the School of Psychology and Speech Therapy, Curtin University, Perth, Australia, and Biostatistician at the Center of Excellence for Eating Disorders, Department of Psychiatry, University of North Carolina at Chapel Hill, North Carolina, USA. SE, PhD, MPsych(Clin). Senior Research Fellow at the School of Psychology and Speech Therapy, Curtin University, Perth, Australia. MH, BSc(Hons)Psych. Research Assistant at CAHS EDP. JM, MPsych(Clin). Specialist Clinical Psychologist at PMH EDP, Perth, Australia. JP, BSc(Nurs). Manager at PMH EDP, Perth, Australia. DF, MB BS. FRACP. Paediatrician at PMH EDP and Professor at the School of Paediatrics and Child Health, The University of Western Australia, Perth, Australia. CS, BSc(Hons)Psych. Research Assistant at CAHS EDP and PhD Candidate at the School of Psychology and Speech Pathology, Curtin University, Perth, Australia.

Acknowledgements

This work was supported by a Department of Health in Western Australia Targeted Research Fund grant (F-AA-16529), a Telethon Institute/Child Adolescent Mental Health Service grant, and a Curtin University Research Allocation Fund grant. Data were collected under protocols approved by the Princess Margaret Hospital for Children Human Research Ethics Committee.

Author details

[1]Eating Disorders Program, Child and Adolescent Mental Health Service, Child and Adolescent Health Service, Roberts Road, Subiaco, Western Australia, Australia. [2]School of Psychology and Speech Pathology, Division of Health Sciences, Curtin University, Kent St, Bentley, Western Australia, Australia. [3]School of Paediatrics and Child Health, Faculty of Medicine, Dentistry and Health Sciences, The University of Western Australia, 35 Stirling Highway, Crawley, Western Australia, Australia. [4]UNC Center of Excellence for Eating Disorders, Department of Psychiatry, Neurosciences Hospital, 101 Manning Drive, Chapel Hill, North Carolina, USA. [5]Princess Margaret Hospital for Children Eating Disorders Program, GPO Box D184, Perth 6840, Western Australia, Australia.

References

1. Madden S, Morris A, Zurynski YA, Kohn M, Elliot EJ: **Burden of eatig disorders in 5-13-year-old children in Australia.** *Med J Aust* 2009, **190**:410–414.
2. Machado PP, Machado BC, Gonçalves S, Hoek HW: **The prevalence of eating disorders not otherwise specified.** *Int J Eat Disord* 2007, **40**:212–217.
3. Reijonen JH, Pratt HD, Patel DR, Greydanus DE: **Eating disorders in the adolescent population.** *J Adolesc Res* 2003, **18**:209–222.
4. Walker T, Watson HJ, Leach DJ, McCormack J, Tobias K, Hamilton MJ, Forbes DA: **Comparative study of children and adolescents referred for eating disorder treatement at a specialist tertiary setting.** *Int J Eat Disord* 2014, **47**:47–53.
5. Birmingham CL, Su J, Hlynsky JA, Goldner EM, Gao M: **The mortality rate from anorexia nervosa.** *Int J Eat Disord* 2005, **38**:143–146.
6. Keel PK, Dorer DJ, Eddy KT, Franko D, Charatan DL, Herzog DB: **Predictors of mortality in eating disorders.** *Arch Gen Psychiatry* 2003, **60**:179–183.
7. Birmingham CL, Treasure J: *Medical management of eating disorders.* Cambridge: Cambridge University Press; 2010.
8. Katzman DK, Kanbur NO, Steinegger CM: **Medical screening and management of eating disorders in adolescents.** In *The Oxford Handbook of Eating Disorders.* Edited by Agras WS. New York: Oxford Universtity Press; 2010:267–291.
9. American Psychiatric Association: *Practice Guidelines for the Treatment of Patients with Eating Disorders.* Washington, DC: American Psychiatric Association; 2006.
10. Smith KB, Humphreys JS, Wilson MGA: **Addressing the health disadvantage of rural populations: How does epidemiological evidence inform rural health policies and research?** *Aust J Rural Health* 2008, **16**:56–66.
11. Preti A, Pinna C, Nocco S, Pilia S, Mulliri E, Micheli V, Consuleo Casta M, Rita Petretto D, Masala C: **Rural/urban differences in the distribution of eating disorder symptoms among adolescents from community samples.** *Aust N Z J Psychiatry* 2007, **41**:525–535.
12. van Son GE, van Hoeken D, Bartelds AI, van Furth EF, Hoek HW: **Urbanisation and the incidence of eating disorders.** *Br J Psychiatry* 2006, **189**:562–563.
13. Australian Institute of Health and Welfare: **Rural, regional and remote health: Indicators of health status and determinants of health.** Edited by Australian Institute of Health and Welfare. Canberra: Australian Institute of Health and Welfare; 2008.
14. Australian Institute of Health and Welfare: **Mental Health Workforce.** Canberra: Australian Institute of Health and Welfare; 2011.
15. Taylor J, Edwards J, Kelly F, Fielke K: **Improving transfer of mental health care for rural and remote consumers in South Australia.** *Health Soc Care Community* 2009, **17**:216–224.

16. McCormack J, Watson HJ, Harris C, Potts J, Forbes D: **A hub and spokes approach to building community capacity for eating disorders in rural western Australia.** *Aust J Rural Health* 2013, **21**:8–12.
17. Kuboki T, Nomura S, Ide M, Suematsu H, Araki S: **Epidemological data on anorexia noervosa in Japan.** *Psychiatry Res* 1996, **62**:11–16.
18. Favaro A, Ferrara S, Santonastaso P: **The spectrum of eating disorder in young women: A prevalence study in a general population sample.** *Psychomatic Med* 2003, **65**:701–708.
19. Watson HJ, McCormack J, Hoiles KJ, Forbes DA, Potts J: **The HOPE (Helping to Outline Paediatric Eating Disorders) Project: development and debut of a paediatric clinical eating disorder registry.** *J Eat Disord* 2013, **1**:30.
20. Australian Bureau of Statistics: *Population by age and sex, regions of Australia: Past and future releases*; 2012.
21. American Psychiatric Association: *Diagnostic and statistical manual of mental disorders (DSM-5).* Washington, DC: American Psychiatric Association; 2013.
22. Fairburn C, Cooper Z: **The Eating Disorder Examination (12th Edition).** In *Binge-eating: Nature, assessment and treatment.* Edited by Fairburn C, Wilson G. New York: Guilford Press; 1993:317–360.
23. Trewin D: **ABS Views on Remoteness.** Edited by Australian Bureau of Statistics. Canberra, ACT: Australian Bureau of Statistics; 2001.
24. Pink B: **Socio-Economic Indexes for Areas (SEIFA).** Edited by Australian Bureau of Statistics. Canberra, ACT: Australian Bureau of Statistics; 2011.
25. Schindeler S, Moore H, Eckstein G, Turner R, Kaldor J, Cerny M: *Rural Health Information Project: Rural Health Classification Systems, New South Wales Department of Health*; 2006.
26. *Centers for Disease Control and Prevention, Epi Info 7 (Version 7.1.0.6) [Computer Program]*; 2012.
27. *Centers for Disease Control and Prevention, Clinical growth charts*; 2010.
28. Peterson CB, Crosby RD, Wonderlich SA, Joiner T, Crow SJ, Mitchell JE, Cardone-Cone AM, Klein M, le Grange D: **Psychometric properties of the eating disorder examination-questionnaire: factor structure and internal consistency.** *Int J Eat Disord* 2007, **40**:386–389.
29. Schouten LJ, Meijer H, Huveneers JA, Kiemeney LA: **Urban–rural differences in cancer incidence in the Netherlands.** *Int J Epidemiol*, **25**(1989–1991):729–736.
30. Australian Institute of Health and Welfare and Australiasian Association of Cancer Registries: *Cancer in Australia: An Overview, 2006.* Canberra: Australian Institude of Health and Welfare; 2006.
31. Lutifiyya MN, Lipsky MS, Wisdom-Behounek J, Inpanbutr-Martinkus M: **Is rural residency a risk factor for overweight and obesity for U.S. children?** *Obesity* 2007, **15**:2348–2356.
32. Firestone R, Punpuing S, Peterson KE, Acevedo-Garcia D, Gortmaker SL: **Child overweight and undernutrition in Thailand: Is there an urban effect?** *Soc Sci Med* 2011, **72**:1420–1428.
33. Fox K, Heaton TB: **Child nutritional status by rural/urban residence: A cross-national analysis.** *J Rural Health* 2012, **28**:380–391.
34. Australian Institute of Health and Welfare: **Australia's Health 2014.** Edited by Australian Institute of Health and Welfare. Canberra: Australian Institue of Health and Welfare; 2014.
35. Stice E, Shaw H: **Eating disorder prevention programs: a meta-analytical review.** *Psychol Bull* 2004, **130**.
36. Lee S, Lee AM, Ngai E, Lee DT, Wing YK: **Rationales for food refusal in Chinese patients with anorexia nervosa.** *Int J Eat Disord* 2001, **29**.
37. Lee S, Ho TP, Hsu LKG: **Fat phobic and non-fat phobic anorexia nervosa: a comparative study of 70 Chinese patients in Hong Kong.** *Psychol Med London* 1993, **23**.
38. Couturier JL, Lock J: **Denial and minimization in adolescents with anorexia nervosa.** *Int J Eat Disord* 2006, **39**:212–216.
39. Binford RB, Le Grange D, Jellar CC: **Eating Disorders Examination versus Eating Disorders Examination-Questionnaire in adolescents with full and partial-syndrome bulimia nervosa and anorexia nervosa.** *Int J Eat Disord* 2005, **37**:44–49.

Internet-based relapse prevention for anorexia nervosa: nine-month follow-up

Manfred Maximilian Fichter[1,2*], Norbert Quadflieg[1] and Susanne Lindner[1]

Abstract

Background: To study the longer term effects of an internet-based CBT intervention for relapse prevention (RP) in anorexia nervosa.

Methods: 210 women randomized to the RP intervention group (full and partial completers) or the control group were assessed for eating and general psychopathology. Multiple regression analysis identified predictors of favorable course concerning Body Mass Index (BMI). Logistic regression analysis identified predictors of adherence to the RP program.

Results: Most variables assessed showed more improvement for the RP than for the control group. However, only some scales reached statistical significance (bulimic behavior and menstrual function, assessed by expert interviewers blind to treatment condition). Very good results (BMI) were seen for the subgroup of "full completers" who participated in all nine monthly RP internet-based intervention sessions. "Partial completers" and controls (the latter non-significantly) underwent more weeks of inpatient treatment during the study period than "full completers", indicating better health and less need for additional treatment among the "full completers". Main long-term predictors for favorable course were adherence to RP, more spontaneity, and more ineffectiveness. Main predictors of good adherence to RP were remission from lifetime mood and lifetime anxiety disorder, a shorter duration of eating disorder, and additional inpatient treatment during RP.

Conclusions: Considering the high chronicity of AN, internet-based relapse prevention following intensive treatment appears to be promising.

Keywords: Anorexia nervosa, Relapse prevention, Internet-based prevention, Online psychotherapy, Risk of relapse, Adherence, Eating disorder, Internet, Follow-up, Maintenance

Background

Anorexia nervosa (AN) is a serious mental disorder with very high rates for chronicity and mortality. In order to reduce chronicity and counteract mortality in AN patients, better and more effective treatments are needed. However, we also need more effective programs for maintaining an improved level of mental health that was achieved through face-to-face therapy; effective relapse prevention over longer periods of time following intensive treatment is truly essential for AN patients. Technological developments of communication media in the past years and decades have brought about new options for clinical research and practice. The development of guidelines for psychotherapy based on empirical results from RCTs (randomly controlled trials) and the development of detailed manuals for use in psychotherapy treatment studies has been very helpful for the next stage of using electronic media and the internet to convey relevant information and interventions to patients suffering from physical or mental disorders.

Internet-based programs can also reach patients or persons at risk who can only be reached with great difficulties by more traditional approaches [1]. There is hardly any limitation in the number of persons who can be reached by an internet-based program. Such programs, however, must not replace traditional service delivery; rather, they should complement and extend the options for medical and psychotherapeutic treatment in situations where there still is a great need [2].

* Correspondence: MFichter@schoen-kliniken.de
[1]Department of Psychiatry and Psychotherapy, University of Munich (LMU), Nussbaumstraße 7, 80336 München, Germany
[2]Schön Klinik Roseneck affiliated with the Medical Faculty of the University of Munich (LMU), 83209 Prien, Germany

There are a significant number of controlled internet-based studies for primary, secondary, and tertiary prevention for physical disorders, mostly delivering interventions for asthma [3], cardiological disorders [4], management of work-related stress [5], the promotion of physical activity to improve health in general [6], and diabetes mellitus [7]. Parallel to these internet-based developments concerning physical disorders, far more than a hundred randomized controlled studies utilize internet-based forms of psychotherapy in a wider sense. Moreover, there have been systematic reviews and meta-analyses concerning internet-based interventions for depression and anxiety disorders combined [8], psychological interventions in general [9], and for depression only [10]. Other controlled studies have dealt with internet-based psychotherapy for posttraumatic stress disorder [11], anxiety disorders [12] including panic disorder and various phobias, and depression [13]. Generally, results of RCTs employing internet-based forms of psychotherapy for physical as well as mental disorders have shown promising results concerning symptom reduction, number of medical consultations, number of sick days, and improvement of coping skills. Internet-based psychotherapeutic approaches can make creative use of a variety of technological options, for example of multiple colors, cartoons or moving animations, and auditory enhancements at crucial points in the process; they can be accompanied by (therapist-guided) internet chat groups, partially or fully automated e-mail and SMS-support [14,15], and standardized telephone contacts to give feedback or encourage participants to use the program conscientiously. Bauer et al. [16], for example, describe successful therapist-guided internet chat groups for relapse prevention following inpatient treatment for mood, personality, and somatoform disorders.

For eating disorders, until recently the few existing studies on internet-based interventions have focused mainly on bulimia nervosa (BN) [15,17-23] and binge eating disorder (BED) [24-27]. Meanwhile, research on internet therapy has expanded. One group addressed users' views and the relevance of individual parts of the program [28,29], while another group compared online versus face-to-face delivery of cognitive behavioral therapy to BN patients [30]. Both studies showed favorable results.

In treatment trials for anorexic and bulimic disorders, cognitive behavior therapy (CBT) has been the most widely used form of treatment. CBT concepts did constitute the main therapeutic approach in our nine-month internet-based relapse prevention program (RP). Two CBT treatment studies for AN inspired our research in this area; however, they both were delivered face-to-face and not via internet: In a one-year trial, Pike et al. [31] found that CBT was superior to nutritional counseling. In a larger controlled study, Carter et al. [32] reported that relapse rates were lower in AN patients receiving the CBT study intervention for maintenance of therapy outcome rather than with treatment as usual (TAU).

Effects of our nine-month internet-based intervention without follow-up data in the intention-to-treat (ITT) sample have already been published elsewhere [33]. The current paper focuses on the nine-month follow-up of an internet-based randomized controlled trial for relapse prevention in adult anorexia nervosa in a sample of program completers. For the current paper we intentionally analyzed the data of participants who received at least four of nine modules of the relapse prevention program and a limited amount of additional treatment (see below) to allow valid conclusions on the use and the effects of such programs. To our knowledge, our RCT on internet-based prevention to reduce the risk of relapse for anorexia nervosa (AN) following intensive (inpatient) treatment is the first such study to address this dangerous eating disorder. Other studies applying internet-based intervention focused on caretakers of AN patients [34,35] or on the parents of female adolescents at risk for AN [36]. Another study targeted young women with body image concerns, offering a prevention program via internet [37]. AN, of all eating disorders, carries the highest rates of chronicity and mortality in adolescent and young women. It is probably *the* psychiatric disorder with the highest mortality in that age group. A controlled treatment trial with AN patients is always a challenge, because AN patients frequently do not perceive the severity of their illness, tend to avoid treatment and frequently take a more passive, not highly motivated role during treatment. Compared to other eating disorders such as bulimia nervosa (BN) and binge eating disorder (BED), very few controlled psychotherapy trials have been conducted for AN. Of the few existing controlled treatment trials for AN, some have revealed enormously high (50 %) relapse rates [38].

The intervention period of intensive treatment with approximately 90 inpatient days was followed by a nine-month follow-up period. The aim of our study was to evaluate the longer-term efficacy of our internet-based CBT relapse intervention program (RP) for AN compared to a control group of AN patients who did not receive additional treatment from us. The main focus of the statistical analyses and data presentation in this paper lies on longer-term maintenance covering the time from the end of the relapse prevention program (T2) until follow-up nine months later (T3). This RCT was registered with the German Registry of Clinical Trials (DRKS00000081) and with Current Controlled Trials (ISRCTN20173615).

Methods

Sample

Participants for this prospective controlled and randomized study entered the study between April 2007 and

September 2009 while treated in one of eight hospitals in Germany providing specialized inpatient services and psychotherapy for eating disorders. The study included one interventional arm (relapse prevention, RP) and one control arm for comparison (controls). Inclusion criteria were a) female gender, b) a minimum age of 16 years, c) anorexia nervosa or subthreshold anorexia nervosa without the requirement of amenorrhea according to DSM-IV criteria, d) easily accessible internet connection available at home, e) at least a 2-point BMI increase during inpatient therapy if the BMI at admission was below 14, or at least one additional BMI point in patients with a BMI above 14 upon admission, f) sufficient motivation for further relapse prevention and for taking part in the study (defined as not having a history of long inpatient stays without a clinically significant weight gain or patient-initiated irregular discharges, no history of forced feeding, good compliance with psychotherapy and routine questionnaires during the index inpatient treatment, and the assumption of sufficient compliance with the RP by the individual's therapist). Individuals with other serious mental or physical impairments, acute or chronic organic or schizophrenic psychosis, marked suicidal ideation and/or behavior, and premature, irregular discharge from inpatient treatment were excluded from the study.

The study protocol was approved by the ethics committee of the Bavarian Medical Association and the ethics committees of other relevant German states. All participants provided informed written consent before they engaged in any research activity.

Figure 1 presents a CONSORT diagram of the patient flow in the study. During the study period a total of 1,802 female patients with anorexia nervosa or subthreshold AN (EDNOS type 1) aged 16 years or above were treated in the participating hospitals. Of these patients, the therapists reported 1,093 to the clinical research study center at Roseneck hospital in Prien; the other patients were either not informed about the study by their therapists or did not consent to being contacted by the study team. Before randomization, a clinical psychologist examined each patient with regard to diagnosis and inclusion or exclusion criteria using questionnaires and telephone or face-to-face interviews during the last weeks of inpatient treatment. Two hundred and fifty-eight individuals expressed interest in the study and met inclusion criteria. At the end of inpatient treatment, 128 participants were randomized into the RP group and 130 participants into the control condition. Randomization was performed at the independent 'Koordinierungszentrum für klinische Studien' (KKS Center), Marburg, Germany.

The control group [a)] received no treatment whatsoever from our team throughout the study following discharge from inpatient treatment; these former patients merely filled out the questionnaires at the relevant time points. For obvious ethical reasons the research team did not interfere in any way with decisions on additional external treatment but left this entirely to the patients' and their physicians' or therapists' discretion. Concomitant in- and outpatient treatments during the intervention and the follow-up periods were carefully documented for both groups (intervention group and controls). During the follow-up period, none of the patients received any intervention or other kind of therapeutic support from our side.

Of the 128 participants randomized into the RP condition, 31 participants (24.2%) *dropped out* from the RP after no or only minimal use of the program. Five other participants in this group reported a high amount of additional treatment during the course of the RP (defined as more than eight weeks of inpatient treatment or

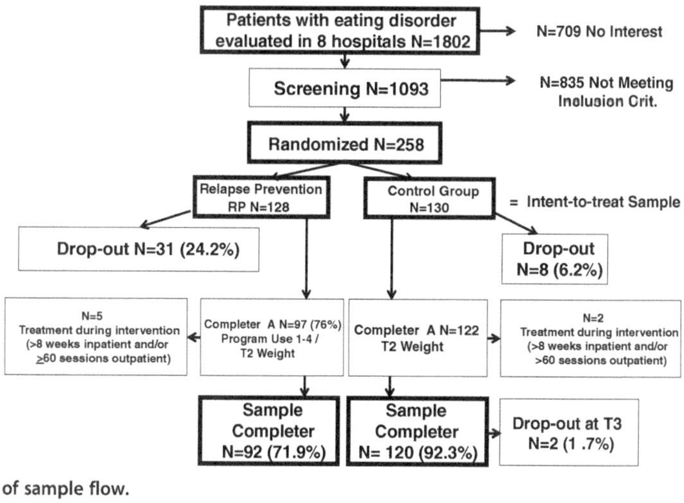

Figure 1 Consort diagram of sample flow.

at least 60 outpatient sessions of psychotherapy). In the control group, eight participants did not provide their body weight at the end of the nine-month "intervention" period (T2), and two others met the criterion of a high amount of additional treatment during that time. A (perceived) lack of time and the avoidance of being confronted with one's own eating attitudes and behaviors constituted the main reasons for not participating in the T2 assessment. Excluding these individuals from statistical analyses resulted in a *completer sample* of 92 participants in the RP group and 120 participants in the control group. At the nine-month follow-up (T3), two participants of the control group did not provide data. Therefore, nine-month follow-up data will be reported on 118 controls and 92 RP participants.

Of the 92 RP completers, 48 patients (52.2%) completed all nine CBT internet modules according to the protocol. Twenty-nine patients (31.5%) were partial users and worked through seven to eight sessions of the RP. Fifteen patients (18.5%) used four to six sessions.

Data presented in this paper are based on the completer sample (see Figure 1). The reasons for this are: 1. Intent-to -treat analyses concerning the intervention effects have been published already [33]. 2. The completer analysis generates valuable information about those who actually used the internet program. This allows us to view the data from a different perspective. 3. AN patients from other treatment studies tended to drop out at high rates, so information on those who (almost) completed our program will be quite useful in order to reduce sample attrition in the future. 4. In addition, results will show that a subgroup of highly motivated AN participants shows a much better outcome than completers of the control group.

Design

For each participant, the study lasted a total of 18 months after inpatient treatment with three observation points: T1 (baseline) at the beginning of the relapse prevention program, which started right at the end of inpatient treatment, T2 (end of intervention after x weeks), and T3 (follow-up) after additional nine months. This paper mainly focuses on the time period from the end of intervention (T2) until the follow-up (T3).

Measures

Body weight was measured by a person blind to the randomization condition (by a nurse from the treating hospital and by a general practitioner near the patients' home at the end of the RP program and at follow-up). The body-mass index (BMI) was created by the formula: body mass in kilogram divided by the square of the person's height in meters.

The Structured Inventory for Anorexic and Bulimic Syndromes Expert Rating (SIAB-EX) [39-43] was conducted to assess changes over time. After finishing the SIAB-EX, the interviewer rated the general severity of the anorexic eating disorder on the Psychiatric Status Rating Scale (PSR) [44]; furthermore, the Morgan Russell Outcome Assessment Schedule (MROAS) [45] focused on additional aspects of AN outcome. Interviewers at T2 (end of intervention) and T3 (follow-up) were blind to the treatment condition of the participants. These interviews were conducted by phone. Psychiatric comorbidity was assessed by the Structured Clinical Interview for DSM-IV Axis I Disorders SCID-I [46,47].

Several self-rating scales completed the questionnaire set: The Eating Disorder Inventory-2 (EDI) [48-51] targets eating specific psychopathology; the Barratt Impulsiveness Scale BIS-11 [52] and the Brief Symptom Inventory (BSI) [53,54] both measure aspects of general psychopathology. Participants also reported on newly occurring pregnancies. Baseline (T1) assessments were conducted right at the end of the inpatient treatment preceding the intervention.

Internet-based intervention

The nine-month web-based CBT relapse prevention program for anorexia nervosa (VIA) after inpatient treatment was developed by our research team and is described in detail elsewhere [33,55]. In short, the program was created according to approved manuals, self-help manuals, and aftercare manuals based on Cognitive Behavioral Therapy (CBT) for anorexia nervosa and related disorders [31,56-62] and adapted to presentation via internet. Participants of the RP group received nine monthly online CBT-based sessions (Chapter 1: Goals and motivation; Chapter 2: Transfer of relevant therapy components conveyed during hospital treatment to everyday life, maintenance of a regular and balanced eating behavior, handling binges and compensatory behaviors; Chapter 3: Body acceptance, Chapter 4: Self-esteem; Chapter 5: Coping with emotions and coping with a variety of feelings and with emotional needs; Chapter 6: Social competence and relationships; Chapter 7: Problem solving; Chapter 8: Depression; Chapter 9: Termination and farewell. An electronic message board for peer support, monthly chat sessions, and automatic short messages complemented the program. Participants could contact the therapist via e-mail. Whenever necessary, the therapist took previously anticipated and then standardized steps to motivate the participants to use the program.

Data analysis

A previous article [33] presented details on the rationale concerning power and sample size. In the current study, means with standard deviations and frequencies for categorical variables are reported, including t-tests for group comparisons, analyses of variance (ANOVA) and

chi^2-tests. Fisher's exact test allowed to compare proportions between groups when any cell count in a 2 x 2 table was less than five. The longitudinal data were suitable for a factorial design with ANOVAs on time point (repeated measures factor) and on intervention condition (RP versus controls, between-subjects factor). Another ANOVA compared groups regarding treatment, and critical distances (Scheffé; 5%) were computed for post-hoc pairwise comparisons. Missing data differed slightly between measures, and for each analysis the number of cases is reported.

Data on body weight and menstrual function led to the exclusion of participants who were pregnant at the time of assessment and who otherwise would have been included in the analyses.

Two-tailed testing was applied throughout. The primary outcome variable according to the study protocol was defined as the mean difference in BMI from randomization to the end of the online intervention [33]. We subsequently extended this definition to the primary outcome at follow-up; the dependent variable thus was the mean difference in BMI from randomization to follow-up over a total time period of 18 months. Due to the fact that this follow-up study on internet-treated AN is the first in its field, no hypotheses concerning course and outcome except for the primary outcome were derived. All additional analyses were exploratory in nature and did not account for multiple testing. P-values below .10 are given in the text to allow an appraisal of relevance.

In (only) four cases at follow-up T3, the general practitioner had not been able to weigh the participants beforehand, and therefore self-reported body weight from the interview was substituted. At the end of the intervention T2, this substitution had been utilized in 3 RP and 16 control participants.

Linear regression analysis on primary outcome (weight change from T1 (baseline) to T3 (follow-up)) identified six predictors in the ITT RP sample published previously [33]. The same predictors were entered in a linear regression analysis on primary outcome defined for T3 (follow-up; BMI at T3 – BMI at T1) including 88 of 92 RP participants in order to gain insight into the longer-term power of predictors of successful relapse prevention.

A range of eating disorder relevant variables known from the literature [63] were employed as predictors at baseline in logistic regression analyses on adherence to the RP. Possible predictors included age, duration of inpatient stay before RP, age at onset of eating disorder, duration of eating disorder, body weight at admission to inpatient treatment and at the beginning of the RP, type of AN (restricting or binge eating/purging type), psychiatric comorbidity, adherence to the RP (using all nine sessions versus others), use of psychiatric drugs during RP, additional inpatient treatment during and after RP, symptom severity of eating disorder, and impulsiveness. Forward selection allowed to reduce the large number of potential predictors.

Full completers who went through all nine sessions of the RP (N = 48) were classified as showing good adherence, and partial completers (N = 44) were classified as showing poor adherence to the RP. Newly defined variables of remitted mental illness were added to the model in order to clarify the earlier finding of lifetime comorbidity being a predictor of adherence [33]. Individuals with a lifetime but no current (at the time of index inpatient treatment) diagnosis of any mental disorder, mood disorder, or anxiety disorder (SCID-I) were defined as remitted.

Adjusted R^2 is reported for linear regression analysis and Nagelkerkes R^2 for logistic regression analysis.

Results

Sample characteristics at baseline

At baseline T1, the 92 RP participants' mean age was 24.0 ± 6.5 SD, their BMI had reached 17.9 ± 1.3. The 118 control participants averaged 24.2 ± 5.7 years, and their BMI had reached 17.8 ± 1.2 at the end of inpatient treatment T1. This treatment had lasted, on the average, 89.5 ± 32.7 (RP) and 90.4 ± 36.4 days (controls). Percentage of AN binge eating/purging type was 43.5% in RP and 46.6% in the control group. At T1 (baseline), groups did not differ significantly on these or most other variables [33].

Course and outcome of body weight

In the RP group, 4 of 92 participants (4.3%) became pregnant between T1 (baseline) and T3 (follow-up), three of them during the course of the RP. During the follow-up period, one of 120 controls (0.8%) became pregnant (chi^2 not significant). For the main analysis of the BMI, we excluded all participants who became pregnant during the 18 months of the study, because pregnancies obviously affect body weight and BMI.

In the completer sample about which we report here, BMI in the RP participants (n = 88) was 17.9 ± 1.3 at T1 (baseline), 18.3 ± 2.8 at T2 (end of intervention) and 18.8 ± 2.6 at T3 (follow-up). In the control group (n = 117), BMI was 17.8 ± 1.2 at T1 (baseline), 17.7 ± 2.1 at T2 (end of intervention) and 18.4 ± 2.6 at T3 (follow-up). There was a statistical trend for group differences at T2 (end of intervention; $t = 1.7$; $p < .10$). RP participants increased their BMI from randomization (T1) to the end of intervention (T2) by 0.47 ± 1.51 BMI points, while controls showed a small weight loss of −0.02 ± 2.05 BMI points. The mean BMI difference from randomization (T1) to the end of the follow-up 18 months later (T3) was 0.86 ± 2.3 BMI points for the RP participants and 0.61 ± 2.6 BMI points in controls (t-tests not significant).

A subgroup of RP participants, namely those who took part in every single session of the nine modules of the RP program (full completers), showed a further increase in BMI during the nine-month follow-up period (Figure 2). RP participants who used fewer than all nine modules of the program showed a course of BMI similar to the controls and significantly different from the better course of the participants who adhered strictly to the intervention protocol. In ANOVA, main effects of group (full versus partial completers versus controls) and time as well as the interaction of group by time were significant (F (group) = 5.92, p = .003; F (time) = 10.58, p = .000; F (group by time) = 3.95, p = .004). Pair-wise comparison of groups showed full completers reached a significantly (p < .05) higher weight compared to the partial users and the control group at T2 (end of intervention) and at T3 (follow-up). Partial completers and the control group did not differ significantly at any time point, with controls showing the lowest weight.

Additional treatment

Data on additional treatment for the same time intervals are presented in Table 1.

Partial RP completers received the highest amount of inpatient treatment during our observation periods, thus differing from both full RP completers and controls who did not differ from each other. No differences were found for intensity of outpatient treatment.

Use of any psychotropic medication during and after the RP was low and did not differ significantly between groups.

Course of symptoms over time

In both groups (RP and controls), scores of all subscales of the *Morgan Russell Outcome Assessment Schedule* (*MROAS*) changed significantly over time (Table 2). Main group effects were found for "Nutritional Status" and "Mental State", indicating a generally better adjustment in RP participants. Although the BMI improved in both groups during the RP and follow-up periods, the expert rating of the patient report on nutritional status deteriorated somewhat at the same time. Separate analyses of the single items of this scale showed this to be primarily due to a deterioration in the item "Dietary Restriction". The items "worry about body weight or appearance" and "body weight" showed only minor variations over time. For the subscale "Menstrual Function", the main group effect was not significant; there was, however, a significant interaction of group by time effects. RP participants showed a lower level of menstrual function on this scale at the beginning of the intervention and reached a menstrual function comparable to the controls at follow-up.

The *Eating Disorder Inventory* (*EDI*) subscale "Maturity Fears" (F = 4.63; p = .010) revealed a significant group by time interaction, and a statistical trend for EDI "Social Insecurity" (F = 2.87; p = .058). Over time, "Maturity Fears" in RP participants (N = 83) increased from 4.04 ± 3.44 (T1) to 4.33 ± 3.95 (T2) and 4.33 ± 3.98 (T3). In controls (N = 107), scores for "Maturity Fears" over time were 4.24 ± 3.94 (T1), 5.89 ± 4.88 (T2) and 5.69 ± 4.98 (T3). For the RP participants (N = 83), the EDI-scores for "Social Insecurity" were 4.69 ± 3.86 (T1), 5.73 ± 3.79 (T2) and 5.19 ± 4.29 (T3); for the control group (N = 106) the corresponding scores were 4.49 ± 3.66 (T1), 6.48 ± 4.20 (T2), and 6.24 ± 4.73 (T3). The same pattern of results but with more deterioration of symptoms in controls, was observed in both subscales. In other subscales of the EDI, ANOVA revealed significant (p < .05) main effects of time but no significant effects of group or group by time interactions.

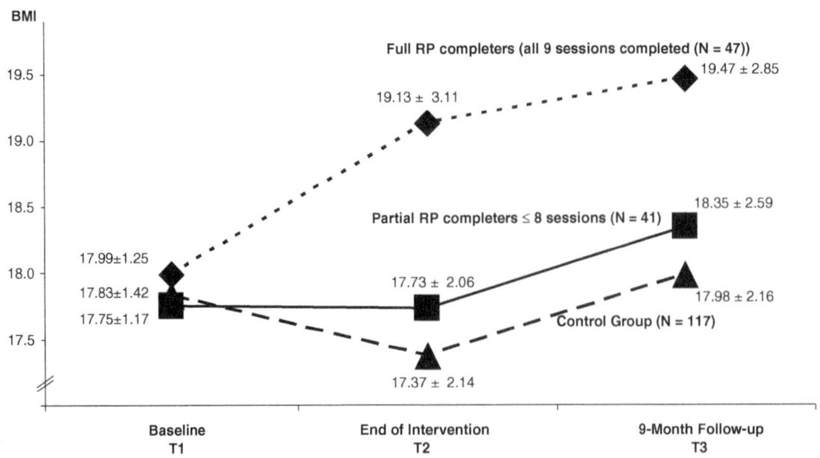

Figure 2 Course of body weight (BMI) in full RP completers, partial RP completers, and controls, excluding participants who were pregnant at the time of assessment. Means and standard deviations are indicated for each data point.

Table 1 Additional treatment between T1 (baseline) and T2 (end of intervention), and between T2 (end of intervention) and T3 (follow-up) in full RP completers, partial RP completers, and control group, excluding participants who were pregnant at the time of assessment

	Full RP completers N = 47 Mean (SD)	Partial RP completers N = 41 Mean (SD)	Control group N = 115 Mean (SD)	Statistics F (df = 2)
Inpatient treatment between T1 and T2 (weeks)	0.16 (0.75)[a]	0.92 (2.21)[b]	0.25 (1.18)[a]	4.2 p = .016
Inpatient treatment between T2 and T3 (weeks)	0.69 (2.68)[a]	3.31 (1.08)[b]	2.05 (5.15)[ab]	2.86 p = .060
Outpatient psychotherapy between T1 and T2 (sessions)	16.13 (12.83)[a]	17.54 (14.76)[a]	17.08 (11.75)[a]	ns
Outpatient psychotherapy between T2 and T3 (sessions)	15.32 (18.00)[a]	19.39 (23.32)[a]	17.10 (16.80)[a]	ns

ns = not significant.
[a, b:] Different letters after the means indicate groups that, according to post hoc-Scheffé-tests, differed significantly (p < 0.05) from one another.

Table 3 presents data for the subscales of the expert interview of the *Structured Inventory for Anorexic and Bulimic Syndromes* (SIAB-EX) over time. Comparing profiles of RP and controls, no specific pattern of change could be identified, but generally, data for RP participants showed slightly more favorable course (lower scores) of recovery.

In ANOVA, the group by time interaction was significant for bulimic symptoms. Breaking down the course of bulimic symptoms into full and partial completers yielded mean values of SIAB-EX bulimic symptoms for full completers (N = 48) of 0.31 ± 0.30 (T1), 0.51 ± 0.65 (T2) and 0.33 ± 0.38 (T3). In partial completers (N = 44), the means were 0.37 ± 0.40 (T1), 0.52 ± 0.67 (T2) and 0.56 ± 0.71 (T3). The ANOVA including full and partial completers and controls (means for controls are presented in Table 3) resulted in F(group) = 2.47, p = .087, F(time) = 12.83, p = .000, and F (group by time) = 2.70, p = .030. A t-test showed significant results (p < .05) for full completers versus controls at T2 and T3, and for partial completers versus controls at T2. Differences for full versus partial completers did not reach significance in t-tests.

Prediction of weight change in RP participants

Entering the same predictors identified in the ITT sample (for a list of predictors see Table 4) in an analysis of the extended primary outcome covering change in BMI from T1 (randomization) to T3 (follow-up) the SIAB-EX subscale compensatory behavior, additional inpatient therapy, and age at onset of eating disorder had no longer-term predictive value for primary outcome, while adherence to the study protocol, the BIS-11 subscale motor impulsiveness, and the EDI subscale ineffectiveness still exerted a significant impact on primary outcome at T3 (Table 4).

Prediction of adherence to the RP protocol

Bivariate comparison of T1 (randomization) variables between individuals with good and poor adherence identified only a small number of significant differences. Patients showing good adherence had experienced a later onset (18.4 ± 7.2 versus 15.2 ± 4.0 years, t = 2.6, p = .011) and a shorter duration (5.9 ± 4.4 versus 8.6 ± 4.8 years, t = 2.8, p = .007) of their eating disorder, plus less additional inpatient treatment during the RP (0.2 ± 0.7 versus 0.9 ± 2.1

Table 2 Morgan Russell Outcome Assessment Schedule (MROAS)

Mean(SD)	Relapse prevention (RP) N = 92			Control group N = 116			Statistics		
	T1 (Discharge Baseline) Mean (SD)	*T2 (End of RP)* Mean (SD)	*T3 9-month follow-up* Mean (SD)	*T1 (Discharge Baseline)* Mean (SD)	*T2 (End of Inter-vention)* Mean (SD)	*T3 9-month follow-up* Mean (SD)	*F (group)*	*F (time)*	*F (group x time)*
Nutritional Status	9.61 (1,4)	8.75 (2,8)	8.93 (8.9)	9.43 (1.6)	8.19 (2.7)	7.99 (2.7)	4.8 p = .029	21.8 p = .000	ns
Menstrual function (N = 87/114)[1]	4.34 (5.3)	6.51 (5.5)	7.94 (5.4)	6.07 (5.7)	7.48 (5.4)	7.54 (5.3)	ns	19.5 p = .000	3.3 p = .037
Mental state (N = 92/115)	8.64 (1.9)	8.35 (2.9)	7.97 (2.0)	7.76 (2.2)	7.57 (3.1)	7.20 (2.0)	12.0 p = .001	4.4 p = .013	ns
Sexual adjustment	7.82 (2.5)	8.90 (2.4)	9.18 (2.8)	7.69 (2.7)	8.81 (2.5)	8.72 (3.0)	ns	27.9 p = .000	ns
Socioeconomic status	9.29 (1.8)	9.74 (2.2)	10.09 (1.8)	9.23 (2.0)	9.79 (2.0)	10.00 (2.0)	ns	15.9 p = .000	ns

[1] Excluding participants who were pregnant at the time of assessment.
ns = not significant.

Table 3 Scales of the Structured Inventory for Anorexic and Bulimic Syndromes-Interview (Expert-rating SIAB-EX) over time

	Relapse prevention (RP) N = 92			Control group N = 116			Statistics		
	T1 (Baseline = Randomization) Mean (SD)	*T2 (End of RP) Mean (SD)*	*T3 (9-month Follow-up) Mean (SD)*	*T1 (Baseline = Randomization) Mean (SD)*	*T2 (End of Intervention) Mean (SD)*	*T3 (9-month Follow-up) Mean (SD)*	*F (group)*	*F (time)*	*F (group x time)*
Body Image and Slimness Ideal (BI)[1](N = 88/105)	1.04 (0.4)	0.97 (0.5)	1.12 (0.6)	1.15 (0.4)	1.11 (0.5)	1.33 (0.6)	6.5 p = .012	12.7 p = .000	ns
General Psycho-pathology and Social Integration (GenPsySoc)	0.61 (0.3)	0.47 (0.4)	0.51 (0.4)	0.69 (0.4)	0.51 (0.4)	0.54 (0.5)	ns	20.8 p = .000	ns
Sexuality (Sex)	2.24 (1.2)	1.68 (1.1)	1.60 (1.2)	2.07 (1.2)	1.80 (0.3)	1.74 (1.4)	ns	18.4 p = .000	ns
Bulimic Symptoms (Bul)	0.34 (0.3)	0.52 (0.6)	0.44 (0.6)	0.33 (0.3)	0.80 (0.9)	0.59 (0.8)	4.1 p = .045	21.1 p = .000	4.2 p = .015
Inappropriate Compensatory Behaviors to Counteract Weight Gain, Fasting and Substance Abuse (Counteract)	0.04 (0.1)	0.16 (0.1)	0.23 (0.1)	0.06 (0.1)	0.20 (0.2)	0.28 (0.2)	7.6 p = .006	146.9 p = .000	ns
Atypical Binges (AtypBinge)	0.04 (0.2)	0.17 (0.3)	0.14 (0.3)	0.08 (0.3)	0.22 (0.4)	0.16 (0.3)	ns	12.9 p = .000	ns

[1] Excluding participants who were pregnant at the time of assessment.
Ns = not significant.

weeks, t = 2.1, p = .044; good and poor adherence respectively). More of any lifetime mental comorbidity was found in patients with good adherence (79.2% versus 59.1% in poor adherence; chi^2 = 4.4, p = .037), and patients with good adherence had reported less current anxiety disorders at index inpatient treatment (12.5% versus 31.8% in poor adherence; chi^2 = 5.0, p = .025). Patients with good and poor adherence did not differ regarding BMI, medication, additional outpatient psychotherapy during the RP, and psychometric measures.

Table 4 Results of multiple linear regression on primary outcome (weight change (BMI) from T1 (baseline) to T3 (follow-up)) in the RP group (replication of ITT analysis [33] for the completer sample[1]) Adjusted R^2 = 0.15; N = 88

Predictor	Regression coefficient	Stand. beta	p
SIAB-EX subscale compensatory behavior T1	- 5.23	- 0.14	.194
BIS-11 motor impulsiveness T1	1.65	0.31	.006
Adherence to RP	1.32	0.28	.010
EDI Ineffectiveness T1	0.15	0.31	.006
Additional inpatient therapy during RP (weeks)	- 0.03	- 0.02	.865
Age at onset of eating disorder	- 0.04	- 0.10	.366

[1] Excluding participants who were pregnant at the time of assessment.
SIAB-EX = Structured Inventory for Anorexic and Bulimic Eating Disorders, Expert Version.
Subscale compensatory behavior is an abbreviation for 'inappropriate compensatory behaviors to counteract weight gain, fasting and substance abuse'.
BIS-11 = Barratt Impulsiveness Scale.
EDI = Eating Disorder Inventory 2.

The final logistic regression model identified four predictors of good adherence (Table 5). Remission from mood and anxiety disorder before the index inpatient treatment increased the probability of good adherence. A longer duration of eating disorder and a longer time in additional inpatient treatment during the course of the RP decreased the probability of good adherence.

Discussion

It still is a difficult task to treat patients with anorexia nervosa successfully. Even intensive in- and outpatient treatments have only limited success in the long run. Therefore, even less must be expected from time-limited, largely automated intervention delivered via DVD or

Table 5 Results of logistic regression analysis on good adherence to the RP

No	predictor	Wald-statistics	Odds ratio	95% CI
1	Remission from lifetime mood disorder at index inpatient treatment	8.4**	5.45	1.73-17.14
2	Remission from lifetime anxiety disorder at index inpatient treatment	4.1*	4.53	1.04-19.73
3	Shorter duration of eating disorder until admission to index inpatient treatment	13.5**	0.79	0.70-0.90
4	Additional inpatient treatment during the course of the RP	4.8*	0.59	0.37-0.94

R^2 = 0.37 (GOF: Chi^2 = 4.5; df = 8; p = .81.)
* = p < .05; ** = p < .01.

internet. Our patients in the RP group mainly received nine monthly internet sessions supported by (largely automated) e-mails and text messages. Much would already be achieved when body weight at discharge from inpatient treatment would only be maintained. In our study, the RP participants showed an even higher BMI than controls at T2 (end of intervention). During the nine-month follow-up period, both groups (RP and controls) achieved an increase in body weight (BMI), and at the end of the follow-up period, the BMI in the RP group was slightly, but non-significantly higher than in the control group. Thus, when we compare RP completers with controls, the significance of the differences in favor of the RP were not maintained over the full 9-month follow-up period.

However, the results look very different when we break down the group of RP completers into full and partial completers. Full RP completers who participated in all 9 monthly internet sessions showed significant improvement during the intervention period and further significant improvement during the nine-month follow-up. On the other hand, the BMI of the partial RP completers did not differ in its course from the control group. All-or-nothing thinking constitutes a frequent attitude in AN patients. The *full RP completers* seemed to have been fully identified with the aims of the study and were eager not to miss any session. They were the most motivated participants and really wanted to achieve something.

In the long run, partial RP completers and controls were also able to increase body weight but less than the full RP completers. During the same time period, partial RP completers and controls (the latter non-significantly) received more additional inpatient treatment after the end of the intervention period. Inpatient treatment is helpful but the health insurance will only pay when there is a need for it such as in the case of relapse. The higher use of inpatient services in partial completers and controls during the follow-up period can therefore be interpreted as an indicator for relapses. Inpatient treatment in these two groups presumably helped them gain weight. This fact, in turn, made it more difficult for the statistical analyses to uncover the true effects of the online relapse prevention program when comparing the three groups (full completers, partial completers and controls).

Two patterns of predictors of adherence to the RP emerged from regression analysis. One pattern was the chronicity of the eating disorder as defined by duration of eating disorder and additional inpatient therapy during the RP period. Both predictors decreased adherence. The other pattern was the experience of remission from a mental disorder other than eating disorder, which actually increased adherence. A recent review found the evidence on predictors of drop-out from internet-based treatment for psychological disorders to be limited and stated a need for more research in this area [64]. Our findings add to the well-established knowledge on the importance of comorbidity when treating eating disorders; they underline the importance of remission from a comorbid mental disorder, shedding new light on possible factors that influence longer-term outpatient adherence favorably.

Symptom severity did not predict adherence to relapse prevention; consequently, this factor probably assumes a differential role in the assessment of general outcome of AN index treatment in contrast to the period of relapse prevention. As our baseline assessment occurred at the end of intensive inpatient treatment, AN severity was certainly much reduced in our sample (BMI values > 17). The study protocol did not provide for any assessment at the beginning of inpatient treatment, and thus no data were available for this interesting research question.

All values of the SIAB-EX interview subscales at T2 (end of intervention) and at T3 (end of follow-up) were less pathological for the RP as compared to the control group, but except for the subscale "Bulimic Symptoms", the differences of symptoms between groups did not reach statistical significance. The course of bulimic symptoms was similar to the course of body weight for full completers, showing more improvement than for the control group. The course of bulimic symptoms for partial completers was similar to that of controls; the difference of the scores for full and partial completers did, however, not reach significance.

At T3 (end of 9-month follow-up period), outcome according to the Morgan Russell Outcome Assessment Schedule was more positive in RP participants. However, group by time interactions only reached statistical significance for the subscale "Menstrual Function".

From the ratings of the clinical interviewers, a pattern of better course and outcome in RP participants emerged. Although statistical significance was rarely reached (for a comment on power and sample size see below), an argument for the positive effect of the RP could be made. The clinical interviewers at T2 (end of intervention) and T3 (follow-up) were blind to the study arm the participant was randomized into, and they did not know data from earlier assessments or patient self-ratings.

The pattern of a better course in RP participants was also found in self-rated maturity fears and social insecurity. However, both scales showed an increase over time in both groups, denoting more fears and insecurity. Chronic AN in itself constitutes a withdrawal from many normal life activities, sometimes lasting for years before initial contact with professionals, and 3 months of inpatient treatment provided a rather protected environment for our study participants. This often combines to years of non-participation in normal life activities. Our post-inpatient assessment period, in contrast, must be considered relatively short in view of the typical history of AN. As normal weight levels are approached, it seems plausible that these young women initially experience *more* fears with regard to entering or reentering a life with adult responsibilities.

Since this is the first internet-based randomized controlled trial for relapse prevention in adult anorexia nervosa, we are only at the very beginning of understanding *predictors for a favorable course* and risk factors for an unfavorable outcome. Only three of six predictors of weight gain during the RP were found to be still relevant for longer-term prediction at follow-up in full and partial completers, after omitting patients who used the RP only marginally or not at all. Short-term predictors related to symptomatic behavior such as compensatory strategies, or additional inpatient treatment and age of onset, were no longer relevant for longer-term prediction. Cognitive characteristics such as "motor impulsiveness", which in this context means more spontaneity, "ineffectiveness" reflecting poor self-esteem, and adherence to the RP, presumably reflecting among other aspects more motivation to change, constitute short and longer-term predictors indicating the importance of more healthy cognitive attitudes for reaching sustained improvement from anorexia nervosa. The finding of more "ineffectiveness" leading to a better outcome does not necessarily contradict this statement. Possibly, participants with lower self-rated self-esteem were more apt to accept therapeutic guidance, even if this variable was no predictor of adherence.

The study has some *limitations*: 1. Anorexia nervosa is a tough illness to treat, and a cure can hardly be expected. Although the sample of 258 AN patients, randomized into the RP and control conditions, may appear sufficiently large, it apparently was not powerful enough to show many consistent, significant results. In many instances the scores at T3 (follow-up) were less pathological for RP when compared to controls. Only on some subscales were the differences at the follow-up statistically significant in favor of the RP participants. Thus, the study, considering the severity of illness and the difficulties of treatment, was most likely underpowered (in spite of moderate drop-out rates). 2. We possess limited knowledge about a possible selection bias concerning the sample. Patients were consecutively admitted to 8 hospitals in Germany specialized in the treatment of eating disorders. However, the hospitals varied in their recruiting rate for the study. Not all eight hospitals offered a behavioral treatment approach; therefore not all patients were equally prepared for a CBT relapse prevention approach. The drop-out rate among those who received the relapse prevention program (N = 31) was higher than among the controls (N = 6). The most likely reason for this differential drop-out rate is that taking part in the intervention took time and meant investing time and effort. In addition, the RP-participants took part in the assessments at several time points. The latter was true for the controls as well, but the controls did not undergo any intervention program from our group from which they might have dropped out. 4. This study mostly presents results from the completer and not the intention-to-treat (ITT) sample. However, we did also analyze key variables for the ITT sample and found only minor differences as compared to the completer analysis. Course of body weight including data shown in Figure 2, and course of the subscales of the Morgan Russell Outcome Assessment Schedule, EDI and SIAB-EX were very similar in the completer and ITT samples. 5. In our study, we can only evaluate the overall global effects of all treatment components. Analyses of our data do not allow to evaluate the impact of single components such as text messages, e-mail support, the internet program module and the largely standardized telephone contacts with the aim of motivating patients to stay with the program. 6. Having used the latest internet technology, it would have been very desirable to also assess issues concerning cost effectiveness of RP as compared to TAU, similar to the work done by the group of Ruth Striegel-Moore on conventionally offered, guided self-help for binge eating [65,66]. However, time and budget restrictions did not allow for inclusion of this important issue. 7. For a small number of participants we could not obtain a measurement of current weight at T2 (end of intervention) or T3 (follow-up) and had to rely on patients' self report of their weight. Therefore it can be argued that self-reported body weight was lower than it actually was. However, analyses of data for those patients who both self-reported their body weight and were also weighed by their GP found correlations of .97 and .98 for the BMI. It therefore appears appropriate to include the few cases with self-reported body weight.

The strength and potential of the study are: 1. It is the first internet-based RCT using a CBT approach for relapse prevention in anorexia nervosa. 2. It is one of the few RCTs that targets health improvement in AN patients who previously had required inpatient treatment. 3. It constitutes the only study reporting on the longer-term effects of such an intervention. We not only have data for the time before and after the intervention, but also presented data on the nine-month follow-up. 4. Randomization was quite successful: At the start (baseline), there was no difference between the RP and the control groups for practically all variables assessed. 5. The drop-out rate in our study, when compared to other AN treatment studies, was quite moderate (!). However, there was a considerable number of partial completers in our RP program. A very high drop-out rate has been a problem in quite a few other randomized controlled trials with anorexia nervosa patients. Halmi et al. [38] published important data on the drop-out problem in the McKnight-Study; the authors decided not to publish the data on the participants of the study because the drop-out rate was extremely high. An RCT on online treatment of bulimic symptoms (not anorexia nervosa) reported a drop-out rate from internet treatment of 26% [22], which is comparable to our drop-out rate. 6. Since change in BMI was of importance in our study, we took great pains to measure height and weight professionally rather than relying on self-report of body weight. BMI upon admission and discharge was measured by hospital nurses blind to the design of the study. The randomization at T1 (baseline) occurred when patients were still in the hospital. At T2 (end of intervention) and at T3 (follow-up), patients lived in their home environment, and body weight was usually measured by the general practitioner blind to the design of the study, who then transmitted the data directly to us.

We found a higher rate of pregnancy in the RP group. Conception is based on many factors, and we did not collect data to explore this issue further. The social and biological aspects of pregnancy in or right after remission from AN merit attention, and future studies should be designed to include these aspects.

Conclusions

In conclusion, our follow-up data indicate that RP as well as controls showed further improvement in body weight (BMI), eating attitudes, and eating behaviors. In the same time period, general psychopathology remained broadly stable on the level achieved at the end of intervention. There was a general tendency for the RP intervention group, as compared to the control group, to show more improvement, but only a limited number of statistical tests actually reached significance. Some areas deteriorated slightly. Considering the chronicity of AN in general, the modest effects of current face-to-face treatments for this disorder and the fact that all our participants presented with a severity of illness that required inpatient treatment, the effects of the relapse prevention program via internet were remarkable. This was especially true for those who made full use of the RP. They reached a significantly higher BMI at follow-up than the controls. Future researchers and clinicians will have the task of predicting which patients they should include in internet-based interventions. Considering our results, it seems rather important to select those who will adhere to the program and will stay with it all the way. For practical purposes based on our data, it would be advisable to offer internet-based relapse prevention programs to patients truly motivated for maintaining the changes achieved through a preceding intensive treatment.

Endnote

[a] In two previous publications [33,55] we used the term "treatment as usual" (TAU) for what we describe as "control group" here. The latter term describes the control condition much better. Patients randomized into the "control group" received no treatment whatsoever within our randomized control trial. Due to ethical considerations, neither the control group nor the RP group could be prevented from seeking additional treatment during the study period but outside the study context. This fact was assessed in detail as an independent variable.

Abbreviations

BSI: Brief symptom inventory; BMI: Body mass index; BIS-11: Barratt impulsiveness scale; EDI: Eating disorder inventory-2; ITT: Intent-to-treat; MROAS: Morgan Russell outcome assessment schedule; PSR: Psychiatric status rating for Anorexia Nervosa; SCID-I: Structured clinical interview for DSM-IV axis I disorders; SIAB-EX: Structured inventory for Anorexic and bulimic syndromes – expert rating.

Competing interests

The authors declare that they have no competing interests.

Authors' contributions

MMF is principal investigator of the study, funded by the German Department of Research and Technology. He originally formulated the topic of the study, developed the main design (RCT), was the primary investigator of the study and general supervisor. He and NQ made substantive intellectual contributions to the conceptual design, statistical analyses, and interpretation of the data. Both took the lead for drafting the manuscript and contributed essentially to all parts of the paper's content. SL also has made significant intellectual contributions to the second part of the study and to the data interpretation; she was involved in drafting the manuscript and contributed substantially. All authors and co-authors approved the final version to be published. Each author participated sufficiently in the work to take public responsibility for his or her respective parts of the article.

Acknowledgements

The study was funded by the German Ministry of Education and Research (Bundesministerium für Forschung und Bildung der Bundesrepublik Deutschland) grant number 01GV0604.
We are grateful to Dipl.-Psych. Kerstin Nisslmüller, Dipl.-Psych. Anne Henneberger and Dipl.-Psych. Henrike Siekmann for their sensitive way of guiding the participants through the study. We thank Dipl.-Psych. Daria Ebneter, Dipl.-Psych. Katrin Görler and Dipl.-Psych Peggy Schmidt who conducted the follow-up interviews, and Dipl.-Psych. Frauke Schmidt of the University of Erlangen who provided the monitoring of the study. The KKS Marburg (Dr. Carmen Schade-Brittinger) contributed the external randomization procedure.
We also thank Dr. Kathleen Pike for her support and for making the treatment manual used by her group available. We thank Susanne Hedlund, Ph.D., for her writing assistance and for providing language help, and Wally Wünsch-Leiteritz, M.D., Bernd Osen, M.D., Thomas Huber, M.D., Sabine Zahn, M.D., Rolf Meermann, M.D., Vitus Irrgang, M.D., and Franz Bleichner, M.D., for their active support in patient recruitment for this multicenter study.

References

1. Moessner M, Bauer S: **Online counseling for eating disorders: reaching an underserved population?** *J Ment Health* 2012, **21**:336–345. doi:10.3109/09638237.2011.643512.
2. Wilson GT, Zandberg LJ: **Cognitive behavioral guided self-help for eating disorders: Effectiveness and scalability.** *Clin Psychol Rev* 2012, **32**:343–357.
3. Runge C, Lecheler J, Horn M, Tews JT, Schaefer M: **Outcomes of a web-based patient education program for asthmatic children and adolescents.** *Chest* 2006, **129**:581–593.

4. Kuhl EA, Sears SF, Conti JB: **Internet-based behavioral change and psychosocial care for patients with cardiovascular disease: A review of cardiac disease-specific applications.** *Heart Lung* 2006, **35:**374–382.
5. Billings DW, Cook RF, Hendrickson A, Dove DC: **A web-based approach to managing stress and mood disorders in the workforce.** *J Occup Environ Med* 2008, **50:**960–968.
6. De Bourdeaudhuij I, Maes L, De Henauw S, De Vriendt T, Moreno LA, Kersting M, *et al*: **Evaluation of a computer-tailored physical activity intervention in adolescents in six European countries: The Activ-O-Meter in the HELENA intervention study.** *J Adolesc Health* 2010, **45**(Suppl 5):458–466.
7. Van Bastelaar KMP, Pouwer F, Cuijpers P, Riper H, Snoek F: **Web-based cognitive-behavioral therapy for depressive symptoms in type 1 and type 2 diabetes: A randomized controlled trial.** *Diabetes Care* 2011, **34**(Suppl 2):320–325.
8. Spek V, Cuijpers P, Nyklicek I, Riper H, Keyser J, Pop V: **Internet-based cognitive-behavior therapy for symptoms of depression and anxiety: A meta-analysis.** *Psychol Med* 2007, **37:**319–328.
9. Barak A, Hen L, Boniel-Nissim M, Shapira N: **A comprehensive review and a meta-analysis of the effectiveness of internet-based psychotherapeutic interventions.** *J Tech Hum Serv* 2008, **26:**109–160.
10. Cuijpers P, Marks IM, Van Straten AM, Cavanagh K, Gega L, Andersson G: **Computer-aided psychotherapy for anxiety disorders: A meta-analytic review.** *Cogn Behav Ther* 2009, 38:66–82.
11. Lange A, Rietdihk D, Hudcovicova M, Van de Ven JP, Schrieken B, Emmelkamp PMG: **Internet therapy: A controlled randomized trial of the standardized treatment of posttraumatic stress through the internet.** *J Consult Clin Psychol* 2003, **71**(Suppl 5):901–909.
12. Rollman BL, Belnap BH, Mazumdar S, Houck PR, Zhu F, Gardner W, *et al*: **A randomized trial to improve the quality of treatment for panic and generalized anxiety disorders in primary care.** *Arch Gen Psychiatry* 2005, **62:**1332–1341.
13. Gerhards SAH, De Graaf LE, Jacobs LE, Severens JL, Huibers MJH, Arntz A, *et al*: **Economic evaluation of online computerized cognitive-behavioral therapy without support for depression in primary care: Randomized trial.** *Br J Psychiatry* 2010, **196**(Suppl 4):310–318.
14. Ljotsson B, Lundin C, Mitsell K, Carlbring P, Ramklint M, Ghaderi A: **Remote treatment of bulimia nervosa and binge eating disorder: A randomized trial of internet-assisted cognitive behavioural therapy.** *Behav Res Ther* 2007, **45:**649–661.
15. Shapiro JR, Reba-Harrelson L, Dymek-Valentine M, Woolson SL, Hamer RM, Bulik CM: **Feasibility and acceptability of CD-ROM-based cognitive-behavioral treatment for binge-eating-disorder.** *Eur Eat Disord Rev* 2007, **15:**175–184.
16. Bauer S, Wolf M, Haug S, Kordy H: **The effectiveness of internet chat groups in relapse prevention after inpatient psychotherapy.** *Psychother Res* 2011, **21:**219–226.
17. Carrard I, Rouget P, Fernandez-Aranda F, Volkart AC, Damoiseau M, Lam T: **Evaluation and deployment of evidence based patient self-management support program for bulimia nervosa.** *Int J Med Inform* 2006, **75:**101–109.
18. Schmidt U, Andiappan M, Grover M, Robinson S, Perkins S, Dugmore O, *et al*: **A randomized controlled trial of the effectiveness of a CD-ROM-based cognitive-behavioral self-care intervention for bulimia nervosa.** *Br J Psychiatry* 2008, **193:**493–500.
19. Fernandez-Aranda F, Nunez A, Martinez C, Krug I, Cappozzo M, Carrard I, *et al*: **Internet-based cognitive-behavioral therapy for bulimia nervosa: A controlled study.** *Cyberpsychol Behav* 2008, **12:**37–41.
20. Sánchez-Ortiz VC, Munro C, Stahl D, House J, Startup H, Treasure J, *et al*: **A randomized controlled trial of internet-based cognitive-behavioral therapy for bulimia nervosa or related disorders in a student population.** *Psychol Med* 2011, **41**(Suppl 2):407–417. Epub 2010 Apr 21.
21. Jacobi C, Völker U, Trockel MT, Barr Taylor C: **Effects of an Internet-based intervention for subthreshold eating disorders: A randomized controlled trial.** *Behav Res Ther* 2012, **50:**90–99.
22. Ruwaard J, Lange A, Broeksteeg J, Renteria-Agirre A, Schrieken B, Dolan CV, Emmelkamp P: **Online cognitive-behavioral treatment of bulimic symptoms: A randomized controlled trial.** *Clin Psychol Psychother* 2012. doi:10.1002/cpp.1767.
23. Wagner G, Penelo E, Wanner C, Gwinner P, Trofaier ML, Imgart H, Waldherr K, Wöber-Bingöl C, Karwautz AFK: **Internet-delivered cognitive-behavioural therapy v. conventional guided self-help for bulimia nervosa: long-term evaluation of a randomized controlled trial.** *Br J Psychiatry* 2013, **202:**135–141.
24. Bedrosian R, Striegel-Moore R, Wang C: **Demographic and clinical characteristics of individuals utilizing an internet-based digital coaching program for recovering from binge eating.** *Int J Eat Disord* 2011, **44**(Suppl 7):639–646.
25. Carrard I, Crépin C, Rouget P, Lam T, Golay A, Van der Linden M: **Randomized controlled trial of guided self-help treatment on the Internet for binge eating disorder.** *Behav Res Ther* 2011, **49:**482–491.
26. Carrard I, Crèpin C, Rouget P, Lam T, Van der Linden M, Golay A: **Acceptance and efficacy of a guided internet self-help treatment program for obese patients with binge eating disorder.** *Clin Prac Epidemiol Mental Health* 2011, **7:**8–18.
27. Graham L, Walton M: **Investigating the use of CD-Rom CBT for bulimia nervosa and binge eating disorder in an NHS adult outpatient eating disorders service.** *Behav Cogn Psychother* 2011, **39:**443–456.
28. Sánchez-Ortiz VC, House J, Munro C, Treasure J, Startup H, *et al*: **"A computer isn't gonna judge you": A qualitative study of users' views of an internet-based cognitive-behavioural guided self-care treatment package for bulimia nervosa and related disorders.** *Eat Weight Disord* 2011, **16:**e93–e101.
29. Sánchez-Ortiz VC, Munro C, Startup H, Treasure J, Schmidt U: **The role of email guidance in internet-based cognitive-behavioral self-care treatment for bulimia nervosa.** *Eur Eat Disord Rev* 2011, **19:**342–348.
30. Bulik CM, Marcus MD, Zerwas S, Levine MD, Hofmeier S, Trace SE, *et al*: **CBT4BN versus CBTF2F: Comparison of online versus face-to-face treatment for bulimia nervosa.** *Contemp Clin Trials* 2012, **33:**1056–1064. doi:10.1016/j.cct.2012.05.008.
31. Pike KM, Walsh BT, Vitousek K, Wilson GT, Bauer J: **Cognitive behavior therapy in the posthospitalization treatment of anorexia nervosa.** *Am J Psychiatry* 2003, **160:**2046–2049.
32. Carter JC, McFarlane TL, Bewell C, Olmsted MP, Woodside DB, Kaplan AS, *et al*: **Maintenance treatment for anorexia nervosa: A comparison of cognitive behavior therapy and treatment as usual.** *Int J Eat Disord* 2009, **42:**202–207.
33. Fichter MM, Quadflieg N, Nisslmüller K, Lindner S, Osen B, Huber T, Wünsch-Leiteritz W: **Does internet-based prevention reduce the risk of relapse for anorexia nervosa?** *Behav Res Ther* 2012, **50:**180–190.
34. Grover M, Naumann U, Mohammad-Dar L, Glennon D, Ringwood S, Eisler I, *et al*: **A randomized controlled trial of an Internet-based cognitive-behavioural skills package for carers of people with anorexia nervosa.** *Psychol Med* 2011, **41:**2581–2591.
35. Grover M, Williams C, Eisler I, Fairbairn P, McCloskey C, Smith G, *et al*: **An off-line pilot evaluation of a web-based systemic cognitive-behavioral intervention for carers of people with anorexia nervosa.** *Int J Eat Disord* 2011, **44:**708–715.
36. Jones M, Völker U, Lock J, Taylor B, Jacobi C: **Family-based early intervention for anorexia nervosa.** *Eur Eat Disord Rev* 2012, **20:**e137–e143.
37. Stice E, Rohde P, Durant S, Shaw H: **A preliminary trial of a prototype internet dissonance-based eating disorder prevention program for young women with body image concerns.** *J Consult Clin Psychol*, **80:**907–916. in print.
38. Halmi KA, Agras WS, Crow S, Mitchell J, Wilson GT, Bryson SW, *et al*: **Predictors of treatment acceptance and completion in anorexia nervosa. Implications for future study designs.** *Arch Gen Psychiat* 2005, **62:**776–781.
39. Fichter MM, Elton M, Engel K, Meyer AE, Mall H, Poustka F: **Structured Interview for Anorexia und Bulimia Nervosa (SIAB): Development of a new instrument for the assessment of eating disorders.** *Int J Eat Disord* 1991, **10:**571–592.
40. Fichter MM, Herpertz S, Quadflieg N, Herpertz-Dahlmann B: **Structured Interview for Anorexic and Bulimic Disorders for DSM-IV and ICD-10: Updated (third) revision.** *Int J Eat Disord* 1998, **24:**227–249.
41. Fichter MM, Quadflieg N: *Strukturiertes Inventar für Anorektische und Bulimische Essstörungen (SIAB).* Göttingen: Hogrefe; 1999.
42. Fichter MM, Quadflieg N: **Comparing self- and expert rating: A self-report screening version (SIAB-S) of the Structured Interview for Anorexic and Bulimic Syndromes for DSM-IV and ICD-10 (SIAB-EX).** *Eur Arch Psychiatry Clin Neurosci* 2000, **250:**175–185.
43. Fichter MM, Quadflieg N: **The Structured Interview for Anorexic and Bulimic disorders for DSM-IV and ICD-10 (SIAB-EX): Reliability and validity.** *Eur Psychiatry* 2001, **16:**38–48.
44. Herzog DB, Keller MB, Lavori PW, Ott IL: **Short-term prospective study of recovery in bulimia nervosa.** *Psychiatry Res* 1988, **23:**45–55.

45. Morgan HG, Hayward AE: **Clinical assessment of anorexia nervosa. The Morgan Russell outcome assessment schedule.** *Brit J Psychiat* 1988, **152:**367–371.
46. First MB, Gibbon M, Spitzer RL: *User's Guide for the SCID-I Structured Clinical Interview for DSM-IV (SCID-I Version 2.0, February 1996 Final Version).* New York: Biometrics Research Department; 1996.
47. Wittchen HU, Wunderlich U, Gruschwitz S, Zaudig M: *Strukturiertes Klinisches Interview für DSM-IV (SKID).* Göttingen, Bern, Toronto, Seattle: Hogrefe; 1997.
48. Garner DM, Olmstead MP: *Eating Disorder Inventory Manual.* New York: Psychological Assessment Resources; 2000.
49. Garner DM, Olmstead MP, Polivy J: **Development and validation of a multidimensional eating disorder inventory of anorexia nervosa and bulimia.** *Int J Eat Disord* 1983, **2:**14–34.
50. Paul T, Thiel A: *Eating Disorder Inventory-2 – German Version.* Göttingen: Hogrefe; 2005.
51. Thiel A, Jacobi C, Horstmann S: **Eine deutschsprachige Version des Eating Disorder Inventory EDI-2.** *Psychother Psychosom Med Psychol* 1997, **47:**365–376.
52. Patton JH, Stanford MS, Barratt E: **Factor structure of the Barratt Impulsiveness Scale.** *J Clin Psychol* 1995, **51:**768–774.
53. Derogatis LR, Melisaratos N: **The Brief Symptom Inventory: An introductory report.** *Psychol Med* 1983, **13:**595–605.
54. Franke GH: *Brief Symptom Inventory von Derogatis.* Göttingen: Hogrefe; 2000.
55. Fichter MM, Quadflieg N, Nisslmüller K, Lindner S, Wünsch-Leiteritz W, Osen B, *et al*: **Internet-basierte Ansätze in der Therapie von Essstörungen (Internet-based approaches for the treatment of eating disorders).** *Der Nervenarzt* 2011, **82:**1107–1117.
56. Kleifield EI, Wagner S, Hoberman H, Halmi K, Wilson T, Agras S, *et al*: *Cognitive Behavioral Treatment (CBT) Manual for Anorexia Nervosa.* McKnight-Foundation Study; 1997.
57. Pike KM, Carter J, Olmsted M: *Cognitive behavioral therapy manual for anorexia nervosa*; 2005. *Manual*, revised February 2005.
58. Treasure J: *Anorexia Nervosa: A Survival Guide for Families, Friends, and Suffers.* East Sussex: Psychology Press; 1999.
59. Schmidt U, Treasure J: *Die Bulimie besiegen: Ein Selbsthilfe-Programm.* Frankfurt/Main, New York: Campus-Verlag; 1996.
60. Jacobi C, Thiel A, Paul T: *Kognitive Verhaltenstherapie bei Anorexia und Bulimia nervosa (2. vollständig überarbeitete Aufl.).* Beltz: Weinheim; 2000.
61. Jacobi C, Paul P, Thiel A: *Essstörungen.* Göttingen: Hogrefe; 2004.
62. Garner DM, Vitousek KM, Pike KM: **Cognitive-behavioral therapy for anorexia nervosa.** In *Handbook of Treatment for Eating Disorders.* London, New York: The Guilford Press; 1997:94–144.
63. Jacobi C, Hayward C, De Zwaan M, Kraemer HC, Agras WS: **Coming to terms with risk factors for eating disorders: Application of risk terminology and suggestions for a general taxonomy.** *Psychol Bull* 2004, **130:**19–65.
64. Melville KM, Casey LM, Kavanagh DJ: **Dropout from Internet-based treatment for psychological disorders.** *Br J Clin Psychol* 2010, **49:**455–471.
65. Striegel-Moore R, Wilson GT, DeBar L, Perrin N, Lynch F, Rosselli F, Kraemer HC: **Cognitive behavioral guided self-help for the treatment of recurrent binge eating.** *J Consult Clin Psychol* 2010, **78:**312–321.
66. Lynch FL, Striegel-Moore RH, Dickerson JF, Perrin N, DeBar L, Wilson GT, Kraemer HC: **Cost-effectiveness of guided self-help treatment for recurrent binge eating.** *J Consult Clin Psychol* 2010, **78:**322–333.

Change in emotion regulation during the course of treatment predicts binge abstinence in guided self-help dialectical behavior therapy for binge eating disorder

Laurel M Wallace[1], Philip C Masson[1], Debra L Safer[2] and Kristin M von Ranson[1*]

Abstract

Background: Dialectical behavior therapy (DBT), which appears to be an effective treatment for binge eating disorder (BED), focuses on teaching emotion regulation skills. However, the role of improved emotion regulation in predicting treatment outcome in BED is uncertain.

Methods: This secondary analysis explored whether change in self-reported emotion regulation (as measured by the Difficulties in Emotion Regulation Scale) during treatment was associated with abstinence from binge eating at post-treatment and 4-, 5-, and 6-month follow-up in individuals who received a guided self-help adaptation of DBT for BED. Participants were 60 community-based men and women with BED who received a self-help manual and six 20-minute support phone calls.

Results: Greater improvement in self-reported emotion regulation between pre- and post-treatment predicted abstinence from binge eating at post-treatment, 4-, 5-, and 6-month follow-up. However, some follow-up results were no longer significant when imputed data was excluded, suggesting that the effect of emotion regulation on binge abstinence may be strongest at 4-month follow-up but decline across a longer duration of follow-up.

Conclusions: This study provides preliminary support for the theoretical role played by improved emotion regulation in achieving binge eating abstinence. If this finding is replicated with larger samples, further research should identify specific techniques to help more individuals to effectively regulate their emotions over a longer duration.

Keywords: Self-help, Dialectical behavior therapy, Emotion regulation, Binge eating disorder

Background

Binge eating disorder (BED) is associated with specific eating disorder psychopathology, notable psychiatric comorbidity, and considerable psychosocial and functional impairment [1,2]. Furthermore, BED is associated with significant medical morbidity and physical health risks [3,4].

The characteristic feature of BED is persistent binge episodes wherein an unusually large quantity of food is eaten within a discrete period of time, while experiencing a sense of loss of control over eating (i.e., objective binge eating episodes [OBEs]). Thus, an important goal of treatment for BED is to reduce the frequency of such episodes and ultimately promote abstinence from binge eating. Research has demonstrated that numerous psychological treatments may be effective in improving binge eating symptoms, including cognitive behavior therapy (CBT; e.g., [5]), interpersonal psychotherapy (IPT; e.g., [6]), and dialectical behavior therapy (DBT; e.g., [7]). However, although these treatments are effective for many individuals, a significant proportion of individuals still fails to benefit from such treatments [8-10]. For example, randomized controlled trials of group CBT [6], group IPT [6], and group DBT [11] for individuals with BED have indicated that approximately 40% of individuals receiving treatment were not binge abstinent for the past month at one-year follow-up. These findings suggest a need to

* Correspondence: kvonrans@ucalgary.ca
[1]Department of Psychology, University of Calgary, 2500 University Drive NW, Calgary, Alberta, Canada
Full list of author information is available at the end of the article

refine available treatments with the aim of helping more individuals. To do so, further research is needed to clarify the processes involved in treatments with some efficacy and determine predictors of positive treatment outcome.

One psychological mechanism that has been hypothesized to be integral to the development and maintenance of binge eating is maladaptive emotion regulation [12-14]. Emotion regulation is defined as "the extrinsic and intrinsic processes responsible for monitoring, evaluating, and modifying emotional reactions, especially their intensive and temporal features, to accomplish one's goals" [15]. In essence, emotion regulation involves the ability to tolerate extreme affect and to regulate one's affect. Binge eating has been described as a maladaptive emotion regulation strategy, wherein binge eating is used to temporarily relieve an aversive emotional state.

Improving emotion regulation is an important goal of DBT as adapted for BED [6]. DBT for BED focuses on understanding and recognizing the link between dysregulated emotions and disordered eating behaviours, and teaching alternative, more adaptive emotion regulation skills. Previous research has demonstrated that DBT is effective in the treatment of BED [7,11]. However, the association of change in emotion regulation with change in binge eating remains uncertain.

Purpose

In this exploratory study, we conducted secondary analyses of a trial of guided self-help DBT for BED aimed at testing the theory that change in emotion regulation within individuals during the course of treatment is associated with treatment outcome at post-treatment and four-, five-, and six-month follow-up. Treatment outcome was defined as abstinence from binge eating (i.e., zero OBEs for the past 28 days), and was measured at multiple points: post-treatment, four-, five-, and six-month follow-up. By including assessment of outcome at multiple points during follow-up, this study investigated whether any association between change in emotion regulation and subsequent binge eating behaviour remained consistent or changed across time.

Guided self-help dialectical behavior therapy for binge eating disorder

A guided self-help adaptation of DBT for BED (see [16]) was developed and evaluated in a randomized wait-list controlled treatment trial [17]. In guided self-help treatment, a health worker guides an individual through a self-help manual. Participants in this treatment trial were randomized to receive treatment immediately (immediate treatment condition) or after a three-month waiting period (delayed treatment condition). The current study utilizes data from this treatment trial. Previously reported results from this trial [17] are briefly summarized here so as to provide background context regarding the efficacy of treatment. These results indicated that, at post-treatment, participants assigned to the immediate treatment condition reported significantly improved scores compared to participants assigned to the delayed treatment condition in terms of higher rates of binge abstinence (40.0% versus 3.3%) and fewer past-month OBEs (6.0 versus 14.4), respectively. Participants in the immediate treatment condition additionally demonstrated improved scores on self-report measures of eating psychopathology, anxiety, depression, and quality of life. Furthermore, these participants demonstrated improved emotion regulation at post-treatment, with better emotion regulation scores than those reported by participants in the delayed treatment condition who had not yet received treatment. The association between emotion regulation and treatment outcome (i.e., binge eating) was not examined. Most improvements were maintained at six-month follow-up. Many participants demonstrated a positive response to guided self-help DBT, yet a significant proportion of participants (70.0%) failed to be binge abstinent at follow-up, which is consistent with results from other treatment trials of DBT for BED (e.g., [7,11]).

Methods

This study received approval from the University of Calgary Conjoint Faculties Research Ethics Board, and informed consent was obtained from all participants prior to participating in the study. A summary of key study variables and procedures is included below; please see Masson and colleagues, 2013 [17] for further details.

Participants

Sixty participants were recruited from the community via local media, with the study described as a treatment for BED that used a self-help book and telephone support. To participate in the study, individuals were required to meet DSM-IV criteria for BED [18] or subthreshold BED criteria, as assessed via the Structured Clinical Interview for DSM-IV Axis I Disorders – Non-Patient Version [19]. Thus, participants were required to have had an OBE at least once a week, on average, over the preceding six months. Diagnostic criteria in DSM-5 largely aligns with this lower threshold [20]. Exclusion criteria included: involvement in concurrent psychotherapy for binge eating; active psychosis; body mass index (BMI) less than 17.5 kg/m^2; use of compensatory behaviors at least once per week over the past three months; any change in dose of psychotropic medication over the past three months; and inability to commit adequate time to assessment and treatment (i.e., approximately two to three hours per week for 16 weeks in total). Of 122 potential participants who inquired about the study and were screened, only three (2.5%) indicated that they were unavailable to commit the required amount of time and/or were unavailable for study dates. All participants spoke English fluently and were 18 years or older. Eighty-eight percent (*n*53) of participants were female and 90.0% (n = 54) were Caucasian. Age ranged from 24 to 67 years (M = 42.8, SD = 10.5) and BMI (based on self-reported height and weight data at pre-treatment assessment) ranged from 22 to 69 kg/m^2 (M = 37.9, SD = 8.8). All participants had graduated from high school or equivalent. Twenty-five percent (n = 15) of participants were taking stable doses of psychotropic medication for mental health issues (primarily depression and/or anxiety symptoms).

Assessment and treatment of both the immediate treatment condition and the delayed treatment condition were conducted identically, with two exceptions. First, participants in the delayed treatment condition began treatment three months after participants in the immediate treatment condition, and therefore completed each assessment (i.e., pre-treatment, post-treatment, and six-month follow-up assessment) three months after participants in the immediate treatment condition had completed the same assessment. Second, participants in the delayed treatment condition completed a baseline assessment at the outset of the study, at the same time that participants in the immediate treatment condition completed a pre-treatment assessment. Thus, participants in the delayed treatment condition were assessed four times (i.e., baseline, pre-treatment, post-treatment, and six-month follow-up), whereas participants in the immediate treatment condition were assessed three times (i.e., pre-treatment, post-treatment, and six-month follow-up). See Table 1. Data from the baseline assessment, which were collected to evaluate treatment efficacy in the randomized wait-list controlled trial, are not considered in the current study.

As all participants in both the immediate treatment and delayed treatment condition completed identical treatment, data from participants in both conditions are pooled together for all analyses in the current study. Between-group mediational analyses are not possible with the current dataset due to small sample size and resultant low statistical power, as well as the unbalanced study design (i.e., as the delayed treatment condition began treatment only three months after the immediate treatment condition began treatment, data are not available to compare to the treatment condition's follow-up data). Preliminary analyses indicated no significant differences between participants in the immediate treatment and delayed treatment condition on OBE frequency or emotion regulation total scores, at pre-treatment, post-treatment, or follow-up; emotion regulation change scores at post-treatment or follow-up; or binge abstinence rates at post-treatment or follow-up (all p's > .1). Lack of group differences in these variables supports our use of pooled data from the immediate treatment condition and the delayed treatment condition in the following analyses.

Assessment and measures

Each assessment included the Difficulties in Emotion Regulation Scale (DERS; [21]) and items from the Eating Disorder Examination (EDE; [22]). As the EDE assesses eating pathology over the three preceding 28-day intervals, administration of the EDE at six-month follow-up assessment provided eating pathology scores for three time periods (i.e., four, five, and six months after treatment completion). In comparison, administration of the DERS at six-month follow-up assessment provided emotion regulation scores for only one time period (i.e., six months after treatment completion).

Eating Disorder Examination

The EDE is a well-established semi-structured interview of eating disorder symptomatology. It has established reliability for the assessment of BED [23], and is considered the gold standard for the assessment of eating disorder psychopathology [24]. Only questions relevant to the differential diagnosis of BED were administered (e.g., questions regarding binge eating frequency, behaviors and feelings associated with binge eating, the use of compensatory behaviors, and self-reported height and weight).

The EDE rater was not involved in treatment delivery and was blind to participants' group assignment at pre-treatment and post-treatment assessment. The rater received training in administration of the EDE prior to the outset of the study and administered the EDE under the

Table 1 Timing of assessments completed by participants in the immediate treatment condition and delayed treatment condition over 12 months

Condition	Study timeline				
	0 months	3 months	6 months	9 months	12 months
Immediate treatment	#1: Pre-treatment assessment	#2: Post-treatment assessment		#3: 6-month follow-up assessment	
Delayed treatment	#1: Baseline assessment[1]	#2: Pre-treatment assessment	#3: Post-treatment assessment		#4: 6-month follow-up assessment

Note. [1]Baseline assessment data were not included in analyses.

supervision of a psychologist. Inter-rater reliability of the EDE binge eating assessment was examined among 12% of the interviews conducted. The original rater's rating of the frequency of binge eating within the last 28 days and consensus coding of two eating disorder researchers were identical (r = 1.0).

Difficulties in Emotion Regulation Scale

The DERS is a 36-item self-report questionnaire designed to assess multiple aspects of emotion regulation. The Total Score was analysed, which is the sum of six subscale scores: Nonacceptance of Emotional Responses, Difficulties Engaging in Goal Directed Behavior, Impulse Control Difficulties, Lack of Emotional Awareness, Limited Access to Emotion Regulation Strategies, and Lack of Emotional Clarity. Higher scores indicate greater difficulty in emotion regulation (*range*=36-180). Based on pre-treatment data, the DERS demonstrated high internal consistency in the current study (α=.95).

Treatment

Treatment was administered via a DBT for BED self-help manual developed for this study and six 20-minute support phone calls. In addition, one in-person, 45-minute orientation session was provided at the outset of treatment wherein the self-help manual was distributed and the basic treatment tenets were discussed. The orientation and all support calls were provided by a doctoral candidate in clinical psychology working under the supervision of a psychologist. The manual was designed to be used over thirteen weeks, and the six support calls were provided approximately every two weeks across this treatment period. Each chapter in the manual had a specific focus and included homework that was intended to be worked on by participants during the week that the chapter was read. Support sessions focused on encouraging participants' use of the manual, answering any questions that participants had about the manual, and problem-solving with participants to determine how they could find the time to use the manual and/or remember strategies discussed in the manual. The manual provided education on three skills modules to aid in regulating emotions (i.e., Mindfulness, Distress Tolerance, and Emotion Regulation), and guided the reader through activities and exercises designed to increase familiarity with these skills and encourage implementation of these skills in daily life.

Statistical analyses

The ability of post-treatment emotion regulation change scores to predict treatment outcome (i.e., binge abstinence) at post-treatment and four-, five-, and six-month follow-up was examined. An emotion regulation change score at post-treatment was created by calculating the difference between each participant's post-treatment DERS total score and his/her pre-treatment DERS total score.

Binary logistic regression analyses were used to examine whether DERS post-treatment change scores (i.e., change in emotion regulation ability) predicted binge abstinence at four-, five-, and six-month follow-up. *T*-tests additionally compared the magnitude of DERS post-treatment change scores between participants who were versus were not binge abstinent at post-treatment, four-, five-, and six-month follow-up.

All statistical analyses were compared to a significance level of $p < .05$.

Missing data

Twenty-one of 60 participants (35.0%) did not fully complete post-treatment assessment (i.e., complete both the EDE and DERS); 27 of 60 participants (45.0%) did not fully complete follow-up assessment. The conservative last observation carried forward method was used in all analyses.

Results

Mean scores for DERS total and subscale scores are presented in Table 2 for descriptive purposes. Only DERS total scores are included in the following results.

Binary logistic regression analyses indicated that DERS change scores at end of treatment predicted binge abstinence at end of treatment ($\chi^2(1)$ = 6.99, $p < .01$; OR = 1.04, CI = 1.01-1.07). DERS change scores at end of treatment also predicted binge abstinence at each follow-up point: four-month ($\chi^2(1)$ = 9.23, $p < .01$; OR = 1.06, CI = 1.02-1.10), five-month ($\chi^2(1)$ = 6.32, $p < .05$; OR = 1.04, CI = 1.01-1.07), and six-month follow-up (χ^2 (1) = 6.43, $p < .05$; OR = 1.04, CI = 1.01-1.07).[a] The odds ratios indicated that for every unit increase in DERS post-treatment change score, there was an approximately 4-6% increase in the odds of being binge abstinent at post-treatment and various follow-up points.

In addition, *t*- tests further demonstrated that participants who were binge abstinent at end of treatment reported greater change in emotion regulation at end of treatment, as compared to individuals who were not binge abstinent at end of treatment. Likewise, participants who were binge abstinent at four-, five-, and six-month follow-up also reported greater change in emotion regulation at end of treatment. Specifically, *t*-tests illustrated that participants who were binge abstinent at post-treatment and each follow-up point demonstrated, on average, approximately three times as much change in DERS scores at end of treatment as individuals who were not binge abstinent at those respective time-points (top of Table 3). Effect sizes (Cohen's *d*) were all approximately large, although the effect size at four-month follow-up (d = 1.01) was notably greater than effect sizes at other time points.

Table 2 Mean emotion regulation scores at pre-treatment, post-treatment, and six-month follow-up (*N*=60)

Difficulties in emotion regulation scale	Pre-treatment *M* (*SD*)	Post-treatment *M* (*SD*)	6-month follow-up *M* (*SD*)
Total score	102.03 (25.39)	84.04 (25.37)	81.76 (26.35)
Nonacceptance of emotional responses	17.29 (6.57)	13.68 (6.10)	13.25 (6.25)
Difficulties engaging in goal directed behavior	16.15 (4.71)	13.58 (4.48)	13.07 (4.65)
Impulse control difficulties	15.90 (6.26)	12.87 (5.32)	12.50 (5.54)
Lack of emotional awareness	18.48 (4.67)	15.78 (4.88)	15.58 (4.78)
Limited access to emotion regulation strategies	20.51 (8.09)	16.59 (7.50)	16.37 (7.85)
Lack of emotional clarity	13.60 (3.95)	11.73 (3.64)	11.20 (3.64)

Post hoc analyses

In post hoc binary logistic regression analyses, we explored whether attrition and use of imputed data affected results. These analyses included only those participants who had completed both the DERS and the EDE at each time point (i.e., 39 participants at post-treatment and 33 participants at each follow-up point). Overall, results from these "completer" analyses trended in the same direction; however, several results were no longer statistically significant. Specifically, DERS post-treatment change scores predicted binge abstinence at four-month follow-up ($\chi^2(1)$ = 5.12, $p < .05$; OR = 1.05, CI = 1.01-1.10). Analyses that examined whether DERS post-treatment change scores predicted binge abstinence at post-treatment ($\chi^2(1)$ = 2.63, $p = .11$; OR = 1.03, CI = 1.00-1.06), five-month follow-up ($\chi^2(1)$=2.71, $p = .10$; OR = 1.03, CI = 1.00-1.06), and six-month follow-up ($\chi^2(1)$ = 3.30, $p = .07$; OR = 1.03, CI = 1.00-1.06) did not reach statistical significance. Likewise, comparison of mean DERS post-treatment change scores between participants who were binge abstinent at post-treatment, four-, five-, and six-month follow-up, and individuals who were not binge abstinent at those respective time points, suggested that participants who were abstinent experienced greater change in emotion regulation from pre-treatment to post-treatment. However, the size of difference in amount of change between participants who were and were not abstinent only reached statistical significance at four-month follow-up (bottom of Table 3). Effect sizes from these analyses were medium at post-treatment, five-, and six-month follow-up, and large at four-month follow-up.

Discussion

This study explored the predictive significance of magnitude of change in emotion regulation during the course of treatment on binge abstinence at post-treatment, four-, five-, and six-month follow-up among individuals who received guided self-help DBT for BED. In analyses of the full sample, the amount of change in emotion regulation over treatment was associated with binge abstinence at post-treatment, four-, five-, and six-month follow-up. Specifically, the amount of change reported in emotion regulation from pre-treatment to post-treatment was almost three times greater among participants who were binge abstinent as compared to participants who were not binge abstinent. These findings support the theoretical notion that improving emotion regulation is associated with binge abstinence. Such findings, if replicated, may help further improve existing therapeutic efficacy and help more individuals to successfully recover from BED.

It is noteworthy that results shifted when only participants who had completed the full assessment at each time-point were included (i.e., completer analyses, with no imputed data included). In these post hoc completer analyses, the amount of change in emotion regulation from pre-treatment to post-treatment was only predictive of binge abstinence at four-month follow-up; results trended toward but did not attain significance at post-treatment, five-, and six-month follow-up. It is possible that the lack of significant differences in these analyses of the completer sample was attributable to low statistical power (i.e., only 33–39 participants were included in these analyses). With a larger sample, the difference in amount of post-treatment change in emotion regulation between participants who were and were not binge abstinent at each time point may have reached statistical significance whether or not data was imputed. However, these findings could also suggest that an association between change in emotion regulation and treatment outcome appears only during the few months subsequent to treatment completion, and is lost over a longer duration of follow-up. Even in analyses of the full sample, the association between change in emotion regulation and binge abstinence was notably stronger at four-month follow-up than any other assessment point, as indicated by both the odds ratio in regression analyses and Cohen's *d* effect sizes in *t*-tests. From this perspective, findings indicate the importance of identifying strategies to strengthen the association between change in emotion regulation and treatment outcome for a longer duration, and/or identifying other factors beyond change in emotion regulation that yield sustained positive treatment outcome. As binge eating is a multiply determined behavior that

Table 3 Mean change in emotion regulat on scores among participants who were binge abstinent versus non-abstinent at each follow-up

	Abstinent at post-treatment			Abstinent at 4-month follow-up			Abstinent at 5-month follow-up			Abstinent at 6-month follow-up		
	Full sample, with imputed data (N =60)											
	Yes	No	t; *Cohen's d*	Yes	No	t; *Cohen's d*	Yes	No	t; *Cohen's d*	Yes	No	t; *Cohen's d*
	(n = 23)	(n = 37)		(n = 26)	(n = 34)		(n = 26)	(n = 34)		(n = 24)	(n = 36)	
DERS post-treatment change	−30.19 (27.20)	−10.39 (19.91)	−3.25*; .83	−31.19 (30.03)	−7.88 (12.97)	−3.70*; 1.01	−28.27 (26.91)	−10.12 (19.96)	−3.00*; .77	−29.12 (28.45)	−10.56 (18.92)	−3.04*; .77
	Treatment completers only, withou: imputed data (N=33-39)											
	Yes	No	t; *Cohen's d*	Yes	No	t; *Cohen's d*	Yes	No	t; *Cohen's d*	Yes	No	t; *Cohen's d*
	(n = 19-23)	(n = 17-18)		(n = 18-20)	(n = 15-17)		(n = 18-20)	(n = 15-17)		(n = 16-18)	(n = 17-19)	
DERS post-treatment change	−31.57 (27.01)	−16.79 (24.98)	−1.75; .57	−38.89 (32.44)	−12.26 (13.75)	−3.16*; 1.07	−34.67 (29.22)	−17.33 (25.87)	−1.79; .63	−36.75 (31.23)	−17.41 (23.22)	−2.03; .70

Note. DERS = Difficulties in Emotion Regulation Scale. *p < .01.

involves numerous interacting variables in its etiology and maintenance, improving emotion regulation may increase the likelihood of binge abstinence but there are likely additional factors that need to be considered in sustaining long-term maintenance of abstinence.

Further research with larger samples is needed. In addition, we encourage research that includes an active comparison group, considers other ways of measuring emotion regulation, and explores additional predictors of treatment outcome.

The current findings need to be interpreted in the context of existing literature. In particular, a randomized controlled trial comparing group DBT to an active comparison group therapy [11] reported significant group differences between OBE frequency and abstinence rates at post-treatment that were not maintained over the 12 month follow-up period. Improvements in in emotion regulation were also similar between treatment groups. In light of these findings, the authors suggested that nonspecific therapeutic factors common to both treatments may account for treatment outcome, rather than specific effects of DBT. When these results are considered alongside results from the current study, it appears that change in emotion regulation *is* important in improving outcome for individuals with BED, although (1) therapeutic approaches other than DBT may also effectively improve individuals' emotion regulation, (2) DBT may not effectively improve emotion regulation and reduce binge eating for all individuals, and/or (3) the importance of improved emotion regulation for reducing binge eating may vary over time. It is also possible that differences in findings across studies regarding the role of emotion regulation in treatment outcome are attributable to differences in study methodology. For example, analyses in the current study focused upon comparing treatment responders versus non-responders, rather than comparing treatment conditions. Recognizing the substantial portion of individuals who do not respond to BED treatment, analyses that consider differences in individual response within a treatment condition may be particularly important. In addition, in the current study we examined *change* in emotion regulation, rather than focusing on *level* of emotion regulation, to test the hypothesis that magnitude of change across treatment in one's ability to regulate his/her emotions is predictive of treatment outcome. Furthermore, guided self-help DBT as provided in the current study involved considerably less direct clinical contact over the course of treatment than either group DBT or the active comparison group therapy (i.e., two hours individual phone contact in guided self-help DBT versus 40 hours face-to-face group contact in DBT and the active comparison group), which may have limited the opportunity for nonspecific therapeutic factors (e.g., therapeutic alliance) to contribute to treatment outcome in the current study.

In sum, results from the current study tend to be consistent with the theoretical notion that improved emotion regulation is associated with better treatment outcome in BED. Notably, in the context of a guided self-help treatment, the present findings showed that individuals with BED can learn adaptive emotion regulation skills in a cost-effective way that does not demand significant time with a therapist. However, further research is needed to better understand inconsistencies in results within this study (e.g., between analyses that did and did not use imputed data) and across studies, and to clarify the duration of time after the end of treatment that this association between change in emotion regulation and treatment outcome is strongest. In addition, research is needed to examine the extent to which nonspecific factors associated with general therapeutic and/or natural recovery processes may additionally contribute to treatment outcome. Finally, research should explore whether improved emotion regulation may be a process that influences treatment outcome in other effective psychological treatments for BED, so as to determine the specificity of the effect. Dismantling studies that identify specific techniques used in DBT that contribute most to improved emotion regulation would also be beneficial, as well as research that identifies other treatment orientations beyond DBT that impact emotion regulation.

Strengths of this study include that it used prospective data collected within a randomized controlled trial. Participants were recruited from the community using very few exclusion criteria, which increases the study's external validity. Measurement of the primary outcome – binge eating – involved a reliably administered, well-established semi-structured diagnostic interview. In addition, measurement of binge eating occurred across multiple points during follow-up. A major limitation of this study is that power to detect significant effects may have been limited by small and unequal cell sizes, particularly in post-hoc analyses that excluded imputed data. Relatedly, attrition and the use of imputed data may have affected results. In addition, a self-report measure was used to assess emotion regulation. In addition, as between-group analyses comparing change in the treatment condition to change in the delayed treatment condition were not possible due to this study's design, findings indicate that change in emotion regulation may be an important process in positive treatment outcome but do not confirm that change in emotion regulation is specific to DBT. Rather, change in emotion regulation could predict positive treatment outcome among other therapeutic orientations, be part of a natural recovery process, or both. Finally, it is possible that change in emotion regulation, as measured by the DERS, is reflective of change in other factors (e.g., change in general psychopathology). If so, the association between change in emotion regulation and subsequent binge abstinence may be accounted for by change in other factors not examined in this study.

Conclusions

Overall, this study suggests that change in emotion regulation by the end of treatment predicts binge abstinence in guided self-help DBT for BED. These findings suggest that emotion regulation is an important skill that predicts positive treatment outcome for BED. However, questions remain regarding the strength of the effect of emotion regulation on outcome at various points across time. Replication and further examination of these exploratory findings with larger samples is needed. Further research that considers how to refine and improve upon treatments for BED should explore the extent to which emotion regulation can be emphasized within treatment protocols, consider additional strategies that can be used to enhance emotion regulation across a range of individuals with BED, and consider other mechanisms that may additionally account for positive treatment outcome at post-treatment and over time.

Endnote

[a]Controversy exists as to whether abstinence from binge eating is the most appropriate criterion of treatment outcome and should be required for remission from BED and other eating disorders [24]. Thus, we also ran a linear regression analysis between DERS post-treatment change scores and OBE frequency scores, thereby assessing treatment outcome among individuals regardless of abstinence status. DERS change scores predicted OBE frequency at post-treatment, four-, five-, and six-month follow-up (p's < .05). Thus analysis of OBE frequency and binge abstinence yielded similar results.

Abbreviations

BED: Binge eating disorder; CBT: Cognitive behavior therapy; DBT: Dialectical behavior therapy; DERS: Difficulties in Emotion regulation scale; EDE: Eating Disorder Examination; IPT: Interpersonal psychotherapy; OBE: Objective binge eating episode.

Competing interests

The authors declare that they have no competing interests.

Authors' contributions

LMW participated in data collection, performed data analysis and interpretation, and drafted the manuscript. PCM participated in development of the DBT for BED treatment manual, designed and coordinated the research trial, participated in recruitment, provided the guided self-help intervention, and participated in manuscript preparation and writing. DS participated in development of the DBT for BED treatment manual as well as manuscript preparation and writing. KvR supervised data collection, data analysis and interpretation, and made substantial contributions to the manuscript. All authors read and approved the final manuscript.

Acknowledgements

The authors thank the Social Sciences and Humanities Research Council of Canada for their financial support.

Author details

[1]Department of Psychology, University of Calgary, 2500 University Drive NW, Calgary, Alberta, Canada. [2]Department of Psychiatry and Behavioral Sciences, Stanford University, Stanford, California, USA.

References

1. Grilo CM, White MA, Masheb RM: **DSM-IV psychiatric disorder comorbidity and its correlates in binge eating disorder.** *Int J Eat Disord* 2009, **42**:228–234.
2. Wilfley DE, Wilson GT, Agras WS: **The clinical significance of binge eating disorder.** *Int J Eat Disord* 2003, **34**(Suppl):96–106.
3. Bulik CM, Reichborn-Kjennerur T: **Medical morbidity in binge eating disorder.** *Int J Eat Disord* 2003, **34**(Suppl):39–46.
4. Grucza RA, Przybeck TR, Cloninger CR: **Prevalence and correlates of binge eating disorder in a community sample.** *Compr Psychiatry* 2007, **48**:124–131.
5. Grilo CM, Masheb RM, Wilson GT: **Efficacy of cognitive behavioral therapy and fluoxetine for the treatment of binge eating disorder: A randomized double-blind placebo-controlled comparison.** *Biol Psychiatry* 2005, **57**:301–309. 25.
6. Wilfley DE, Welch RR, Stein RI, Spurrell EB, Cohen LR, Saelens BE, Dounchis JZ, Frank MA, Wiseman CV, Matt GE: **A randomized comparison of group cognitive-behavioral therapy and group interpersonal psychotherapy for the treatment of overweight individuals with binge-eating disorder.** *Arch Gen Psychiatry* 2002, **59**:713–721.
7. Telch CF, Agras WS, Linehan MM: **Dialectical behavior therapy for binge eating disorder.** *J Consult Clin Psychol* 2001, **69**:1061–1065.
8. Agras WS, Telch CF, Arnow B, Elderedge K, Detzer MJ, Henderson J, Marnell M: **Does interpersonal therapy help patients with binge eating disorder who fail to respond to cognitive-behavioral therapy?** *J Consult Clin Psychol* 1995, **63**:356–360.
9. Brownley KA, Berkman ND, Sedway JA, Lohr KN, Bulik CM: **Binge eating disorder treatment: A systematic review of randomized controlled trials.** *Int J Eat Disord* 2007, **40**:337–348.
10. Wilson GT, Grilo CM, Vitousek KM: **Psychological treatment of eating disorders.** *Am Psychol* 2007, **62**:199 216.
11. Safer DL, Robinson AH, Jo B: **Outcome from a randomized controlled trial of group therapy for binge eating disorder: Comparing dialectical behavior therapy adapted for binge eating to an active comparison group therapy.** *Behav Ther* 2010, **41**:106–120.
12. Heatherton TF, Baumeister RF: **Binge eating as escape from self-awareness.** *Psychol Bull* 1991, **110**:86–108.
13. Polivy J, Herman CP: **Etiology of binge eating: Psychological mechanisms.** In *Binge eating: Nature, assessment and treatment.* Edited by Fairburn CG, Wilson GT. New York: Guilford Press; 1993:173–205.
14. Wiser S, Telch CF: **Dialectical behavior therapy for binge-eating disorder.** *J Clin Psychol* 1999, **55**:755–768.
15. Thompson RA: **Emotion regulation: A theme in search of a definition.** *Monogr Soc Res Child Dev* 1994, **59**:25–52.
16. Safer DL, Telch CF, Chen EY: *Dialectical Behavior Therapy for Binge Eating and Bulimia.* New York: Guilford Press, 2009.
17. Masson PC, von Ranson KM, Wallace LM, Safer DL: **A randomized wait-list controlled trial of dialectical behaviour therapy guided self-help for binge eating disorder.** *Behav Res Ther* 2013, **51**:723–728.
18. American Psychiatric Association: *Diagnostic and statistical manual of mental disorders*, Text Revision. 4th edition. Washington, DC: American Psychiatric Association; 2000.
19. First MB, Spitzer RL, Gibbon M, Williams JBW: *Structured Clinical Interview for DSM-IV-TR Axis I Disorders, Research Version, Non-patient Edition (SCID-I/NP).* New York: Biometrics Research, New York State Psychiatric Institute; 2002.
20. American Psychiatric Association: *Diagnostic and statistical manual of mental disorders.* 5th edition. Washington, DC: American Psychiatric Association; 2013.
21. Gratz KL, Roemer L: **Multidimensional assessment of emotion regulation and dysregulation: Development, factor structure, and initial validation of the Difficulties in Emotion Regulation Scale.** *J Psychopathol Behav Assess* 2004, **26**:41–54.
22. Fairburn CG, Cooper Z, O'Connor M: **Eating Disorder Examination (16.0D).** In *Cognitive Behavior Therapy and Eating Disorders.* Edited by Fairburn CG. New York: Guilford Press; 2008.

23. Grilo CM, Masheb RM, Lozano-Blanco C, Barry DT: **Reliability of the Eating Disorder Examination in patients with binge eating disorder.** *Int J Eat Disord* 2004, **35**:80–85.
24. Berg KC, Peterson CB, Frazier P, Crow SJ: **Psychometric evaluation of the Eating Disorder Examination and Eating Disorder Examination-Questionnaire: a systematic review of the literature.** *Int J Eat Disord* 2011, **45**:428–438.

Adolescent risk factors for purging in young women: findings from the national longitudinal study of adolescent health

Eric M Stephen[1], Jennifer Rose[1*], Lindsay Kenney[1], Francine Rosselli-Navarra[2] and Ruth Striegel Weissman[1]

Abstract

Background: There exists a dearth of prospective adolescent eating disorder studies with samples that are large enough to detect small or medium sized effects for risk factors, that are generalizable to the broader population, and that follow adolescents long enough to fully capture the period of development when the risk of eating disorder symptoms occurring is highest. As a result, the purpose of this study was to examine psychosocial risk factors for purging for weight control in a nationally representative sample of adolescents. Data were extracted from the restricted-use data sets of the National Longitudinal Study of Adolescent Health (Waves I-III), selecting females with valid demographic and purging information (N = 5,670).

Results: The prevalence of purging was 0.88% at Wave II and 0.56% at Wave III. In multivariable multinomial logistic regressions, purging at Wave II was predicted by parental poverty and low levels of self-esteem at Wave I; purging at Wave III was predicted by body mass index and the frequency of delinquent behaviors at Wave I.

Conclusions: Individuals with high body mass index, individuals with low self-esteem, and individuals in families experiencing economic hardship appear specifically at risk for the development of purging behaviors in later years and may benefit from more targeted prevention efforts.

Keywords: Eating disorders, Risk factors, Purging behavior, Weight control, Adolescent

Background

The etiologies of eating disorders and their core symptoms are best characterized by multifactorial models involving biological, psychological, interpersonal, and cultural variables [1]. Experts have also noted, however, that the research is limited by the dearth of prospective studies with samples large enough to detect small or medium sized effects, the inclusion of demographically limited samples, and the lack of follow-up periods that are long enough to fully capture the period of development when the risk of the onset of eating disorder symptoms is highest [1,2].

The present study focused on purging (vomiting or abusing laxatives) to lose weight or keep from gaining weight as a clinically relevant symptom and as a possible proxy for the presence of an eating disorder. Purging behaviors have received increasing scientific attention not only in the context of a full syndrome eating disorder but also as symptoms of clinical relevance in their own right [3-5]. Only a few studies have explored risk factors for purging using longitudinal designs, and most of these studies have focused on just one risk factor. For example, two studies of adolescent girls found that eating dinner [6] or eating meals with their families [7] was associated with a decreased risk for onset of purging or extreme weight control behaviors.

Due to skip patterns used in most epidemiological studies of adults, information about purging behaviors typically was collected only in individuals who scored positively on the core symptom of anorexia nervosa (refusal to maintain a minimum adequate body weight) or bulimia nervosa (recurrent episodes of purging and binge eating) [8]. In contrast, studies of adolescents typically have measured disordered eating symptoms among all participants, thus affording the opportunity to explore correlates of these behaviors. Results show marked

* Correspondence: jrose01@wesleyan.edu
[1]Department of Psychology, Wesleyan University, 207 High Street, Middletown, CT 06459, USA
Full list of author information is available at the end of the article

gender differences in the incidence and prevalence of purging [9]. For example, in a community sample of over 13,000 boys and girls (ages 9 to 14 years), one-year incidence of purging was 1.3% in girls and 0.3% in boys [6]. In a school-based sample of over 2,500 boys and girls, "extreme weight control behaviors" (which included purging) were also reported to be more common in girls than boys [10]. The present study capitalized upon the availability of data collected as part of the National Longitudinal Study of Adolescent Health (Add Health), which affords the unique opportunity to examine the prevalence and incidence of, as well as risk factors for, purging in a nationally representative sample of United States' (US) youth. Because of the low base rate of males who purged in our sample (only 0.55% of young men reported purging at any wave of study whereas 1.96% of young women reported purging), we excluded male participants from our sample.

Our approach to and selection of potential risk factors was informed by Kraemer and colleagues' conceptual framework and by a corresponding review paper of the empirical studies of risk factors for eating disorders [2,11]. Specifically, to test whether a variable confers risk (rather than merely representing a correlate), data are needed that were either collected prior to occurrence of the behavior or are of a nature where one may reasonably infer that, even when collected after occurrence, the data are not contaminated by the outcome in question (e.g., gender, race/ethnicity). Therefore, in our study, we defined occurrence, or "incidence cases", as participants who reported purging at a subsequent wave of study, controlling for purging behaviors at Wave I. Given our interest in identifying adolescent risk factors for purging, we limited our sample to adolescent girls who, at study entry (Wave I), were age 18 or younger.

Our study included a considerable range of potential adolescent risk factors including demographic variables, early onset menarche, body image concerns, adverse childhood experiences, coping, and health or mental health problems [2]. We hypothesized that, after controlling for age, race, parental education, and purging at Wave I, higher scores on each of these risk factor constructs (and, in the case of self-esteem, lower scores) would confer greater risk for the occurrence of purging behaviors in young adult women.

Methods

Participants

The sample comprised 5,670 female participants whose data were extracted from the restricted-use Add Health survey Waves I (1994–1995), II (1996), and III (2001–2002). Add Health has been following over 20,000 American adolescents starting in grades 7–12 over the course of fourteen years, with four waves of data collection throughout this time period (Wave IV did not collect data about purging and, therefore, was not used for the present study). The initial sample was established by sampling students from 132 schools in the United States. Due to oversampling of some population subgroups, Add Health investigators developed sampling weights to be used in statistical analyses so findings can be generalized to be representative for region, urbanicity, and ethnicity. Further details about the Add Health study design can be found elsewhere [12,13].

Inclusion criteria for the present study were those participants who were reported as female at all three waves (in a few instances, gender information was not consistent across study waves), had valid age information, were age 18 or younger at Wave I, reported responses to purging behaviors at Wave I, and had valid data required for applying sampling weights (see Data Analysis section). Of the total 10,480 girls included in Add Health at Wave I, 5,670 met the inclusion criteria required for our analyses (54% Wave I sample, 75% of Wave II sample, and 71% of Wave III sample). Most of the girls that we excluded did not have information needed for applying sample weights at all waves. However, because we used the sample weights developed by Add Health in our statistical models to account for attrition and oversampling, our findings are representative of young women in the United States.

The mean age at study entry was 15.15 (SD = 1.57); about one-third (30.97%) of the weighted sample was non-White. Highest parental education was reported by participants' parents or guardians as follows: less than high school, 11.65%; high school diploma or equivalent, 32.10%; some college, 22.38%; and college degree or more, 33.87%. All results reflect adjustment for sampling strategy [13,14].

Instruments and procedures

The Add Health survey measures a wide range of psychological and physical health issues and behaviors, a subset of which was used in this study. Some constructs (e.g., depressive symptoms) were measured using unequal numbers of items across waves; in such cases, we followed the practice of prior investigators of using only those items that were administered in all three waves, and we calculated Cronbach's alpha based on the unweighted sample included in the present study.

Because, by definition, exposure to a risk factor must occur prior to occurrence of the dependent variable of interest, predictor variables collected at Wave I were used to investigate purging at Wave II and Wave III. Attention-deficit hyperactivity symptoms and childhood abuse were the only predictor variables used in this study that were collected at Wave III, as they were measured retrospectively at Wave III with a focus on experiencing them in early childhood.

Demographic information

Following work by Brown and colleagues, [15] participants' self-reported race/ethnicity was coded into a binary variable representing White vs. non-White, and highest parental education achieved by either parent or adult guardian was coded as an ordinal variable representing less than high school, high school or equivalent, some college, and college graduate or postgraduate education. Age was recorded as age at last birthday. (Age at Wave I needed to be calculated because only birth year and birth month were available in Wave I. To calculate age, information given on birth date was subtracted from date of interview).

Body image and eating behaviors

Body Mass Index (BMI) was calculated by dividing weight (in pounds) by the product of height (in inches) squared times the value 703 [16]. Weight perception was measured using a single item "How do you think of yourself in terms of weight?" with response choices ranging from "1 = very underweight" to "5 = very overweight". Purging status was determined based on participants' responses to the question of whether, in the past 7 days, the participant had been trying to lose or maintain weight. If the respondent answered yes, Add Health asked a series of follow up questions to determine what method the individuals were using to lose or maintain weight. Participants could select multiple options that were provided, including diet, exercise, vomiting, diet pill use, laxative use, or other. Those who reported that they had, in the last 7 days, tried to lose or maintain weight through the use of vomiting and/or laxative misuse were coded as purging. Questions did not address frequency of occurrence. Diet pill use in the absence of purging was coded as present if respondents reported use of diet pills but denied vomiting or laxative use.

Classification of participants as current purgers

A three-level polyotomous variable was created to classify current purging. The first group was comprised of participants who did not report purging at either Wave II or Wave III. The second group was comprised of those reported purging at Wave II. Finally, all individuals who did not report purging at Wave II but did report purging at Wave III were coded into the third group. A small number of individuals reported purging at both Waves II and III (0.04% of the weighted sample), and were placed into the Wave II group.

Reproductive health related variables

Early onset menarche was coded as present in girls reporting having their first menstrual period before age 11 years [17]. Pregnancy was coded as present if the respondent reported having been pregnant, including any pregnancy that ended in abortion, stillbirth, miscarriage, or live birth after which the baby died.

Self-esteem

Four questions based on Rosenberg's Self-Esteem Scale [18] were used to measure self-esteem, including "You have many good qualities", "You have much to be proud of", "You like yourself just the way you are", and "You feel you are doing things just right". Participants rated each item on a scale from 1 to 5, and, consistent with Kort-Butler et al., [19] a total score was calculated by adding across the items, where higher numbers indicate higher self-esteem. (Cronbach's alpha = 0.80).

Active coping

Four questions were used to measure active coping, including "When you have a problem to solve, the first thing you do is get as many facts about the problem as possible", "When you are attempting to find a solution to a problem, you usually try to think of as many different ways to approach the problem as possible", "When making decisions, you generally use systematic methods for judging and comparing alternatives", and "After carrying out a solution to a problem, you usually try to analyze what went right and what went wrong". Each item was rated on a scale from 1 to 5; a total score was created by summing across the items, and higher scores reflected more active coping. [15] (Cronbach's alpha = 0.75).

Mental health related variables

Depressive symptoms were measured using a modified version of the Center for Epidemiologic Studies-Depression (CES-D) scale [20]. Participants rated symptom frequency in the past week on a scale from 0 (never or rarely) to 3 (most of the time). In the present study we used the nine items that were asked at all three waves, and created a total score for Wave I. [21] (Cronbach's alpha = 0.81). In addition, participants were asked, "During the last 12 months, how many times did you actually attempt suicide?" A binary variable (attempted suicide) was created contrasting those who had not attempted suicide during the past 12 months with those who had attempted suicide one or more times. Participants were asked (no/yes) whether, in the past 12 months, they had "received psychological or emotional counseling" (psychological counseling). Attention-deficit/hyperactivity Disorder (ADHD) was measured in Wave III. Participants were asked to "Think back to when you were between 5 and 12 years of age. For each of the following statements, which answer best describes your behavior when you were that age?" A list of all but one of the symptoms for ADHD as described in the 4th edition of the Diagnostic and Statistical Manual for Mental Disorders (DSM-IV) [22] was then presented, and participants rated how frequently the symptoms were experienced ("never or rarely", "sometimes", "often", or "very often"). The impulsivity symptom "often interrupts or intrudes on others" was not measured in Add Health. Consistent with McClernon and colleagues, [23] each symptom was coded as present if the frequency rating was "often" or "very often". Two severity subscales were created by summing the nine binary inattention symptoms (ADHD-IN; Cronbach's alpha = 0. 80) and the eight binary hyperactivity-impulsivity items (ADHD-HI; Cronbach's alpha = 0.72).

Delinquency

Seven questions measuring delinquent behavior were available at each wave. Specifically, participants were asked "In the past 12 months, how often did you: (1) damage property that didn't belong to you; (2) steal something worth more than $50; (3) go into a house or building to steal something; (4) use or threaten to use a weapon to get something from someone; (5) sell marijuana or other drugs; (6) steal something worth less than $50; (7) take part in a fight where a group of your friends was against another group". Consistent with previous studies, responses to each individual question were dichotomized by recoding the original 4-point Likert format (never, one or two times, three or four times, five times or more) into never versus ≥ 1. The recoded items were then summed, generating a Delinquency Scale total score with a range from 0 to 7. [24] The reliability of this scale was modest (Cronbach's alpha = 0.61).

Childhood adversity

Family poverty was measured using a parent's responses to three questions (no = 0, yes = 1): receiving public assistance, aid to families with dependent children, or food stamps; responses were summed for a total family poverty score with higher scores indicating greater economic hardship (Cronbach's alpha = 0.86). Binary variables were created indicating whether the participant had experienced these events for at least one parent: never lived with parent and parental death. In Wave III, participants were asked to retrospectively report (no/yes) whether, before the 6th grade, they had experienced childhood abuse (from parents or other adult caretakers): "not taking care of your basic needs, such as keeping you clean or providing food and clothing?" (childhood neglect) or "slapped, hit or kicked you?" (childhood physical abuse).

Data analysis

All data analyses were performed using Stata 12.1 [24]. As part of Add Health's survey design, certain demographic subgroups were sampled with unequal probability. In order to generate nationally representative estimates, therefore, Add Health investigators developed a weighting system which includes a stratum variable to adjust for geographic stratification, a cluster variable to adjust for the primary sampling unit (PSU; i.e. the school identifier), and a weight variable (using Wave III weights) to adjust for the oversampling of certain demographic characteristics within each PSU [13,25]. All analyses and estimates were performed using the weighted sample.

For each hypothesized risk or protective factor, multinomial logistic regression analysis was conducted, adjusting for the potentially confounding effects of age, race, parental education, and purging at Wave I. In the next step, a multivariable multinomial regression model was tested including only those risk or protective factors that had been shown to significantly differ ($p < 0.05$) between any two groups within the univariable comparisons.

Results

Prevalence and incidence of purging across the three waves

Unweighted frequencies and weighted proportions for purging are provided in Table 1. Regarding the weighted sample, the prevalence of purging was 0.40% at Wave I. The prevalence of current purging, as it was defined above, was 0.88% at Wave II and 0.56% at Wave III.

Risk factors for the development of current purging

As shown in Table 2, among the variables pertaining to body image and eating behavior, overweight self-perception was found to be significantly associated with purging at Wave II: a significantly higher percentage of young women with purging at Wave II reported that they felt overweight at Wave I compared to those who were not purging at Wave II. Purgers at Waves II and III had significantly higher BMI at Wave I. However, BMI at Wave I did not predict differences in the likelihood of purging between Waves II and III. Using diet pills as weight control was not

Table 1 Sample demographic characteristics (n = 5670)

Variable	N	Unweighted %	Weighted %
Purging occurrence, Wave II	58	0.54%	0.88%
Purging occurrence, Wave III	36	0.33%	0.56%
Race Other Than White	2507	44.22%	30.97%
Education			
Less than HS	689	12.15%	11.65%
HS diploma	1625	28.66%	32.10%
Some college	1155	20.37%	22.38%
College diploma	1953	34.44%	33.87%
	Unweighted mean	Unweighted SD	
Age[1]	15.15	1.57	

[1]Weighted descriptives unavailable for quantitative variables.

Table 2 Association of risk and protective factors with likelihood of purging at Waves II and III

Variable	Purging behavior	Coefficient	Std. error	p-value	CI
Weight perception (Likert)	Wave II	**1.01**	**0.37**	**0.01**	**0.28, 1.74**
	Wave III	0.54	0.49	0.27	−0.42, 1.50
	Wave III - Wave II	−0.47	0.60	0.44	−1.65, 0.72
Body mass index	Wave II	**0.09**	**0.03**	**0.00**	**0.03, 0.14**
	Wave III	**0.09**	**0.04**	**0.02**	**0.01, 0.16**
	Wave III - Wave II	0.00	0.05	0.99	−0.09, 0.09
Diet pill use	Wave II	1.16	0.97	0.24	−0.76, 3.08
	Wave III	1.24	1.06	0.25	−0.86, 3.34
	Wave III - Wave II	0.08	1.40	0.95	−2.68, 2.85
Menses onset < age 11 years	Wave II	0.37	0.47	0.43	−0.56, 1.29
	Wave III	0.13	0.74	0.87	−1.34, 1.60
	Wave III - Wave II	−0.24	0.89	0.79	−1.99, 1.52
Teenage pregnancy	Wave II	−0.83	0.94	0.38	−2.69, 1.04
	Wave III	−0.41	0.95	0.67	−2.28, 1.47
	Wave III - Wave II	0.42	1.34	0.75	−2.22, 3.06
Self-esteem scale	Wave II	**−0.22**	**0.06**	**0.00**	**−0.33, -0.11**
	Wave III	−0.01	0.09	0.90	−0.20, 0.17
	Wave III - Wave II	**0.21**	**0.10**	**0.04**	**0.00, 0.42**
Depressive symptoms scale	Wave II	**0.12**	**0.03**	**0.00**	**0.07, 0.18**
	Wave III	**0.09**	**0.03**	**0.01**	**0.02, 0.15**
	Wave III - Wave II	−0.04	0.04	0.31	−0.12, 0.04
Attempted suicide	Wave II	**1.14**	**0.47**	**0.02**	**0.21, 2.07**
	Wave III	0.25	0.66	0.71	−1.05, 1.54
	Wave III - Wave II	−0.90	0.81	0.27	−2.49, 0.70
Had psychological counseling	Wave II	**1.05**	**0.36**	**0.01**	**0.33, 1.77**
	Wave III	0.25	0.66	0.70	−1.05, 1.56
	Wave III - Wave II	−0.79	0.78	0.31	−2.34, 0.75
Delinquency scale	Wave II	**0.25**	**0.10**	**0.02**	**0.04, 0.45**
	Wave III	−0.32	0.28	0.26	−0.88, 0.24
	Wave III - Wave II	−0.57	0.29	0.06	−1.15, 0.01
Inattentiveness scale[3]	Wave II	0.11	0.09	0.23	−0.07, 0.29
	Wave III	0.03	0.14	0.84	−0.25, 0.30
	Wave III - Wave II	−0.08	0.18	0.65	−0.43, 0.27
Hyperactive/impulsive scale[3]	Wave II	**0.15**	**0.06**	**0.02**	**0.03, 0.26**
	Wave III	−0.04	0.15	0.80	−0.34, 0.27
	Wave III - Wave II	−0.18	0.17	0.29	−0.53, 0.16
Active coping scale	Wave II	−0.05	0.06	0.41	−0.18, 0.07
	Wave III	−0.08	0.07	0.25	−0.21, 0.06
	Wave III - Wave II	−0.03	0.09	0.77	−0.21, 0.15
Never lived with parent (s)	Wave II	**1.42**	**0.53**	**0.01**	**0.37, 2.46**
	Wave III	0.38	0.77	0.63	−1.15, 1.91
	Wave III - Wave II	−1.04	0.93	0.27	−2.88, 0.81
Parental poverty	Wave II	**0.42**	**0.19**	**0.03**	**0.05, 0.78**
	Wave III	−0.14	0.43	0.75	−1.00, 0.71

Table 2 Association of risk and protective factors with likelihood of purging at Waves II and III *(Continued)*

	Wave III - Wave II	−0.56	0.40	0.17	−1.35, 0.24
Not eating with parent	Wave II	−0.21	0.40	0.60	−1.00, 0.58
	Wave III	0.35	0.49	0.47	−0.61, 1.31
	Wave III - Wave II	0.56	0.66	0.40	−0.75, 1.87
Parent died	Wave II	−0.18	0.64	0.78	−1.44, 1.08
	Wave III	0.49	0.74	0.51	−0.97, 1.95
	Wave III - Wave II	0.66	0.95	0.49	−1.22, 2.54
Childhood neglect[3]	Wave II	0.46	0.56	0.41	−0.64, 1.56
	Wave III	−0.62	0.84	0.47	−2.29, 1.05
	Wave III - Wave II	−1.08	1.02	0.29	−3.10, 0.94
Childhood physical abuse[3]	Wave II	−0.42	0.44	0.35	−1.29, 0.45
	Wave III	0.64	0.51	0.21	−0.37, 1.65
	Wave III - Wave II	1.06	0.71	0.14	−0.35, 2.46

Note: All risk factor variables were measured at Wave I except those marked [3]; the latter were measured at Wave III via self-reported retrospective recall. Those reported in bold are significant at $p<0.05$.

associated with purging at Waves II or III, nor was early-onset menarche or teenage pregnancy.

Several significant effects were found in the mental health domain. Those who purged at Wave II had lower levels of self-esteem at Wave I; interestingly, those who purged at Wave III had higher levels of self-esteem at Wave I than those who purged at Wave II, but self-esteem was not associated with purging at Wave III. Higher scores on the depressive symptom scale at Wave I were significantly associated with purging at Wave II as well as purging at Wave III. Those who purged at Wave II were more likely to have attempted suicide, received psychological counseling, or engaged in delinquent behaviors at Wave I. Regarding the measures of ADHD symptoms, no significant associations were found for the inattentiveness scale; however, participants who purged at Wave II high higher levels of hyperactivity/impulsiveness at Wave I than those who did not. Finally, no significant relationships were found regarding the active coping scale variable.

Of the measures of childhood adversity, having never lived with one (or both) parent (s) and parental poverty were associated with an increased likelihood of purging at Wave II. Not eating with parents, losing a parent to death, childhood neglect, and childhood physical abuse were not significantly associated with purging.

Table 3 shows the multivariable multinomial regression model that included only variables that had a significant relationship with purging at Wave II and/or Wave III. In this model, suicide attempts, body image, depression symptoms, hyperactivity, having psychological counseling, and never having lived with one or both parents were not significantly associated with purging at either wave.

However, parental poverty and self-esteem were associated with an increased likelihood of purging at Wave II. Specifically, those who purged at Wave II had higher levels of parental poverty and lower self-esteem. BMI was not significantly associated with purging at Wave II, but those who purged at Wave III had significantly higher BMI levels at Wave I.

Contrary to what we had hypothesized, it was found that those who purged at Wave III had significantly lower rates of delinquent behavior at Wave I. Additionally, those who purged at Wave III had lower rates of delinquency than those who purged at Wave II.

Discussion

The overall aim of this study was to examine a broad range of potential adolescent risk factors for developing purging behaviors in a nationally representative sample of U.S. young adult women. Demographic variables did not differentiate risk for the development of purging behaviors. In univariable analyses, several childhood variables were identified to increase risk for purging. Higher BMI, suicide attempts, overweight self-perception, parental poverty, depression symptoms, hyperactivity-impulsivity, delinquent behaviors, low self-esteem, and never having lived with one (or both) parent (s) were associated with purging at Wave II. Higher BMI and depressive symptoms were associated with purging at Wave III. Finally, lower levels of self-esteem were associated with an increased likelihood of purging at Wave II compared to Wave III.

Of the demographic variables controlled for in our study, purging at Wave I was the only variable that was associated with purging at either follow-up time point. Neither participants' age, race/ethnicity, nor highest level of parental education was found to be associated with

Table 3 Multivariable comparison of purging at waves II and III using measures significant at univariable level

Variable	Purging behavior	Coefficient	Std. error	p-value	CI
Weight perception (Likert)	Wave II	0.19	0.47	0.68	−0.74, 1.13
	Wave III	−0.43	0.63	0.49	−1.67, 0.81
	Wave III - Wave II	−0.63	0.74	0.40	−2.09, 0.84
Body mass index	Wave II	0.05	0.04	0.23	−0.03, 0.12
	Wave III	**0.09**	**0.04**	**0.01**	**0.02, 0.16**
	Wave III - Wave II	0.04	0.06	0.45	−0.07, 0.16
Depressive symptoms scale	Wave II	0.07	0.04	0.06	0.00, 0.15
	Wave III	0.09	0.05	0.06	0.00, 0.19
	Wave III - Wave II	0.02	0.06	0.78	−0.11, 0.14
Hyperactive/impulsive scale[3]	Wave II	0.09	0.08	0.25	−0.06, 0.24
	Wave III	−0.11	0.16	0.49	−0.41, 0.20
	Wave III - Wave II	−0.19	0.18	0.29	−0.56, 0.17
Delinquency scale	Wave II	0.17	0.12	0.15	−0.06, 0.41
	Wave III	**−0.89**	**0.37**	**0.02**	**−1.63, -0.15**
	Wave III - Wave II	**−1.07**	**0.38**	**0.01**	**−1.83, -0.31**
Self-esteem scale	Wave II	**−0.18**	**0.07**	**0.01**	**−0.32, -0.04**
	Wave III	−0.10	0.10	0.31	−0.29, 0.09
	Wave III - Wave II	0.08	0.12	0.48	−0.15, 0.31
Had psychological counseling	Wave II	0.73	0.39	0.06	−0.04, 1.49
	Wave III	−0.21	0.91	0.82	−2.00, 1.59
	Wave III - Wave II	−0.93	1.02	0.36	−2.95, 1.09
Attempted suicide	Wave II	−0.04	0.60	0.95	−1.22, 1.15
	Wave III	0.50	0.76	0.51	−1.00, 2.01
	Wave III - Wave II	0.54	0.92	0.56	−1.28, 2.37
Parental poverty	Wave II	**0.44**	**0.21**	**0.04**	**−0.29, -2.35**
	Wave III	−0.17	0.47	0.72	−1.10, 0.75
	Wave III - Wave II	−0.61	0.44	0.17	−1.47, 0.25
Never lived with parent (s)	Wave II	1.03	0.67	0.12	−0.29, 2.35
	Wave III	−0.31	1.17	0.79	−2.63, 2.01
	Wave III - Wave II	−1.34	1.30	0.30	−3.92, 1.23

Note: All risk factor variables were measured at Wave I except those marked [3]; the latter were measured at Wave III via self-reported retrospective recall. Those reported in bold are significant at p<0.05.

purging at Wave II or III. The lack of age differences across the two groups is not particularly surprising given the fact that the Add Health sample has a restricted age range. Consistent with a growing literature that reports that girls or women from various racial/ethnicity backgrounds are equally likely to develop disordered eating, [26,27] our results suggest that purging may be a problem across various racial or ethnic groups. Our finding that highest level of parental education, an indicator often used in the literature as a proxy for parental socioeconomic status, did not differ when comparing purging groups warrants comment in light of our result that family poverty did differentiate the two groups. Both variables were measured using parent/guardian self-report. While parental education does not appear to increase risk for purging, experiencing economic hardship may elevate such risk as will be discussed in more detail below.

Regarding the purging variable, it was found that those who reported purging at Wave I were less likely to also report purging at Wave II or III, and purging at Wave I was not associated with a difference in the likelihood of purging between Wave II and III. It is possible that this inverse relationship is a byproduct of how purging was measured in this study, given that the variable only reflected purging behavior over the last seven days. More frequent longitudinal assessments might better capture the extent to which purging behavior is stable between adolescence and young adulthood.

Additionally, our study confirmed several risk factors for purging that have been shown to predict risk for eating disorders in previous studies, and identified previously understudied time varying effects for several of these variables. For example, self-perception of being overweight significantly predicted purging at Wave II but not at Wave III. Research consistently has found that body image concern (operationalized in a variety of ways in different studies) contributed to increased risk for eating disorder symptoms [2,28] and, therefore, has been targeted as a key risk factor to be addressed in prevention programs [29]. However, our results suggest that this may only be a risk factor over a certain time range. Given the stability of these risk factors over time, it's surprising that some Wave I predictors that showed significant relationships at Wave II did not predict Wave III purging behaviors. Again, more intensive longitudinal data collection would be useful to more clearly determine how risk factors may affect the likelihood of purging between adolescence and young adulthood.

Similarly, consistent with previous studies, low self-esteem, [28] depression, [28,30,31] and impulsivity [32-34] were significantly associated with increased risk for purging. In addition, we found significant relationships between purging and self-reported suicide attempts as well as between purging and having received psychological counseling. In a series of case control studies, Fairburn and colleagues found that "parental separation" (e.g., due to prolonged illness) and "parental loss" (e.g., due to death) were risk factors for developing an eating disorder [35,36]. In our study, never having lived with one (or both) parent (s) was a risk factor for purging, but having lost a parent to death was not. We cannot answer whether these discrepant findings are a function of methodological differences (e.g., case–control design versus longitudinal design; differences in how the target groups were defined). As noted by Fairburn and colleagues (35), parental separation and loss are also risk factors for other psychiatric problems. Therefore, these parental risk factors may be indirectly associated with the development of eating disorders. For example, parental separation or loss may increase the risk of developing psychiatric problems, which in turn, could increase the likelihood of eating disorders. Future research that examines the nature of the association between these parental factors and eating disorders is important to determine how parental separation and loss might influence eating disorder risk in terms of being mediated or moderated by other risk factors, such as depression. Finally, in our sample, family poverty was found to be predictive of purging onset. This bolsters emerging literature that suggests a relationship between socioeconomic hardship and unhealthy weight control behaviors [37].

Several limitations need to be acknowledged. Although Add Health is a large epidemiological study, the sample still was not large enough to test hypotheses about risk factors for purging in young adult men. Therefore, our findings should not be generalized to boys or men. As is common in large-scale epidemiological studies, key study variables were measured using self-report questionnaires, which tend to be less reliable than interview based measures. Childhood abuse variables as well as the ADHD-IN and -HI scales were collected retrospectively and were, therefore, subject to recall errors. Additionally, because frequency information was not available for the purging behaviors, we were unable to study severity of the behaviors. Interval censoring may also be an issue, given that questions only addressed purging in the last seven days, which did not allow us to identify whether those reporting purging during those days were new onset purgers or whether they may have purged prior to the assessment period. As a result, purging is likely to be underestimated.

Finally, information was not available regarding binge eating behaviors or other extreme weight control behaviors, such as extreme dietary restrictions or excessive exercise. Further studies would be needed to compare our results regarding purging to these similar unhealthy behaviors.

These limitations were offset by several strengths. The study involved a community sample, thus not featuring the limitations inherent in studies of patient samples. The relatively large sample size afforded us the opportunity to use multivariable modeling of risk factors for purging, a relatively uncommon yet clinically important behavior. As well, Add Health collected data on numerous psychosocial variables, allowing us to explore factors that have been considered in psychopathology research regarding other disorders but less so in studies of eating disorders. Finally, our study covered a considerable period of time (8 years) from adolescence into early adulthood.

Conclusions

This study prospectively examined risk factors for young adult purging in a large nationally representative sample of adolescent females. Results provided support for several risk factors for purging that have been shown to predict risk for eating disorders in previous studies. Future research on the development of purging behavior might include measures of economic adversity and self-esteem to better predict purging in young adults.

Competing interests

The authors have no conflicts of interest to report.

Authors' contributions

EMS conducted all analyses, contributed to methodology selection, and provided data interpretation to the manuscript. JR supervised the design of analyses and contributed to interpretation of data and revisions to drafts of the manuscript. LK contributed to the conception of the study as well as the drafting of the manuscript. FR made significant revisions to the original manuscript for intellectual content. RSW made substantial contributions to the original manuscript and supervised all data analysis and interpretation. All authors read and approved the final manuscript.

Acknowledgements
This research was supported by Academic Research Enhancement Award DK092768-01A1 (Striegel) from the National Institute of Diabetes, Digestive, and Kidney Disease. The Add Health study is directed by Kathleen Mullan Harris and designed by J. Richard Udry, Peter S. Bearman, and Kathleen Mullan Harris at the University of North Carolina at Chapel Hill. It is funded by grant P01-HD31921 from the Eunice Kennedy Shriver National Institute of Child Health and Human Development, along with funding from 23 other federal agencies and foundations. Data were collected under protocols approved by the Institutional Review Boards of the University of North Carolina at Chapel Hill, and the Miriam Hospital.

Author details
[1]Department of Psychology, Wesleyan University, 207 High Street, Middletown, CT 06459, USA. [2]Department of Psychology, Manchester Community College, Great Path MS#4, Manchester, CT, USA.

References

1. Striegel-Moore RH, Bulik CM: **Risk factors for eating disorders.** *Am Psychol* 2007, **62**(3):181–198.
2. Jacobi C, *et al*: **Coming to terms with risk factors for eating disorders: application of risk terminology and suggestions for a general taxonomy.** *Psychological bulletin* 2004, **130**(1):19–65.
3. Piran N, Robinson SR: **Patterns of associations between eating disordered behaviors and substance use in two non-clinical samples: a university and a community based sample.** *J Health Psychol* 2011, **16**(7):1027–1037.
4. Keel PK, Striegel-Moore RH: **The validity and clinical utility of purging disorder.** *Int J Eat Disord* 2009, **42**(8):706–719.
5. Ackard DM, Fulkerson JA, Neumark-Sztainer D: **Psychological and behavioral risk profiles as they relate to eating disorder diagnoses and symptomatology among a school-based sample of youth.** *Int J Eat Disord* 2011, **44**(5):440–446.
6. Haines J, *et al*: **Family dinner and disordered eating behaviors in a large cohort of adolescents.** *Eat Disord* 2010, **18**(1):10–24.
7. Fulkerson JA, *et al*: **Family meal frequency and weight status among adolescents: cross-sectional and 5-year longitudinal associations.** *Obesity* 2008, **16**(11):2529–2534.
8. Hudson JI, *et al*: **The prevalence and correlates of eating disorders in the National Comorbidity Survey Replication.** *Biol Psychiatry* 2007, **61**(3):348–358.
9. Baker JH, *et al*: **Pubertal development predicts eating behaviors in adolescence.** *Int J Eat Disord* 2012, **45**(7):819–826.
10. Neumark-Sztainer D, *et al*: **Dieting and disordered eating behaviors from adolescence to young adulthood: findings from a 10-year longitudinal study.** *J Am Diet Assoc* 2011, **111**(7):1004–1011.
11. Kraemer HC, *et al*: **Coming to terms with the terms of risk.** *Arch Gen Psychiatry* 1997, **54**(4):337–343.
12. Harris KM, *et al*: *The National Longitudinal Study of Adolescent Health: Codebooks*; 2009. Available from: http://www.cpc.unc.edu/projects/addhealth/codebooks.
13. Chantala K, Tabor K: *Strategies to perform a design-based analysis using the Add Health data*; 2010. [cited 2012 September 12]; Available from: http://www.cpc.unc.edu/projects/addhealth/data/guides/weight1.pdf.
14. Tourangeau R, Shin H: *National Longitudinal Study of Adolescent Health: Grand sample weight*; 1999. [cited 2012 October 26]; Available from: http://www.cpc.unc.edu/projects/addhealth/data/guides/weights.pdf.
15. Elder GH, Meadows SO, Brown JS: **Race-ethnic inequality and psychological distress: depressive symptoms from adolescence to young adulthood.** *Developmental Psycholology* 2007, **43**(6):1295–1311.
16. Centers for Disease Control and Prevention: *About BMI for Adults*; 2013. [cited 2013 August 27]. Available from: http://www.cdc.gov/healthyweight/assessing/bmi/adult_bmi/.
17. Stunkard AJ, Grace WJ, Wolff HG: **The night-eating syndrome; a pattern of food intake among certain obese patients.** *Am J Med* 1955, **19**(1):78–86.
18. Rosenberg A: *Society and the adolescent self-image*. Princeton, New Jersey: Princeton University Press; 1965.
19. Kort-Butler LA, Hagewen KJ: **School-based extracurricular activity involvement and adolescent self-esteem: a growth-curve analysis.** *J Youth Adolesc* 2011, **40**(5):568–581.
20. Radloff LS: **The CES-D Scale: A Self-Report Depression Scale for Research in the General Population.** *Applied Psychological Measurement* 1977, **1**(3):385–401.
21. Adkins DE, Wang V, Elder GH Jr: **Structure and Stress: Trajectories of depressive dymptoms across adolescence and young adulthood.** *Soc Forces* 2009, **88**(1):31.
22. American Psychiatric Association: *Diagnostic and Statistical Manual of Mental Disorders*. 4th edition. Washington, DC: American Psychiatric Association Press; 1994.
23. McClernon FJ, *et al*: **Interactions between genotype and retrospective ADHD symptoms predict lifetime smoking risk in a sample of young adults.** *Nicotine Tob Res* 2008, **10**(1):117–127.
24. Aalsma MC, *et al*: **The impact of delinquency on young adult sexual risk behaviors and sexually transmitted infections.** *J Adolesc Health* 2010, **46**(1):17–24.
25. Sysko R, Walsh BT: **Does the broad categories for the diagnosis of eating disorders (BCD-ED) scheme reduce the frequency of eating disorder not otherwise specified?** *Int J Eat Disord* 2011, **44**(7):625–629.
26. Alegria M, *et al*: **Prevalence and correlates of eating disorders in Latinos in the United States.** *Int J Eat Disord* 2007, **40**(Suppl):S15–S21.
27. Javaras KN, *et al*: **Co-occurrence of binge eating disorder with psychiatric and medical disorders.** *J Clin Psychiatry* 2008, **69**(2):266–273.
28. Stice E, *et al*: **An 8-year longitudinal study of the natural history of threshold, subthreshold, and partial eating disorders from a community sample of adolescents.** *J Abnorm Psychol* 2009, **118**(3):587–597.
29. Stice E, *et al*: **Dissonance and healthy weight eating disorder prevention programs: long-term effects from a randomized efficacy trial.** *J Consult Clin Psychol* 2008, **76**(2):329–340.
30. Sysko R, *et al*: **A latent class analysis of psychiatric symptoms among 125 adolescents in a bariatric surgery program.** *International journal of Pediatric Obesity* 2011, **6**(3–4):289–297.
31. Jacobi C, *et al*: **Who is really at risk? Identifying risk factors for subthreshold and full syndrome eating disorders in a high-risk sample.** *Psychol Med* 2011, **41**(9):1939–1949.
32. Hoffman ER, *et al*: **Understanding the association of impulsivity, obsessions, and compulsions with binge eating and purging behaviours in anorexia nervosa.** *Eur Eat Disord Rev* 2012, **20**(3):e129–e136.
33. Marmorstein NR, *et al*: **Longitudinal associations between externalizing behavior and dysfunctional eating attitudes and behaviors: a community-based study.** *J Clin Child Adolesc Psychol* 2007, **36**(1):87–94.
34. Slane JD, Burt SA, Klump KL: **The road less traveled: associations between externalizing behaviors and eating pathology.** *Int J Eat Disord* 2010, **43**(2):149–160.
35. Fairburn CG, *et al*: **Risk factors for anorexia nervosa: three integrated case–control comparisons.** *Arch Gen Psychiatry* 1999, **56**(5):468–476.
36. Fairburn CG, *et al*: **Risk factors for bulimia nervosa. A community-based case–control study.** *Arch Gen Psychiatry* 1997, **54**(6):509–517.
37. Oddy WH, Forbes D, Allen KL, SM B: **Factors for full- and partial-syndrome early adolescent eating disorders: a population-based pregnancy cohort study.** *Journal of the American Academy of Child & Adolescent Psychiatry* 2009, **48**(8):800–809.

The presence, predictive utility, and clinical significance of body dysmorphic symptoms in women with eating disorders

Deborah Mitchison[1*], Rocco Crino[2] and Phillipa Hay[3,4]

Abstract

Background: Both eating disorders (EDs) and body dysmorphic disorder (BDD) are disorders of body image. This study aimed to assess the presence, predictive utility, and impact of clinical features commonly associated with BDD in women with EDs.

Methods: Participants recruited from two non-clinical cohorts of women, symptomatic and asymptomatic of EDs, completed a survey on ED (EDE-Q) and BDD (BDDE-SR) psychopathology, psychological distress (K-10), and quality of life (SF-12).

Results: A strong correlation was observed between the total BDDE-SR and the global EDE-Q scores ($r = 0.79$, $p < 0.001$). Multivariate analyses demonstrated that participants with probable EDs ($n = 61$) and BDD ($n = 23$) scored higher on 28 of the 30 BDDE-SR items compared to healthy controls ($n = 173$; all $p < 0.05$), indicating greater severity of BDD symptoms. BDD participants also scored higher than ED participants on 15 of the 30 BDDE-SR items (all $p < 0.05$). The remaining 15 items that ED and BDD participants scored similarly on (all $p > 0.05$) measured appearance checking, reassurance-seeking, camouflaging, comparison-making, and social avoidance. In addition to these behaviors, inspection of sensitivity (Se) and specificity (Sp) revealed that BDDE-SR items measuring preoccupation and dissatisfaction with appearance were most predictive of ED cases (Se *and* Sp > 0.60). Higher total BDDE-SR scores were associated with greater distress on the K-10 and poorer quality of life on the SF-12 (all $p < 0.01$).

Conclusions: Clinical features central to the model of BDD are common in, predictive of, and associated with impairment in women with EDs. Practice implications are that these features be included in the assessment and treatment of EDs.

Keywords: Eating disorder, Body dysmorphic disorder, Comorbidity, Symptoms, Community-based study, Distress, Impairment

Background

The presence, predictive utility, and clinical significance of body dysmorphic symptoms in women with eating disorders

The eating disorders (EDs) and body dysmorphic disorder (BDD) are disorders of body image [1]. While the main concern is with overall body shape and/or weight in the EDs, in BDD the primary concerns vary widely, and commonly include concerns with facial features, skin, and hair [2]. It has been suggested that BDD and the EDs might be better clustered under an encompassing 'body image disorder' [3]. However, the current hierarchical organization of the Diagnostic and Statistical Manual for Mental Disorders (DSM-IV-TR) [4] stipulates that a diagnosis of BDD cannot be provided if symptoms are *"better accounted for by another mental disorder (e.g., dissatisfaction with body shape and size in Anorexia Nervosa"* (p510 [4]). Discussions about the validity of this hierarchy have also raised questions such as whether the EDs are in fact a variant of BDD [5].

* Correspondence: d.mitchison@uws.edu.au
[1]School of Psychology and Social Science, University of Western Sydney, Sydney, NSW, Australia
Full list of author information is available at the end of the article

Studies have reported that between 39 to 88% of patients in an ED treatment setting concurrently meet diagnostic criteria for BDD [6-8]. Conversely, it has also been found that 32.5% of a clinical BDD sample had a lifetime diagnosis of an ED [9]. The higher proportion of cases of BDD in ED than vice versa is expected due to the wider array of appearance concerns in BDD [4]. This high comorbidity would suggest that there may be underlying similarities in the predisposition to both EDs and BDD. It is possible however that comorbid cases would be more likely to seek treatment [10], and this may be due to implied greater severity. Further, the majority of people with EDs and BDD may not present for treatment of their body image problems [11-13], and because of this, research using non-clinical samples may provide a more representative account of comorbidity.

Based on its phenomenological similarity to obsessive compulsive disorder (OCD), BDD has been considered an OCD 'spectrum' disorder, and its classification (see DSM-5 draft criteria) [14], assessment (e.g. the Yale-Brown Obsessive Compulsive Scale) [15], and recommended treatment (i.e. exposure and response prevention) [16] have been aligned to that of OCD. As such, the cognitive behavioral therapy (CBT) model of BDD has focused on compulsive acts (e.g. checking, fixing, and camouflaging the imagined defect in appearance; making mental comparisons to others' bodies) in response to obsessive preoccupation with appearance [17,18]. As far as is known, previous research has not explored the relevance of this model to an ED sample, however elements of the model may be applicable. For instance, 'fixing behaviors' is also a commonly recognized feature in models of EDs [19]. While 'fixing' presents in BDD primarily through behaviors such as excessive cosmetic surgery and grooming, patients with EDs may attempt to 'fix' perceived fatness through extreme dieting and compulsive exercising and purging. Another behavioral BDD feature is excessive body-checking, which has been suggested to be present in up to 92% of ED patients [20,21], for example in the form of mirror examining, weighing, measuring, and skin-pinching. Finally, although it has received little attention in the field of EDs, preoccupation with appearance may be more predictive of EDs in comparison to other cognitive constructs such as body image perception and body dissatisfaction [22]. Camouflaging, reassurance-seeking, comparison-making, and social avoidance are also likely to present in and maintain pathology in ED patients, although research is yet to firmly establish this.

Clinically severe BDD symptomatology may be present in people with EDs, regardless of comorbidity. For instance, studies have found that participants with EDs scored similarly to participants with BDD on measures of body dissatisfaction, checking, appearance evaluation, appearance fixing, body image distress and preoccupation, but lower on measures of negative self-evaluation, avoidance of activities, overvaluation of appearance, body image disturbance, and quality of life impairment [23,24]. These studies were limited by a lack of investigation into specific maintaining factors, as they tended to group symptoms into broader constructs. The samples used were also from clinical settings, which may limit generalisability [11-13].

Aims

The aim of this study was to examine the extent to which symptoms theoretically associated with BDD are experienced by, predictive of, and associated with impairment in women with probable EDs. It was hypothesized that participants with probable EDs would report more severe BDD symptoms than healthy control participants, although less severe BDD symptoms than participants with probable BDD. It was also hypothesized that a number of items on the Body Dysmorphic Disorder Examination Self Report (BDDE-SR) [25] would have high specificity and/or sensitivity in predicting probable ED cases, particularly those items measuring checking and fixing. Finally, it was hypothesized that the presence of clinical BDD symptoms would be associated with greater impairment in quality of life and greater psychological distress in participants with EDs.

Methods

Participants

The present study was nested within a larger project (The Women's Eating and Health Literacy longitudinal study), which includes two cohorts. The data is sourced from the ninth-year survey follow-up of these cohorts.

Cohort 1

Participants from the first cohort were originally from the Health and Well-Being of Female Australian Capital Territory (ACT) Residents Study [26]. At baseline, 10 000 women were randomly selected from the ACT electoral roll, between the ages of 18 and 42, and invited to complete a self-report questionnaire regarding socio-demographic information, ED symptoms, psychological distress, and quality of life. Of the 5255 (52.6%) participants who returned the survey, 324 met screening criteria for an ED (global EDE-Q score > 2.5 and endorsement of any ED behaviour; see *Eating Disorders Examination Questionnaire* under *Measures* below) and were interviewed using the EDE [27]. The interview identified 185 participants with ED symptoms of 'clinical severity', and 122 of these consented to participate in the longitudinal study. Clinical severity was determined using the EDE and was denoted by the presence of extreme weight/shape concerns; and/or current regular (defined as at least weekly over the past three months) binge eating; and/or regular use of any extreme weight control behaviours (i.e. self-induced vomiting, laxative use, diuretic use, fasting or severe food restriction, compulsive exercise).

Cohort 2

The second cohort was a convenience sample derived from a parallel longitudinal survey of women with disordered eating recruited through advertisements in four universities and colleges of higher education in the Australian states of Queensland and Victoria [28]. Recruitment was via central university email, posters on student bulletins and in residence halls, and direct approach in the university common areas. For individuals approached via email, participants were given the option of completing an electronic survey. For all other participants, hard copies were provided with reply-paid envelopes. The survey included questions on socio-demographic information, ED health literacy, ED psychopathology (EDE-Q, see *Measures* below), and health-related quality of life. Seven hundred and six participants returned the surveys and agreed to be part of the longitudinal study. Because of the recruitment strategy it was not possible to determine the response rate. Two hundred and twenty-one were identified as having ED symptoms of clinical severity. This was defined using the criteria used above for cohort 1, however also included participants who identified themselves as currently having a problem like that of a fictional woman with bulimia nervosa (described in a vignette in the survey). At baseline the mean global score on the EDE-Q score for cohort 2 as a whole was 1.74, with a standard deviation of 1.34. This is slightly higher than community norms for the EDE-Q [29], which reflects that this sample included participants with a range in ED pathology.

The ED symptomatology from baseline to five-year follow-up of these cohorts has been previously described. In both cohorts, symptomatology was mostly reflective of eating disorder not otherwise specified (EDNOS), with regular binge eating and less regular purging behaviour [30].

For the present study, participants were grouped into one of three groups: ED-only (identified as having a probable ED, see under EDE-Q below), BDD (identified as having probable BDD, see under BDDE-SR below), or Healthy Controls (identified as not having a probable ED or BDD, and also not reporting ED behaviors or extreme weight/shape concerns according to the EDE-Q, see below).

Measures

The survey package sent for the ninth year follow-up included questions on demographic information including marital and employment status, educational level obtained, and self-reported height and weight. A number of measures of psychopathology, quality of life, and health service utilisation were also included. For the present study, completed responses to the following specific measures were used.

The eating disorder examination questionnaire (EDE-Q)

The EDE-Q [29] has been validated in community and clinical samples of people with EDs. The questionnaire, which assesses ED pathology over the past month, yields four sub-scales: dietary restraint, eating concerns, weight concerns, and shape concerns. A global score is also computed as the average of the four subscales. The frequency of specific behaviours is also assessed, including objective and subjective binge eating, various types of purging, and compulsive exercise. Norms for Australian women have been reported previously [31]. The four subscales have good reliability (α-coefficients $\geq$ 0.8) and moderate predictive validity (sensitivity = 0.8, specificity = 0.8) in identifying probable ED cases [31]. Cronbach's α in the present study was 0.95.

Probable ED cases were defined in the current study using the EDE-Q and according to criteria used in a previous study [32]. These criteria included the presence of extreme weight/shape concerns (score $\geq$ 4 on Q21 and/or Q22) and any current regular ED behaviour. ED behaviours included objective binge eating, subjective binge eating, purging (self-induced vomiting, laxative use, or diuretic use), compulsive exercise (Q14 - Q20), and dietary fasting (Q2). For binge eating and purging 'regular' was defined as at least once weekly over the past four weeks; for dietary fasting and exercising 'regular' was defined as at least thrice weekly over the past four weeks.

The body dysmorphic disorder examination, self report (BDDE-SR)

The BDDE-SR [25] is a measure of body dysmorphic symptoms. It has three parts. The first asks the participant to nominate, rank, and describe five body parts that they are most dissatisfied with. Part two asks participants to list and rate the frequency of various remedies ever used to 'fix' the body part most dissatisfied with. The final part, and the focus of the analysis below, includes 28 likert-type items (scale from 0 to 6) and 2 dichotomous yes/no items based on the body part rated as being most dissatisfied with. These questions cover a range of BDD clinical symptoms such as preoccupation and dissatisfaction with, and overvaluation of appearance; social concern, anxiety, and avoidance; and checking, camouflaging, reassurance-seeking, and comparison-making behaviours. Unpublished data report male and female community and clinical norms; and for the community sample, test-retest reliability as r = 0.90 and internal consistency as Cronbach's α = 0.94 [22,29]. A total score is computed based on the 28 likert items and ranges from 0 to 168, with higher scores indicating greater pathology. Cronbach's α in the present study for the 28 likert items was 0.95.

Criteria for a probable BDD case have been specified by the authors of the BDDE-SR (available upon request) as a score ≥ 4 on an item measuring preoccupation with the imagined defect (Q6); *and* a score ≥ 4 on either of two items measuring social concern (Q7, Q8); *and* a score ≥ 4 on an item measuring overvaluation of appearance (Q12); *and* a score ≥ 4 on an item measuring negative evaluation of self due to the imagined defect (Q13); *and* a score ≥ 4 on any of 5 items measuring distress and impairment (Q4, Q17, Q18, Q19, Q21).

Kessler psychological distress scale (K-10)

The K-10 [33] is a measure of general psychological distress. It was developed specifically for general population samples. The K-10 includes 10 likert-type items that assess the frequency (scale from 1 to 5) with which various depressive and anxiety symptoms are experienced. Thus total scores may range from 10 to 50, with higher scores indicating greater distress. A score greater than 20 is indicative of a clinically significant mood disorder. Chronbach's α for the K-10 total score in this study was 0.91.

Medical outcomes study (12 item) short-form (SF-12)

The SF-12 [34] is a standardized measure of health-related quality of life. It has been used extensively in research interested in the impairment associated with physiological and psychological health conditions, and good psychometric properties have been demonstrated, including in an Australian population sample [34,35]. The questionnaire has 12 items that contribute to two weighted scales, a Physical Component Summary Scale (PCS) and a Mental Component Summary Scale (MCS), each of which have a mean of 50 and standard deviation of 10. Higher scores indicate higher levels of functioning. Cronbach's α's in the present study were 0.83 for the total 12 items, 0.81 for the 6 items contributing to the PCS, and 0.80 for the 6 items contributing to the MCS.

Procedure

The study was reviewed and approved by the human research ethics committee at the University of Western Sydney (ethics approval number: H9283). All participants were either posted or emailed (depending on previously stated preferences) the survey. Surveys were then sent again to non-responding participants two, three, and four months later in order to maximise response rate.

Data analysis

Descriptive statistics were computed to assess the prevalence of probable ED and BDD cases based on the EDE-Q and BDDE-SR criteria stipulated above. Three groups of participants were then separated for further analysis. The first group included participants who had a probable ED, but who did not have probable BDD ('ED-only group'). BDD was excluded from this first group so as to not confound analyses aiming to assess the presence of BDD symptoms in participants with EDs. The second group included all participants who had probable BDD ('BDD group'). The final and third group included participants who were identified as not having current BDD or an ED, or any current regular ED behaviours or weight/shape concerns ('healthy control group').

Body mass index (kg/m^2; BMI) was computed. Chi-square tests for categorical demographic variables (education, marital status) and analyses of variance (ANOVAs) for non-categorical demographic variables (age, body mass index) were carried out to compare the three groups.

The Pearson correlation (r_p) for the EDE-Q global and BDDE-SR total scores was computed. An analysis of covariance (ANCOVA), covarying for BMI (as this differed significantly between the groups, see below), was computed to compare the total score of the BDDE-SR between the three groups. This was followed by a multivariate ANOVA (MANOVA) covarying for BMI to compare groups on each of the 30 items in the third part of the BDDE-SR. The purpose of these analyses was to address the research question of whether participants with EDs experience BDD symptoms, and to what extent in comparison to participants with BDD and healthy controls.

Two-by-two cross-tabulation tables were examined to assess the specificity and sensitivity of the 30 BDDE-SR items to predict ED-only cases. Sensitivity was defined as the proportion of ED-only cases who scored high (≥ 4) on a BDDE-SR item. Specificity was defined as the proportion of cases with no probable ED who did not score high (≥ 4) on a BDDE-SR item. The cut-off of ≥ 4 on items has been suggested by the authors of the BDDE-SR to indicate clinical severity [25]. The purpose of these analyses was to examine the predictive utility of BDD symptoms in probable ED cases.

Finally, three multiple linear regressions with backward method were conducted using data from the ED-only group, to assess the association between BDD symptoms and distress and impairment. A separate regression was conducted for each dependent variable: the K-10, the SF-12 MCS subscale, and the SF-12 PCS subscale. The total score on the BDDE-SR was entered in each regression as the predictor of interest, and the EDE-Q global score was entered as a covariate predictor.

Results

Demographic analyses

Three hundred and twelve participants returned the survey for this study, 53 from cohort 1 and 259 from cohort 2. Overall, this represented a total response rate of 51.7% ($N = 312$) of the participants with whom we had current contact details. Sixty-one participants were identified as 'ED-only', 23 as 'BDD', and 173 as 'healthy controls'. The remaining 55 respondents who reported sub-threshold ED or BDD symptoms were not included in this study.

As can be seen from Table 1, no significant differences between groups in terms of age, highest education level achieved, and marital status were observed. A significant main effect was found for BMI. Post-hoc pairwise analyses using the Bonferroni adjusted significance value for multiple comparisons revealed that the ED-only group had a significantly higher BMI on average than both the BDD ($p = 0.00$) and the healthy controls ($p = 0.00$) groups. The pairwise comparison between the BDD and the healthy controls group was not significant ($p = 1.00$).

Presence of body dysmorphic symptoms in probable eating disorders cases

Higher global EDE-Q scores were associated with higher total BDDE-SR scores ($r_p = 0.79$, $p < 0.001$).

A significant main effect of group was observed on the BDDE-SR total score, $F(2, 216) = 83.68$, $p < 0.001$, $\eta_p^2 = 0.44$. Pairwise comparisons demonstrated that the BDD group had significantly higher total scores (M = 95.61, SD = 12.73) on average than both the ED-only (M = 78.22, SD = 30.65; $p = 0.00$) and healthy control (M = 37.78, SD = 21.47; $p < 0.001$) groups; and that the ED-only group had significantly higher scores than the healthy control group ($p < 0.001$).

Table 2 displays the means for each item score on the BDDE-SR and results of the pairwise analyses between the three comparison groups. A significant main effect of group was observed on all items (all $p < 0.05$), except for item 1 ($p = 0.10$), which asked participants to rank how much they believed that their particular concern with appearance was common in others (see Table 3 for a descriptive list of all BDDE-SR items). Pairwise comparisons revealed that the healthy control group scored significantly lower on all items in comparison to the BDD and ED-only groups, except for item 1 as mentioned above, and item 16a (which asked participants whether they ever had times that they did not think their appearance was 'so bad'). On this item, scores did not differ between healthy controls and the ED-only group, however the BDD group did score higher than the controls. On 15 of the 30 items, participants in the BDD group scored significantly higher than participants in the ED-only group. On the other 15 items however, there was no significant difference in the scores between the BDD and ED-only groups. These findings indicate that participants with BDD or EDs experienced a greater severity/frequency of BDD symptoms than healthy controls; and that participants with BDD experienced some, but not all, BDD symptoms to a greater extent than participants with EDs only.

Predicting probable eating disorder cases

As seen in Table 3, 4 items (4, 6, 23, and 26) had particularly high sensitivity and specificity in predicting probable ED cases. These measured dissatisfaction with overall appearance, preoccupation with an imagined defect in appearance, camouflaging through posturing to

Table 1 Demographic characteristics of the ED-only, BDD, and healthy control groups

Demographic	BDD (n = 23)	ED-only (n = 61)	Healthy controls (n = 173)		
		M (SD)		F (df)	p
Age	41.14 (9.73)	38.85 (10.54)	37.42 (10.93)	1.37 (2, 252)	0.27
Body Mass Index	24.88 (3.55)	30.37 (9.43)	25.68 (5.25)	12.33 (2, 236)	<0.001
		n (%)		χ^2 (df)	p
Education Level				7.73 (12)	0.81
High school	6 (26.1)	11 (18.0)	20 (11.6)		
Non graduate higher education	2 (8.7)	9 (14.8)	20 (11.6)		
Graduate	10 (43.5)	22 (36.1)	87 (50.3)		
Post graduate	5 (21.7)	19 (31.1)	46 (26.6)		
Marital Status				3.83 (8)	0.87
Single	10 (43.4)	18 (29.5)	58 (33.5)		
Married / Defacto	13 (56.6)	43 (70.5)	115 (66.5)		

ED = eating disorder, *BDD* = body dysmorphic disorder.

Table 2 Results from the MANOVA and pairwise comparisons comparing BDDE-SR item scores between diagnostic groups

BDDE-SR item	ED-Only (*n* = 61)	BDD (*n* = 23)	Healthy controls (*n* = 173)			
		M (SD)		*F* (*df*:2, 213)	*p*	η_p^2
1.	3.00 (1.33)	3.17 (1.04)	2.59 (1.34)	2.36	0.10	0.02
2.	4.06 (1.83)*	5.33 (1.24)*	2.85 (2.01)	20.89	< 0.001	0.16
3.	4.35 (0.99)*†	5.28 (0.67)*	3.08 (1.23)	44.22	< 0.001	0.29
4.	3.83 (1.36)* †	4.44 (0.92)*	2.19 (1.24)	44.56	< 0.001	0.30
5.	1.43 (1.73)*	1.67 (1.57)*	0.80 (1.19)	5.94	0.00	0.05
6.	3.85 (1.84)* †	5.11 (0.76)*	1.62 (1.78)	49.93	< 0.001	0.32
7.	3.37 (1.90)* †	4.11 (1.37)*	1.66 (1.54)	29.26	< 0.001	0.22
8.	3.56 (1.83)* †	4.72 (0.83)*	1.68 (1.47)	46.90	< 0.001	0.31
9a.	3.02 (2.07)* †	4.39 (1.42)*	1.12 (1.38)	49.77	< 0.001	0.32
9b.	3.20 (1.97)* †	4.22 (1.26)*	1.28 (1.47)	42.40	< 0.001	0.29
10a.	1.20 (1.14)* †	1.72 (1.45)*	0.74 (0.93)	8.48	< 0.001	0.07
10b.	2.31 (1.86)*	2.94 (1.47)*	0.99 (1.32)	22.30	< 0.001	0.17
11a.	0.83 (1.37)* †	1.28 (1.45)*	0.23 (0.65)	12.42	< 0.001	0.10
11b.	1.35 (1.88)* †	1.89 (1.94)*	0.21 (0.67)	23.85	< 0.001	0.18
12.	3.37 (1.31)* †	4.39 (0.50)*	1.65 (1.24)	65.05	< 0.001	0.38
13.	3.19 (1.63)* †	4.61 (0.70)*	0.95 (1.06)	111. 80	< 0.001	0.51
14.	2.39 (1.81)* †	2.89 (1.60)*	0.74 (1.03)	37.92	< 0.001	0.26
15.	2.89 (1.62)*	2.72 (1.60)*	1.24 (1.48)	19.36	< 0.001	0.15
16a.	1.33 (0.48)	1.44 (0.51)*	1.19 (0.39)	3.51	0.03	0.03
16b.	1.48 (0.50)* †	1.61 (0.50)*	1.12 (0.33)	19.49	< 0.001	0.16
17.	1.50 (1.75)*	1.39 (1.42)*	0.32 (0.87)	15.90	< 0.001	0.13
18.	1.39 (1.75)*	1.39 (1.42)*	0.23 (0.70)	24.46	< 0.001	0.19
19.	2.26 (2.00)*	2.50 (1.54)*	0.59 (1.16)	28.69	< 0.001	0.21
20.	2.57 (2.07)*	2.78 (1.73)*	0.88 (1.50)	20.54	< 0.001	0.16
21.	1.91 (1.95)*	1.61 (1.75)*	0.46 (1.08)	15.92	< 0.001	0.13
22.	4.31 (2.05)*	4.61 (1.65)*	2.83 (2.23)	11.59	< 0.001	0.10
23.	4.04 (2.01)*	3.94 (1.83)*	1.92 (1.97)	21.37	< 0.001	0.17
24.	2.56 (2.03)* †	3.44 (1.82)*	0.89 (1.51)	28.37	< 0.001	0.21
25.	3.24 (2.15)*	3.67 (2.45)*	1.33 (1.85)	23.14	< 0.001	1.18
26.	4.09 (1.84)*	5.00 (1.19)*	2.11 (1.87)	118.61	< 0.001	0.25

ED = eating disorder, *BDD* = body dysmorphic disorder, *BDDE-SR* = body dysmorphic disorder examination, short form, * Significant difference ($p < 0.05$) with healthy control group; † significant difference ($p < 0.05$) with BDD group.

hide an imagined defect in appearance, and comparison-making between self and others based on area of imagined defect in appearance. These results suggest that these symptoms are unlikely to present in non-ED cases and are likely to be present in ED cases.

Clinical significance of body dysmorphic symptoms

As can be seen in Table 4, the BDDE-SR emerged as a significant predictor of the K-10 and the PCS subscale on the SF-12, and in each of these regressions the EDE-Q global score was not a significant predictor. However the BDDE-SR did not emerge as a significant predictor of scores on the MCS subscale on the SF-12, whereas the EDE-Q global score did. These findings indicate that the presence of BDD symptoms is associated with greater psychological distress and physical health-related quality of life impairment in participants with probable EDs.

Discussion

Investigations into the models of similar body image disorders to ascertain their applicability to EDs have not been rigorously pursued. This has had clinical implications,

Table 3 Sensitivity and specificity of BDDE-SR items in predicting ED-Only cases (n = 61)

BDDE-SR item	Sens. (%)	Spec. (%)
1. Belief that imagined defect is common	37.7	72.7
2. Checking the imagined defect	65.6	58.3
3. Dissatisfaction with the imagined defect	82.0	53.5
4. Dissatisfaction with overall appearance †	63.9	71.9
5. Reassurance-seeking behavior	13.1	94.4
6. Preoccupation and distress associated with the imagined defect †	62.3	75.7
7. Social anxiety with strangers due to the imagined defect	45.9	76.2
8. Social anxiety with familiar people due to the imagined defect	54.1	74.3
9a. Belief that others notice the imagined defect	41.0	84.0
9b. Distress when others are believed to notice the imagined defect	50.0	81.7
10a. Frequency of comments made by others	3.3	95.2
10b. Distress caused by others' comments	26.2	88.3
11a. Belief that treated differently because of defect	8.2	96.5
11b. Distress caused by being treated differently by others	14.8	96.1
12. Undue importance placed on appearance in self-evaluation	42.4	80.9
13. Negative evaluation of self based on imagined defect	42.6	87.8
14. Belief of being negatively evaluated by others due to the imagined defect	36.1	90.4
15. Rating of self-attractiveness	32.8	84.8
16a. Fluctuation in thinking/feeling *	34.4	74.0
16b. Ever believed not defected *	50.0	76.8
17. Avoidance of being around strangers	14.8	96.1
18. Avoidance of being around familiar people	14.8	98.7
19. Avoidance of physical contact	27.9	92.2
20. Restricting amount of contact during physical contact	39.3	88.3
21. Avoidance of physical activities	21.3	94.8
22. Camouflaging the imagined defect through dressing/grooming	77.0	52.0
23. Camouflaging the imagined defect through posturing/body movements †	68.9	70.3
24. Avoidance of looking at body	32.8	88.3
25. Avoidance of others seeing the body part unveiled	52.5	82.1
26. Comparing imagined defect to others' body parts †	67.2	71.4

ED = eating disorder, *BDDE-SR* = body dysmorphic disorder examination, short form, Sens. (sensitivity) = % of people with a probable eating disorder who endorsed the item, Spec. (specificity) = % of people without a probable eating disorder who did not endorse the item, † items with sensitivity and specificity > 60%; *items were yes/no dichotomous questions, where sensitivity was defined as % of participants with a probable eating disorder who answered 'no' and specificity was the % of participants without a probable eating disorder who answered 'yes'.

since assessment and treatment are generally guided by disorder-specific models [19,27,29]. Consequently, while disorders can share similarities, such as the EDs and BDD; their treatments are notably distinct - transdiagnostic CBT for the EDs [19] versus exposure and response prevention for BDD [16]. This study aimed to explore the applicability of symptoms associated with the model of BDD [17] to EDs in terms of presence, predictive utility, and association with distress and impairment.

In terms of presence, as hypothesized, this study found that almost all BDD symptoms measured by the BDDE-SR were more common in participants with EDs and BDD than in control participants. This supports findings from previous research [23,24]. It was also hypothesized that BDD participants would report more severe BDD symptoms than ED participants. While this was supported generally, with BDD participants having higher total BDDE-SR scores; closer inspection however revealed no significant differences on half of the BDDE-SR items that measured specific features between ED and BDD participants.

Items on which BDD participants tended to score higher than ED participants measured cognitive features such as dissatisfaction and preoccupation with appearance, overvaluation of appearance, and negative evaluation of self based on appearance. This is in

Table 4 Multiple linear regressions with body dysmorphic and eating disorder symptoms as predictors of distress and impairment in participants with a probable ED (n = 61)

Dependent	Significant predictors	B	SE (B)	β	t	p	R^2_{adj}
1. K-10	BDDE-SR Total	0.16	0.02	0.66	6.39	0.00	0.42
	EDE-Q Global	*n.s.*					
2. SF-12 MCS	BDDE-SR Total	*n.s.*					
	EDE-Q Global	−3.87	1.31	−0.40	−2.96	0.01	0.14
3. SF-12 PCS	BDDE-SR Total	−0.12	0.03	−0.52	−4.05	0.00	0.25
	EDE-Q Global	*n.s.*					

ED = eating disorder, R^2_{adj} = variance in the dependent variable accounted for by the predictor variables, adjusting for statistical shrinkage, K-10 = Kessler psychological distress scale, *SF-12* = Medical outcomes study short form, *PCS* = Physical component summary scale, *MCS* = Mental component summary scale, *EDE-Q* = Eating disorders examination questionnaire.

partial support of previous research that also found greater negative evaluation of self [23] and overvaluation of appearance [24] associated with BDD versus EDs. In contrast however, Rosen and Ramirez [23] found that preoccupation with appearance was similar between participants with EDs and BDD. In the present study, scores on an item assessing whether participants ever "thought their appearance was basically normal" also suggested that BDD participants had a greater level of distorted beliefs regarding ugliness [25] compared to ED participants. Indeed previous research has suggested that around 50% of patients with BDD may have preoccupations of delusional intensity [36].

On the other hand, the items on which BDD and ED participants scored similarly tended to measure the frequency of mental and behavioral acts such as appearance checking, reassurance-seeking, camouflaging, comparison-making, and social avoidance. This supports previous research findings that checking is common in patients with EDs [20,21]. It also expands on the work of Rosen and Ramirez [23], who found that a construct of checking, reassurance-seeking, and comparison-making was equally common in EDs and BDD; our findings indicate that this is true for each of these symptoms separately.

The ability to predict 'caseness' is also important in considering the key clinical features associated with disorders. This study found that the vast majority of the BDDE-SR items had high specificity to ED cases, suggestive that BDD symptoms may not be commonly observed in people without an ED in the general community. Fewer items had high sensitivity to ED cases, meaning that not all people with EDs experience BDD-type features. The items that did have relatively high sensitivity to ED cases measured checking, camouflaging, and comparison-making behaviors; as well as preoccupation and dissatisfaction with appearance. All of these items also had reasonably high specificity, and thus there is a strong case that these symptoms are particularly predictive of people with EDs.

The DSM defines syndromes as being clinically meaningful if they are associated with significant distress and/or impairment in important areas of functioning (e.g. criterion B in Body Dysmorphic Disorder) [4]. This study found that the presence of BDD symptoms in participants with a probable ED was a significant predictor of and explained a large proportion of the variance in scores on the K-10 and the physical component subscale of the SF-12, independent of the severity of ED symptoms. Given that the K-10 and SF-12 are indicators of psychological distress and practical limitations in important areas of functioning, respectively, these findings indicate that BDD symptoms are in fact clinically significant for people with EDs. It was of interest to note that while BDD symptoms were a significant predictor of scores on the physical component subscale, this was not true for the mental component subscale of the SF-12. Rather, mental health scores appeared to be accounted for by ED severity, as indicated by scores on the EDE-Q.

Strengths and limitations

An important strength of this study was the assessment of specific BDD symptoms (e.g. checking behavior, preoccupation with appearance), as opposed to whole psychological constructs (e.g. body image disturbance). This enabled a detailed analysis of the applicability of BDD on a symptom-level, complementing previous diagnostic-level research [6-9]. Another strength was the use of non-clinical cohorts, which, given the low rates of treatment-seeking in people with body image disorders [11-13], allowed for a more representative study than previous research using clinical treatment samples. Previous population-based research has shown that the average age of people who report regular ED behaviors is between 34 and 48 years [37]. The average age of participants with probable EDs in the current study was 39 years, and thus appears to be in line with findings from the broader population. Participants in clinical studies however do tend to be younger, which may indicate that caution should be taken in generalizing the current findings to patients in a treatment setting. Future replication with a younger sample would clarify this.

The relative limitations of this study include foremost the validity of the BDD group. While participants in this group were all cases of probable BDD, 15 of these 23 participants also had a comorbid probable ED. Thus a possible explanation for the greater severity in this group could have been the comorbidity. However this would have been a greater problem for interpreting the data if the aim of this study had been to assess ED symptoms in a BDD sample. Attempts to limit comorbidity confounds were undertaken in the current study by ensuring that the ED group did not include participants with comorbid BDD; and this was critical given the aim of the study was to assess BDD symptoms in participants with EDs. Furthermore the analyses of predictive utility and impact on distress and impairment in this study did not include participants from the BDD group, and thus greater confidence can be afforded for these results. Nonetheless a stronger study in future would make comparisons between non-comorbid groups of participants with EDs and BDD. It would also be of interest in future research to compare the relative presence and function of BDD symptoms across ED diagnoses.

Other limitations relate to analysis. Appearance-fixing behaviours were not included in the 28 likert items of the BDDE-SR. This type of behavior is known to be present in both BDD (e.g. cosmetic surgery, grooming;) [17] and the EDs (e.g. dieting, exercising, purging) [19] and it would have been of interest to compare the two diagnostic groups, especially given previous equivocal findings [24]. Finally, space limitations precluded the inclusion of analyses to examine the impact of each BDDE-SR item separately on distress and impairment. Future studies should report on this.

Clinical implications

The findings of this study indicate that people with EDs may respond similarly to perceived fatness as people with BDD may respond to perceptions of defectiveness in other appearance domains (such as nose size or hair coverage). In particular symptoms that were most prevalent and predictive included preoccupation and dissatisfaction with appearance; and checking, camouflaging, comparison-making, reassurance-seeking, and social avoidance behaviours. This has implications for the assessment and treatment of people with EDs. If these symptoms are indeed common and predictive in people with EDs, as this study suggests, then it is imperative that these symptoms be probed and identified in clinical assessment. Further, if these symptoms are identified as maintaining distress and impairment, then they should also be targeted in treatment interventions.

The presence of BDD symptomatology in probable ED cases and the high correlation between ED and BDD pathology demonstrated in this study might provide support for the proposal of a 'body image disorder' [3] that encompasses both BDD and the EDs. However, apart from shared symptomatology, other factors are also important in clustering disorders into higher-order classes. It has been argued for instance that EDs should not be alongside BDD in the OCD 'spectrum' disorders, on the basis that the gender bias, poorer response to treatment, and lack of familial link to OCD in the EDs sets them apart from the other spectrum disorders [5].

Conclusions

In conclusion, this study, which aimed to assess the applicability of BDD symptoms to EDs, found that a number of specific symptoms traditionally associated with BDD are also common in and predictive of ED cases. Furthermore, BDD pathology as a whole was found to be associated with greater psychological distress and impairment in quality of life in participants with EDs. While future research is needed to validate these findings in community samples free of cross-comorbidity, implications for current clinical practice are to broaden the focus of ED assessment and treatment practices to also cover body dysmorphic symptoms.

Competing interests

The authors declare that they have no competing interests.

Authors' contributions

DM = design, analysis, interpretation, manuscript preparation. RC = design, interpretation, manuscript preparation, review. PH = recruitment, interpretation, manuscript preparation, and review. All authors read and approved the final manuscript.

Acknowledgments

A scholarship was provided to Ms Deborah Mitchison from SARRAH - Services for Australian Rural and Remote Allied Health. Further funding for direct research costs was provided to Ms Mitchison from the University of Western Sydney, School of Medicine. Funding for the initial recruitment and first 5 years of follow-up of participants was provided by The Canberra Hospital Private Practice Fund, Australian Capital Territory (ACT) Health, and Community Care and ACT Mental Health (for participants from The Health and Well-Being of Female ACT Residents Study); and by two mental health project grants from the Australian Rotary Health Research Fund (for participants recruited from tertiary educational institutional campuses).

Author details

[1]School of Psychology and Social Science, University of Western Sydney, Sydney, NSW, Australia. [2]School of Psychology, Charles Sturt University, Bathurst, NSW, Australia. [3]School of Medicine and Centre for Health Research, University of Western Sydney, Sydney, NSW, Australia. [4]School of Medicine, James Cook University, Townsville, QLD, Australia.

References

1. Rosen JC, Reiter J: **Development of the body dysmorphic disorder examination.** *Behav Res Ther* 1996, **34**(9):755–766.

2. Veale D, Boocock A, Gournay K, Dryden W, Shah F, Willson R, Walburn J: **Body dysmorphic disorder, A survey of fifty cases.** *Br J Psychiatry* 1996, **169**(2):196–201.
3. Cororve MB, Gleaves DH: **Body dysmorphic disorder: a review of conceptualizations, assessment, and treatment strategies.** *Clin Psychol Rev* 2001, **21**(6):949–970.
4. American Psychiatric Association: *Diagnostic and Statistical Manual for Mental Disorders Fourth Edition, Text Revision edition.* Washington DC: American Psychiatric Association; 2000.
5. Grant J, Phillips KA: **Is anorexia nervosa a subtype of body dysmorphic disorder? Probably not, but read on.** *Harv Rev Psychiatry* 2004, **12**(2):123–126.
6. Dingemans AE, van Rood YR, de Groot I, van Furth EF: **Body dysmorphic disorder in patients with an eating disorder: Prevalence and characteristics.** *Int J Eat Disord* 2012, **45**(4):562–569.
7. Rosen JC, Reiter J, Orosan P: **Assessment of body image in eating disorders with the Body Dysmorphic Disorder Examination.** *Behav Res Ther* 1995, **33**(1):77–84.
8. Grant J, Kim SW, Eckert ED: **Body dysmorphic disorder in patients with anorexia nervosa: Prevalence, clinical features, and delusionality of body image.** *Int J Eat Disord* 2002, **32**(3):291–300.
9. Ruffolo JS, Phillips KA, Menard W, Fay C, Weisberg RB: **Comorbidity of body dysmorphic disorder and eating disorders: severity of psychopathology and body image disturbance.** *Int J Eat Disord* 2006, **39**(1):11–19.
10. Mackenzie CS, Reynolds K, Cairney J, Streiner DL, Sareen J: **Disorder-specific mental health service use for mood and anxiety disorders: associations with age, sex, and psychiatric comorbidity.** *Depress Anxiety* 2012, **29**(3):234–242.
11. Evans EJ, Hay PJ, Mond J, Paxton SJ, Quirk F, Rodgers B, Jhajj AK, Sawoniewska MA: **Barriers to help-seeking in young women with eating disorders: a qualitative exploration in a longitudinal community survey.** *Eat Disord: The Journal of Treatment & Prevention* 2011, **19**(3):270–285.
12. Grant J, Kim S, Crow S: **Prevalence and clinical features of body dysmorphic disorder in adolescent and adult psychiatric inpatients.** *J Clin Psychiatry* 2001, **62**(7):517–522.
13. Hart L, Granillo M, Jorm A, Paxton S: **Unmet need for treatment in the eating disorders: a systematic review of eating disorder specific treatment seeking among community cases.** *Clin Psychol Rev* 2011, **31**:727–735.
14. American Psychiatric Association: *DSM-5 development: Obsessive-compulsive and related disorders.* 2012. Retrieved 6th September, 2012.
15. Phillips KA, Hollander E, Rasmussen SA, Aronowitz BR, DeCaria C, Goodman WK: **A severity rating scale for body dysmorphic disorder: development, reliability, and validity of a modified version of the Yale-Brown Obsessive Compulsive Scale.** *Psychopharmacol Bull* 1997, **33**(1):17–22.
16. National Institute for Clinical Excellence: *Obsessive-compulsive disorder: core interventions in the treatment of obsessive-compulsive disorder and body dysmorphic disorder*; 2005.
17. Veale D: **Advances in a cognitive behavioural model of body dysmorphic disorder.** *Body Image* 2004, **1**(1):113–125.
18. Veale D, Gournay K, Dryden W, Boocock A, Shah F, Willson R, Walburn J: **Body dysmorphic disorder: A cognitive behavioural model and pilot randomised controlled trial.** *Behav Res Ther* 1996, **34**(9):717–729.
19. Fairburn CG, Cooper Z, Shafran R: **Cognitive behaviour therapy for eating disorders: a "transdiagnostic" theory and treatment.** *Behav Res Ther* 2003, **41**(5):509–528.
20. Reas DL, Grilo CM, Masheb RM, Wilson GT: **Body checking and avoidance in overweight patients with binge eating disorder.** *Int J Eat Disord* 2005, **37**(4):342–346.
21. Shafran R, Fairburn CG, Robinson P, Lask B: **Body checking and its avoidance in eating disorders.** *Int J Eat Disord* 2004, **35**(1):93–101.
22. Mazzeo SE: **Modification of an existing measure of body image preoccupation and its relationship to disordered eating in female college students.** *J Couns Psychol* 1999, **46**(1):42–50.
23. Rosen JC, Ramirez E: **A comparison of eating disorders and body dysmorphic disorder on body image and psychological adjustment.** *J Psychosom Res* 1998, **44**(3–4):441–449.
24. Hrabosky JI, Cash TF, Veale D, Neziroglu F, Soll EA, Garner DM, Strachan-Kinser M, Bakke B, Clauss LJ, Phillips KA: **Multidimensional body image comparisons among patients with eating disorders, body dysmorphic disorder, and clinical controls: a multisite study.** *Body Image* 2009, **6**(3):155–163.
25. Rosen JC, Reiter J: *The body dysmorphic disorder examination: Self report (BDDE-SR).* University of Vermont: Department of Psychology; 1994. Unpublished instrument.
26. Mond JM, Hay PJ, Rodgers B, Owen C, Beumont PJV: **Validity of the Eating Disorder Examination Questionnaire (EDE-Q) in screening for eating disorders in community samples.** *Behav Res Ther* 2004, **42**(5):551–567.
27. Fairburn CG, Cooper Z: **The Eating Disorder Examination.** In *Binge Eating: Nature, Assessment and Treatment*, Volume 12th Ed. Edited by Fairburn CG, Wilson G. New York: Guildford Press; 1993.
28. Mond JM, Hay PJ, Paxton SJ, Rodgers B, Darby A, Nillson J, Quirk F, Owen C: **Eating disorders 'mental health literacy' in low risk, high risk and symptomatic women: implications for health promotion programs.** *Eat Disord: The Journal of Treatment & Prevention* 2010, **18**(4):267–285.
29. Fairburn CG: **Eating Disorder Examination Questionnaire.** In *Cognitive behaviour therapy and eating disorders.* New York: Guilford Press; 2008.
30. Hay PJ, Buettner P, Mond J, Paxton SJ, Quirk F, Rodgers B: **A community-based study of enduring eating features in young women.** *Nutrients* 2012, **4**(5):413–424.
31. Mond JM, Hay PJ, Rodgers B, Owen C: **Eating Disorder Examination Questionnaire (EDE-Q): Norms for young adult women.** *Behav Res Ther* 2006, **44**(1):53–62.
32. Mond JM, Myers TC, Crosby RD, Hay PJ, Rodgers B, Morgan JF, Hubert Lacey J, Mitchell JE: **Screening for eating disorders in primary care: EDE-Q versus SCOFF.** *Behav Res Ther* 2008, **46**(5):612–622.
33. Kessler R, Andrews G, Colpe L, Hiripi E, Mroczek D, Normand S-L, Walters E, Zaslavsky A: **Short screening scales to monitor population prevalences and trends in non-specific psychological distress.** *Psychol Med* 2002, **32**(06):959–976.
34. Ware JEJ, Kosinski M, Keller SD: **A 12-item short-form health survey: construction of scales and preliminary tests of reliability and validity.** *Med Care* 1996, **34**(3):220–233.
35. Sanderson K, Andrews G: **The SF-12 in the Australian population: cross-validation of item selection.** *Aust N Z J Public Health* 2002, **26**(4):343–345.
36. Phillips KA, McElroy SL: **Insight, overvalued ideation, and delusional thinking in body dysmorphic disorder: theoretical and treatment implications.** *J Nerv Ment Dis* 1993, **181**(11):699–702.
37. Hay PJ, Mond J, Buttner P, Darby A: **Eating disorder behaviors are increasing: findings from two sequential community surveys in South Australia.** *PLoS One* 2008, **3**(2):e1541.

12

What can we learn from the history of male anorexia nervosa?

Chengyuan Zhang

Abstract

The eating disorders literature has focussed on females and little is known of the male experience. The overall image this has generated suggests a young woman in conflict with socio-cultural pressures which associate thinness with beauty. Historical studies have examined anorexia nervosa from an entirely female focus while ignoring how diagnostic categories have shaped approaches to the male body. This paper will track the case of the male with anorexia nervosa through changing theories of causation and treatment approaches, from when the condition first emerged in 1873 to the present. In doing so, we gain a valuable new insight into how anorexia nervosa has been historically gendered and the far-reaching implications this has had for diagnosis and treatment of the male sufferer.

Similarities between the sexes helped to establish male anorexia as a distinct category. However, this shifted focus away from important differences, which have yet unexplored implications in the assessment, diagnosis and management of disordered eating. Throughout history, there has been constant pressure to give a precise definition to anorexia nervosa, despite being fraught with medical uncertainties. This has resulted in inevitably harmful generalisations rooted in the dominant epidemiology. This paper reveals that anorexia nervosa is a truly global phenomenon which cannot be adequately constructed through exclusive studies of the female. There is consequently a pressing need to address the dearth of research examining eating disorders in males.

Keywords: Anorexia nervosa, Eating disorder, History of psychiatry

Background

Anorexia nervosa is currently viewed as an almost exclusively female disorder and women account for 90% of those diagnosed. However, an estimated 3 in 10 cases occur in males who are often overlooked, underdiagnosed and understudied in research [1]. Ever since the clinical term was first coined by Sir William Gull in 1874, anorexia nervosa has been bound to an inherently female nosology. Over-simplistic explanations throughout history, from hysteria, ovarian failure and oral impregnation to the thin female ideal, have resulted from the assumption of a unilaterally female epidemiology. These have produced treatment approaches which, throughout history, have persistently neglected to consider the important differences between men and women struggling with disordered eating.

Correspondence: chengyuan.zhang09@imperial.ac.uk
Imperial College London; South Kensington Campus, SW7 2AZ, Exhibition Road, London, UK

A historical perspective

In an address to the Clinical Society on 'Anorexia Hysterica (Apepsia Hysterica)' in 1873, Sir William Gull described a disease 'occurring mostly in young women between the ages of fifteen and twenty-three, and characterised by extreme emaciation' [2]. Gull made no mention of males and despite introducing the term 'Anorexia Nervosa' a year later, the condition became intimately tied to hysteria, an inherently female diagnosis [3]. The main treatment approach was separation from the family, as the 'thin-blooded emotional' female was seen as 'a vampire who sucks the blood of the healthy people about her' [4]. Yet, while still dominant in the years before and after the First World War, this orientation would be challenged from two different quarters: new psychiatric approaches, partly stemming from interest in war-related conditions, notably shell-shock, and in the socio-genic role of the family, began to explore 'male anorexia'; and the new science of endocrinology sought to establish a biochemical basis for anorexia, igniting dynamic debate over the existence of male forms of the disorder.

The first medical definitions of anorexia nervosa left little room for identifying male sufferers. Increasingly, however, anorexia nervosa was being reframed as a psychiatric problem linked to dysfunction within the family. This made it possible to conceive of a male form of anorexia. In 1931, a group of eminent British physicians attributed male cases to 'an authoritarian father, and a weak (crushed) mother' and being 'homosexualist' [5]. This family-oriented explanation derived from preconceptions of hysteria and a focus on the mother-daughter relationship within families of adolescent girls. However, there was a lack of knowledge surrounding male family dynamics which has persisted to the present [6]. Despite this, males with anorexia nervosa were viewed as effeminate homosexuals who, like their female counterparts, needed to be isolated from their families.

One of the first challenges to earlier models centred on hysteria came in 1914 through descriptions of Simmonds' disease, an endocrine disorder of the pituitary gland which closely resembled anorexia nervosa, with amenorrhoea as a key symptom of both conditions [7]. Physicians searched for an endocrine cause of amenorrhoea, erasing male cases altogether by connecting anorexia nervosa with 'primary ovarian failure' [8]. Oestrogen injections were given to stimulate menstrual periods, generating a focus on amenorrhoea which became embedded within diagnostic categories until DSM-5 [9]. However, during the course of successive DSM revisions, studies have repeatedly questioned the diagnostic relevance of amenorrhoea, demonstrating that it reflects nutritional status rather than psychopathology [10-12]. Furthermore, the absence of an analogous criterion for men built a gender bias into the first definitions of the disorder.

By the 1940s, a new approach rooted in Freudian psychoanalysis had seized the ground. Anorexia nervosa was framed as a female sexual neurosis where food was associated with impregnation and obesity with pregnancy [13]. Amenorrhoea was now seen as a direct psychological consequence of pregnancy fantasies and constipation symbolised the child in the abdomen [13]. Despite aims of developing a singular explanation for anorexia nervosa, psychosexual approaches focussed on female sexual dysfunction, which was targeted aggressively by psychotherapy. Oestrogen treatment continued, not to compensate for any ovarian failure, but for 'ovarian deficiencies' linked to the 'anorectic's psychic state' [7].

However, neither oestrogen injections nor psychotherapy produced positive results, and these ideas were increasingly challenged [14]. Hilde Bruch championed new approaches to the disorder in the 1960s, finding the same core features in male and female cases, including an endocrine dysfunction 'gauged by urinary output of testosterone' comparable to amenorrhoea [15,16]. These findings, embodied by DSM-III in 1980, redefined anorexia nervosa, with 'distortion of body image' and 'fear of ugliness' as its primary features [15,17]. However, attention to similarities between the sexes shifted focus away from important differences. As a result, treatment approaches generated exclusively by studies on female subjects went unchallenged when applied often inappropriately to their male counterparts.

Subsequently, second-wave feminism around the 1980s framed anorexia nervosa as evidence of a misogynistic society which objectified the female body and devalued female experiences. This helped to establish a psychotherapeutic approach targeting female body image issues within 'a culture that praises thinness and fragility in women' [18,19]. To this day, psychotherapy does not comprehensively address the disorder in males. Feminist analyses have disregarded the male as an unlikely candidate for the diagnosis. As psychologist Julie Hepworth argues, male cases provided 'a discursive problem because the dominant explanation of anorexia nervosa specifically links it with an ideology of femininity' [20]. In light of feminist socio-cultural framing, males are still often excluded from clinical research, despite the same core psychopathology in both sexes. Additionally, the widely used Eating Disorders Inventory-3, developed from and validated in female populations to predict eating disorders, has drawn criticism for its lower reliability in men [21]. Given men are already underdiagnosed, there is a pressing need to construct a validated male-specific assessment tool.

Lessons for the future

Insufficient attention has been given to reasons why males develop the disorder. Feminists have framed the disorder as one which is socially produced by patriarchical social structures; what happens to non-dominant males within a patriarchy is never specified. While gender has been a key 'category of analysis' [22], it has been used asymmetrically, concentrating on how anorexia nervosa has been gendered as 'female' while ignoring how it shaped approaches to the male body. Within this framework, feminists have assumed that men are also subject to many of the same social pressures of aestheticism as women, without separate study of the male subject [23].

Yet, feminist concern with how gender shapes social and medical categories is critical to better understanding male anorexia nervosa and, crucially, to its acceptance as a condition. Women and men are 'defined in terms of one another' and anorexia nervosa cannot therefore be adequately constructed by entirely separate study of the female [22]. This approach has historically created a string of stigmatising suppositions which have all failed to fully encapsulate the condition. Early female victims were cruelly force-fed to combat an emaciation thought to result from emotional excesses or inappropriate sexual fantasies of oral conception and pregnancy. Men were either missing from medical discourses or feminised as homosexuals. Whilst homosexuality is currently a specific risk factor for anorexia nervosa in men, 'most men with body image disorders are straight and most gay men do not have body image disorders' [24,25]. Diagnostic categories have repeatedly been created out of assumptions, supported by examples which affirm the definition whilst ignoring exceptions which the dominant rule cannot explain.

Currently, this approach stigmatises sufferers as young women trapped in a vicious cycle to achieve a thin-ideal. This view has fundamentally shaped the identity and status of male sufferers who bear the added burden of a feminised diagnosis. Yet, the literature reveals crucial differences between male and female experiences of eating disorders which may have unexplored treatment implications [26]. It has recently been suggested that muscle dysmorphia, which shares a similar concern for body image, food intake and exercise, may be classified as an eating disorder with a predominantly male epidemiology [27]. The similarities that can be drawn with anorexia nervosa emphasise a need to understand male experiences of body image disturbance and the impact constructions of masculinity and femininity have on the sufferer [28].

Whilst anorexia nervosa and bulimia nervosa are strongly associated with the female sex, several epidemiological studies have found binge eating to be equally common in men and women [29]. Emerging evidence also suggests that binge eating may be more debilitating for men [30]. However, few studies on binge eating have included men despite this equal gender distribution. The way in which anorexia nervosa has been historically constructed as a 'woman's illness' has enduring implications in the way we currently view eating disorders in general. At present, men are less likely to receive treatment and are treated for fewer days [31]. We must therefore decouple the experience of eating disorders from feminised cultural imagery in order to break down the barriers men face in recognising their symptoms and seeking help [32]. There is a need to explore specifically and in detail what it is like to inhabit a male body in the context of anorexia nervosa. Only then can we appropriately clarify fact from fiction – what anorexia nervosa really is and what it is not – to improve the way we assess, diagnose and treat all groups of people.

Competing interests

The author declares that he has no competing interests.

Acknowledgements

I would like to thank Michael Bresalier, Julie Hipperson and Emily Mayhew for their helpful comments on earlier drafts of this article.

References

1. Andersen AE: **Eating disorders in males.** In *In Eating disorders and obesity: a comprehensive handbook.* 2nd edition. Edited by Fairburn GC, Brownell KD. New York: Guildford Press; 2002:210–214.
2. Anonymous: **Clinical Society of London. Friday, 24 October.** *Med Times Gaz* 1873, **2:**534–535.
3. Gull WW: **Anorexia nervosa (apepsia hysterica, anorexia hysterica).** *Trans Clin Soc Lond* 1874, **7:**180–185.
4. Mitchell SW: *Fat and blood: and how to make them.* Philadelphia: J. B. Lippincott & co.; 1878.
5. Langdon-Brown W, Crookshank FG, Young JC, Gordon G, Bevan-Brown J: *Anorexia nervosa: a discussion.* London: The C. W. Daniel Company; 1931.
6. May AL, Kim JY, McHale SM C, Crouter A: **Parent-adolescent relationships and the development of weight concerns from early to late adolescence.** *Int J Eat Disord* 2006, **39**(8):729–740.
7. Brumberg JJ: *Fasting girls: The history of anorexia nervosa.* New York: Vintage Books; 2000.
8. Nicolle G: **Pre-Psychotic Anorexia: (Section of Psychiatry).** *Proc R Soc Med* 1939, **32**(3):153–162.
9. American Psychiatric Association: *Diagnostic and Statistical Manual of Mental Disorders.* 5th edition. Washington, DC: American Psychiatric Association; 2013.
10. Cachelin FM, Maher BA: **Is amenorrhea a critical criterion for anorexia nervosa?** *J Psychosom Res* 1998, **44**(3–4):435–440.
11. Roberto CA, Steinglass J, Mayer LE, Attia E, Walsh BT: **The clinical significance of amenorrhea as a diagnostic criterion for anorexia nervosa.** *Int J Eat Disord* 2008, **41**(6):559–563.
12. Attia E, Roberto CA: **Should amenorrhea be a diagnostic criterion for anorexia nervosa?** *Int J Eat Disord* 2009, **42**(7):581–589.
13. Waller JV, Kaufman MR, Deutsch F: **Anorexia nervosa: A psychosomatic entity.** *Psychosom Med* 1940, **2:**3–16.
14. Kay DWK: **Anorexia nervosa: a study in prognosis.** *Proc R Soc Med* 1953, **46**(8):669–674.
15. Bruch H: **Perceptual and conceptual disturbances in anorexia nervosa.** *Psychosom Med* 1962, **24:**187–194.
16. Beumont PJV, Beardwood CJ, Russell GFM: **The occurrence of the syndrome of anorexia nervosa in male subjects.** *Psychol Med* 1972, **2**(3):216–231.
17. American Psychiatric Association: *Diagnostic and Statistical Manual of Mental Disorders.* 3rd edition. Washington, DC: American Psychiatric Association; 1980.
18. Orbach S: *Fat is a feminist issue.* London: Paddington Press; 1978.
19. Orbach S: **Accepting the symptom: A feminist psychoanalytic treatment of anorexia nervosa.** In *Handbook of psychotherapy for anorexia nervosa and bulimia.* Edited by Garner DM, Garfinkel PE. New York, London: The Guildford Press; 1985:83–104.
20. Hepworth J: *The social construction of anorexia nervosa.* London: SAGE Publications; 1999.
21. Stanford SC, Lemberg R: **A clinical comparison of men and women on the Eating Disorder Inventory-3 (EDI-3) and the Eating Disorder Assessment for Men (EDAM).** *Eat Disord* 2012, **20**(5):379–394.
22. Scott JW: **Gender: A useful category of historical analysis.** *Am Hist Rev* 1986, **91:**1053–1075.
23. Bordo SR: *The male body: A new look at men in public and in private.* New York: Farrar, Straus and Giroux; 1999.
24. Russell CJ, Keel PK: **Homosexuality as a specific risk factor for eating disorders in men.** *Int J Eat Disord* 2002, **31**(3):300–306.
25. Morgan J: *The invisible man: A self-help guide for men with eating disorders, compulsive exercise, and bigorexia.* New York: Routledge; 2008.
26. Fichter M, Krenn H: **Eating disorders in males.** In *Handbook of eating disorders: Theory, treatment and research.* 2nd edition. Edited by Treasure J, Schmidt U, van Furth E. Chichester: Wiley Blackwell; 2003.
27. Murray SB, Rieger E, Touyz SW, De la Garza Garcia Lic Y: **Muscle dysmorphia and the DSM-V conundrum: where does it belong? A review paper.** *Int J Eat Disord* 2010, **43**(6):483–491.
28. Murray SB, Rieger E, Karlov L, Touyz SW: **Masculinity and femininity in the divergence of male body image concerns.** *J Eat Disord* 2013, **1:**11.
29. Striegel RH, Bedrosian R, Wang C, Schwartz S: **Why men should be included in research on binge eating: results from a comparison of psychosocial impairment in men and women.** *Int J Eat Disord* 2012, **45**(2):233–240.
30. Mitchison D, Mond J, Slewa-Younan S, Hay P: **Sex differences in health-related quality of life impairment associated with eating disorder features: a general population study.** *Int J Eat Disord* 2013, **46**(4):375–380.

31. Striegel-Moore RH, Leslie D, Petrill SA, Garvin V, Rosenheck RA: **One-year use and cost of inpatient and outpatient services among female and male patients with an eating disorder: evidence from a national database of health insurance claims.** *Int J Eat Disord* 2000, **27**(4):381–389.
32. Räisänen U, Hunt K: **The role of gendered constructions of eating disorders in delayed help-seeking in men: a qualitative interview study.** *BMJ Open* 2014, **4**(4):e004342.

Mapping the evidence for the prevention and treatment of eating disorders in young people

Alan P Bailey[1,2*], Alexandra G Parker[1,2], Lauren A Colautti[1,2], Laura M Hart[3], Ping Liu[1,2] and Sarah E Hetrick[1,2]

Abstract: Eating disorders often develop during adolescence and young adulthood, and are associated with significant psychological and physical burden. Identifying evidence-based interventions is critical and there is need to take stock of the extant literature, to inform clinical practice regarding well-researched interventions and to direct future research agendas by identifying gaps in the evidence base.

Aim: To investigate and quantify the nature and distribution of existing high-quality research on the prevention and treatment of eating disorders in young people using evidence mapping methodology.

Method: A systematic search for prevention and treatment intervention studies in adolescents and young adults (12–25 years) was conducted using EMBASE, PSYCINFO and MEDLINE. Studies were screened and mapped according to disorder, intervention modality, stage of eating disorder and study design. Included studies were restricted to controlled trials and systematic reviews published since 1980.

Results: The eating disorders evidence map included 197 trials and 22 systematic reviews. Prevention research was dominated by trials of psychoeducation (PE). Bulimia nervosa (BN) received the most attention in the treatment literature, with cognitive behavioural therapy (CBT) and antidepressants the most common interventions. For anorexia nervosa (AN), family based therapy (FBT) was the most studied. Lacking were trials exploring treatments for binge eating disorder (BED) and eating disorder not otherwise specified (EDNOS). Relapse prevention strategies were notably absent across the eating disorders.

Conclusions: Despite substantial literature devoted to the prevention and treatment of eating disorders in young people, the evidence base is not well established and significant gaps remain. For those identified as being at-risk, there is need for prevention research exploring strategies other than passive PE. Treatment interventions targeting BED and EDNOS are required, as are systematic reviews synthesising BN treatment trials (e.g., CBT, antidepressants). FBTs for AN require investigation against other validated psychological interventions, and the development of relapse prevention strategies is urgently required. By systematically identifying existing interventions for young people with eating disorders and exposing gaps in the current literature, the evidence map can inform researchers, funding bodies and policy makers as to the opportunities for future research.

Keywords: Eating disorders, Treatment, Prevention, Evidence mapping, Adolescent, Young adult

Introduction

Adolescence and young adulthood is recognized as a period of heightened risk for the development of eating disorders. International epidemiological studies estimate 75% of anorexia nervosa (AN) and bulimia nervosa (BN) cases and 50% of binge eating disorder (BED) and eating disorder not otherwise specified (EDNOS) cases onset before the age of 22 [1,2]. Eating disorders are recognised as a significant public health issue with Australian data indicating that they represent the second leading cause of disability due to mental disorder in females aged 10–24 years [3]. The psychological, social and physical ramifications of eating disorders are severe [4,5]. A recent meta-analysis showed mortality rates to be twice as high in those with BN and EDNOS and close to six times higher in people with AN when compared to expected population mortality rates [6]. Suicide contributes significantly to these high

* Correspondence: alan.bailey@unimelb.edu.au
[1]Orygen Youth Health Research Centre, Centre for Youth Mental Health, The University of Melbourne, Locked Bag 10, Parkville, Melbourne, Victoria 3052, Australia
[2]Centre of Excellence in Youth Mental Health, headspace National Youth Mental Health Foundation Ltd, Level 2, South Tower, 485 La Trobe Street, Melbourne, Victoria 3000, Australia
Full list of author information is available at the end of the article

mortality rates, with rates of suicide elevated among those with eating disorders [7-9]. Comorbidity with depression, anxiety and substance use disorders is common [10-13], adding significantly to the burden. Additionally, the estimated financial cost associated with disability-adjusted life years attributable to eating disorders is higher than that of depression and anxiety combined [14].

Given the severity and burden associated with eating disorders, and the particular vulnerability across the adolescent and young adult period, there is pressing need to both develop, and encourage the uptake of, evidence-based prevention and intervention strategies with this population. Despite the need, and consistent with mental health research generally [15], evidence-based interventions are far from universally delivered in the clinical management of eating disorders [16-19]. For example, cognitive behavioural therapy (CBT) is recognised as an empirically supported intervention and the 'treatment of choice' for BN [20-22], yet surveys of clinicians indicate a majority do not use CBT as their primary psychological treatment choice [23,24]. This highlights a significant evidence-practice gap.

A commonly cited barrier to incorporating evidence into daily clinical practice is the time and resources required to navigate the large volume of extant research literature (e.g., [25]). This points to the need for translational tools that make these vast bodies of literature accessible, digestible and usable. One such approach to knowledge translation and exchange is evidence mapping; an established methodology for collating and summarising the literature in a manner that enables the breadth of the research activity in a particular field to be explored (e.g., [26-28]). Evidence maps are based on an explicit research question relating to the field of enquiry, which drives the search for, and collection of, appropriate studies utilising explicit, systematic and reproducible methods [29-32]. The key difference from a systematic review is that the purpose of evidence mapping is to provide a broad overview of existing research, with the view to identifying evidence, and therefore does not include an in-depth quality appraisal and synthesis of the findings [30]. The end-user may be: 1) Researchers or research funding bodies who can utilise the gaps in the evidence highlighted in the evidence map to drive their research agenda; 2) Policy makers who can use the evidence map to inform policy decisions; and 3) Clinicians who can quickly and easily access information about interventions.

This paper presents the results of an evidence map we conducted on eating disorders in adolescents and young adults. The extent, range and nature of high-quality clinical research interventions for eating disorders in this population is summarised, gaps in the evidence base are identified and opportunities for future research are discussed. This process of taking stock of the evidence is an essential first step in collating the breadth of research activity in an area before further exploring the effectiveness of interventions.

Methods and materials

The eating disorder evidence map was produced as part of a larger evidence-mapping project undertaken by the Centre of Excellence (CoE) in Youth Mental Health (part of headspace; the Australian National Youth Mental Health Foundation). A detailed description of the methodology for evidence mapping has been published elsewhere [31]; methods specific to the eating disorder map are provided below.

Creating a map based on broad clinical questions relating to the field of enquiry

After consultation with expert youth mental health researchers and clinicians working within the eating disorders field at Orygen Youth Health Research Centre and headspace, the questions and scope of the mapping project were defined. This process revealed two critical questions:

i. What evidence exists regarding interventions for eating disorders in the youth population?
ii. What areas are, and are not, well researched?

Defining key variables, specifying characteristics to be mapped and developing inclusion and exclusion criteria

Based on these explicit questions, the characteristics of studies to be included in the map were defined, which included specifying the population, stage of eating disorder, measured outcomes and study design.

Population

Included trials were required to have participants with a mean age between 12 and 25 years as their sample, or where the author specified an adolescent and/or young adult population. Studies with both adult and adolescent participants were included if the mean age of any intervention group was 25 years or under. Studies that recruited participants on the basis of physiological or medical conditions (e.g., changes in eating behaviours induced by brain tumour) were excluded.

Stage of eating disorder and outcomes

Prevention, treatment intervention and relapse prevention studies were all included. Prevention trials were categorised as universal or at-risk prevention. Universal interventions were those delivered to a designated population regardless of their risk (e.g., all school students); whereas at-risk prevention interventions were those delivered to either members of a population with an established risk factor for the development of an eating disorder (e.g., athletes) or individuals with signs or symptoms of a disorder such that participants were recruited on the basis of elevated risk factors or sub-threshold presentations of an eating disorder [33].

Studies including those with an established eating disorder diagnosis, classified by the diagnostic and statistical manual of mental disorders (DSM) [34] or the international classification of diseases (ICD) [35], were included where the treatment intervention was "anything delivered for the purpose of relieving symptomatology or improving functioning of the target disorder" [31]. These intervention studies were classified as 'established eating disorder'.

Relapse prevention studies were included if the authors specified the intervention was designed to prevent relapse, or to maintain improvements in individuals with eating disorders who had previously responded to treatment.

Finally, included trials had to measure a specific eating disorder outcome, for example body mass index (BMI), eating disorder symptom measure, binge/purge frequency.

Study design

Our map utilised evidence from randomised controlled trials (RCT), controlled clinical trials (CCT), systematic reviews and meta-analyses, as these are considered the most robust study designs for examining the effectiveness of interventions [36]. Definitions of review types are not consistent and many different terms are used, at times interchangeably [29], therefore we included those reviews providing both a systematic search strategy and the relevant data-bases searched. Additionally reviews had to meet the criteria outlined above. Studies published in English from 1980 to December 2012 were included.

Searching the literature

Search strategies appropriate for each of the MEDLINE, PSYCINFO and EMBASE databases were devised using terms such as "eating disorder", "controlled trial" and "review". Additional terms identified by experts were also included.

Searches targeted the pre-defined inclusion criteria by combining terms describing: type of eating disorder, study methodology and stage of eating disorder (the full search strategy is available upon request to the corresponding author). Search strategies were revised after a random sample of 100 citations was examined and after cross-checking that the search strategy retrieved 20 articles known to meet the inclusion criteria.

Screening and positioning the relevant evidence within the map (charting)

Two authors independently screened 100 references randomly selected from the search results to determine the consistency of applying the inclusion/exclusion criteria (inter-rater reliability > 0.90 was achieved). Two authors then screened all retrieved references and where a title or abstract reported a trial that appeared to be eligible for inclusion, the full article was obtained and assessed against the inclusion and exclusion criteria.

Studies meeting the inclusion criteria were coded by one author and double coded independently by a second author. Discrepancies were discussed and consensus reached. Studies were coded according to: 1. Type of eating disorder; 2. Type of intervention; 3. Stage of eating disorder; and 4. Study design. Type of eating disorder was coded as AN, BN, EDNOS or BED, according to author report of participant classification. Type of intervention was classified as psychological, biological and service/delivery improvement. Stage of eating disorder was coded as universal prevention, at-risk, established eating disorder and relapse prevention. Study designs were coded as RCT/CCT (hereafter referred to as 'trials') and systematic review/meta analysis (hereafter referred to as 'reviews').

Studies that evaluated the effectiveness of more than one type of intervention or eating disorder classification were double coded for each intervention and classification, thus the sum of trials from each coded section is greater than the total number of included studies. The primary reference for each study was established with secondary publications indicated as such. This process prevented counting one trial multiple times and misrepresenting the number of studies in a particular area. In addition to these codes, a qualitative description of the interventions used in each trial was recorded. For the purposes of this paper, where a review was available and included in the map, a short synthesis of the main findings has been provided.

Review

Included trials

Database searches were conducted in February of 2013 and our strategies identified 8,856 references, of which 229 met the predefined inclusion criteria based on title, abstract and full text screening (see Figure 1). The 229 publications included in the final map consisted of 22 reviews, 197 trials and 10 follow-up studies. A list of citations for all included studies in the map is available on request or from our online searchable database (see [37]).

Interventions for prevention

A total of 52 universal prevention studies were identified (46 trials; 6 reviews). Of the 46 trials, psychoeducation based programs were the most common (n = 26), followed by cognitive dissonance (n = 6) and cognitive behavioural based (n = 5) programs. The remaining trials investigated non-specific psychological strategies such as media literacy training, writing tasks and school-based prevention programs.

A total of 46 prevention studies for at-risk populations were identified (40 trials; 6 reviews). Of the trials,

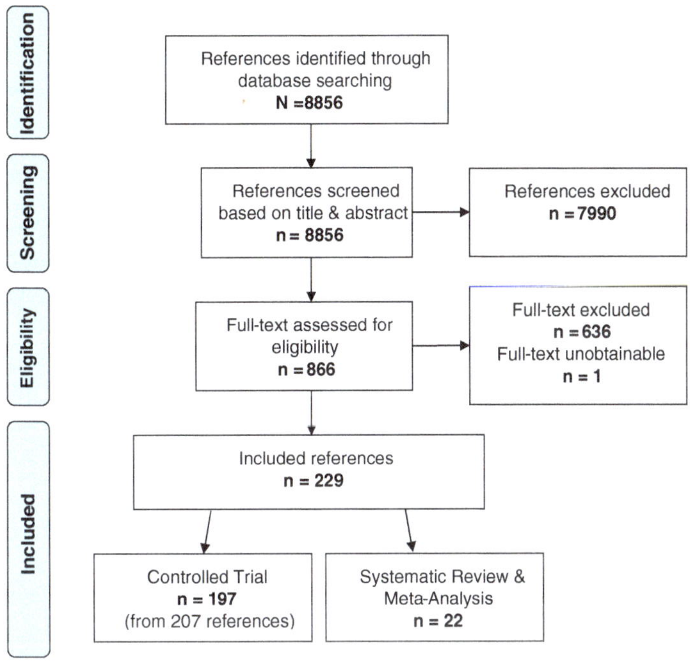

Figure 1 Flow chart of included studies.

psychoeducation based (n = 12) and cognitive dissonance based (n = 12) programs were most common, followed by cognitive-behavioural based programs (n = 7). Other non-specific psychological intervention trials included multicomponent school based programs, media literacy training, writing tasks, relaxation and yoga. Table 1 displays the complete distribution of identified studies for prevention in both universal and at-risk populations.

Reviews summarising prevention programs for both universal and at-risk populations indicate the evidence for their effectiveness is modest and not without significant limitations [38-43]. Meta-analyses of controlled trials indicate prevention programs generally produce large effects on outcomes related to eating disorder knowledge, and only small net effects for other important prevention targets such as reducing exhibited risk factors, changing attitudes and

Table 1 Distribution of included prevention studies

	Intervention	Trial	AN	BN	BED	EDNOS	ED	Review
Universal prevention								
Psychological	Cognitive dissonance	6					6	
	Psychoeducation based	26					26	
	Cognitive/Behavioural based	5					5	1
	Psychological - other	14	1				13	1
	Psychological - general							4
At-risk prevention								
Psychological	Cognitive dissonance	12					12	
	Psychoeducation based	12		2			10	
	Cognitive/Behavioural based	7		1			6	1
	Motivational interviewing	1		1	1	1		
	Psychological - other	18		3	2		13	1
	Psychological - general							4

Legend: AN=anorexia nervosa, BN=bulimia nervosa, BED=binge eating disorder, EDNOS=eating disorder not otherwise specified, ED=eating disorder general.

reducing eating pathology. This has prompted the search for and identification of moderating factors that may lead to larger prevention effects, for example targeting high-risk populations versus universal, utilising active programs delivered in interactive formats versus passive didactic programs (e.g., psychoeducation) and multisession programs versus single session (see [39,42]). Promising preventative effects are generally exhibited directly following program delivery and over the immediate short-term, however little work has been done investigating whether effects are sustained long-term. This lack of follow-up testing combined with the limited use of standardised eating pathology measures and diagnostic criteria makes it difficult to accurately conclude on the preventative effects of most evaluated programs.

Interventions for an established eating disorder

A total of 129 studies investigating interventions for established eating disorders were identified (see Table 2), of which 77 involved psychological interventions (67 trials; 10 reviews), 54 involved biological interventions (47 trials; 7 reviews).

Psychological interventions for established eating disorders

Of the identified studies investigating psychological interventions, the most common strategy for diagnosed

Table 2 Distribution of included disorder established treatment studies

	Intervention	Trial	AN	BN	BED	EDNOS	Review
Psychological	Cognitive & behavioural therapies	27	3	22	2	5	
	Psychoeducation	10	6	6			
	Family based therapy (FBT)	15	12	5		2	5
	Supportive therapy	3	1	3			
	Psychodynamic/Psychoanalysis	5	1	3			1
	Motivational interview/enhancement	4	2	3	1	3	
	Exposure therapy	2		2			
	Interpersonal therapy	2		2			
	Dialectical behavioural therapy	1		1			
	Eye movement desens. & reprocessing	1	1	1		1	
	Psychological - other	27	14	18	2	6	
	Psychological - general						4
Biological	SSRI	15	4	9	1	1	
	TCA	10	3	8			
	SNRI	1				1	
	MAOI	1		1			
	Appetite moderator	6	1	5	1		
	Anticonvulsant	1		1			
	Typical antipsychotic	1	1				2
	Atypical antipsychotic	6	6			1	3
	Lithium	2	1	1			
	Antidepressant - other (trazodone)	1		1			
	Opioid antagonist (naltrexone)	1		1			
	Neutraceutical (inositol)	1		1	1		
	Transcranial magnetic stimulation	1		1			
	Re-feeding	2	2				
	Biological - other	4	3	1			
	Biological - general						4
Service	Service/Delivery improvement	6	3	4		1	

Legend: AN=anorexia nervosa, BN=bulimia nervosa, BED=binge eating disorder, EDNOS=eating disorder not otherwise specified, SSRI=selective serotonin reuptake inhibitor, TCA=tricyclic antidepressant, SNRI=serotonin norepinephrine reuptake inhibitor, MAOI=monoamine oxidase inhibitor.

AN was family based therapy (FBT, 12 trials; 5 reviews). For diagnosed BN, trials were dominated by cognitive behavioural therapy (CBT, n = 22) with a smaller number investigating FBT (n = 5). Psychological intervention trials for EDNOS and BED were scarce in comparison. Table 2 displays the complete distribution of identified studies by type of psychological intervention and type of disorder.

Included reviews of psychological interventions for diagnosed eating disorders were restricted to syntheses of family based therapies (FBT) for AN, with one review also including BN [44-50]. FBT as defined in this paper and summarised in included reviews refers to any intervention where the family constitutes a core intervention component. The most commonly evaluated models include the Maudsley Model [51] and its variants and a highly similar modality called behavioural family systems therapy [52]. Reviews highlight the growing evidence base for FBT in AN, providing summaries of RCTs which support its position in clinical guideline recommendations as a first line treatment. Evidence indicates that FBTs are generally effective with reviews indicating up to half of adolescents receiving the intervention achieving remission. A smaller subset of studies has noted higher rates of remission at follow-up for FBT compared to individual level interventions. FBT also appears to be more effective for younger adolescents and those with a shorter duration of illness, however the majority of trials only report mean participant ages in the 12–18 range. It should be noted that these findings come only from a small number of trials with small sample sizes, where risk of bias is notable. Nonetheless, syntheses from the included reviews provide mostly supportive conclusions for FBT as an effective treatment for AN in young people.

A single recently published review of FBTs investigated this modality in BN [47], summarising two extant RCTs. The first trial found higher remission rates for FBT versus individual supportive therapy at post-treatment and 6 months [53]; the second trial found higher binge abstinence rates for CBT guided self-care versus FBT at post-treatment but no differences at 6 months [54]. FBT is promising but requires further verification in BN before stronger recommendations about its effectiveness can be made. No reviews of other psychological interventions for BN were identified. Similarly reviews for BED and EDNOS were absent.

Biological interventions for established eating disorders

Of the identified studies investigating biological interventions, medications were the most common. For diagnosed BN, selective serotonin reuptake inhibitors (SSRI, n = 9) and tricyclic antidepressants (TCA, n = 8) were the most investigated. For diagnosed AN, antipsychotics (7 trials; 3 reviews) were the most common, followed by SSRIs (n = 4). Biological interventions for EDNOS and BED were almost non-existent. Table 2 displays the complete distribution of identified studies by type of biological intervention and type of disorder.

Included reviews synthesised findings from controlled medication trials and were restricted to investigations of antipsychotics in AN [55-57] and general medication reviews including analyses of antidepressants for AN and BN [58,59]. Reviews of controlled medication trials for EDNOS and BED in our population were absent.

Antipsychotics for AN were synthesized by meta analysis (mean age 22 years across 8 RCTs [56]), with findings indicating no advantage over placebo or treatment as usual in terms of weight gain or symptom improvement.

General medication reviews did not identify any trials investigating antidepressants in adolescents (12–18 years) [58,59]. While trials exist in the younger adult population (18–25 years), these were lost within broad adult level syntheses. For adult AN, the use of both TCAs and SSRIs has not produced encouraging results [58], with safety issues and lack of effectiveness data making translation to younger populations problematic. For adult BN, SSRIs have produced positive findings with moderate effects on binge/purge frequency and reviews indicate their potential utility with young people [58,59]. However this needs to be balanced with the lack of current efficacy and safety data in this younger population, particularly given the controversy surrounding the use of SSRIs with adolescents and young adults in the depression field (see [60]). The lack of trials in adolescents and the urgent need to systematically synthesise existing young adult trials means medication management recommendations are currently restricted to broad adult level evidence.

Interventions for relapse prevention

Research into relapse prevention among young people with eating disorders is limited. Only six trials were identified; five trials in AN (n = 3 CBT; n = 1 psychoeducation; n = 2 SSRI) investigating relapse prevention strategies following successful inpatient weight restoration, and one trial in BN investigating SSRIs delivered after successful psychotherapy (see Table 3). No systematic reviews were identified.

Discussion

The results of the evidence map highlight areas that have received research attention while simultaneously exposing numerous opportunities for research in the area of eating disorder intervention. Gaps in the current evidence base are discussed with a focus on specific research opportunities.

Research opportunities for prevention

Prevention literature is heavily dominated by education based programs and while providing information on

Table 3 Distribution of included relapse prevention studies

	Intervention	Trial	AN	BN	BED	EDNOS	Review
Psychological	Cognitive & behavioural therapies	3	3				
	Psychoeducation	1	1				
Biological	SSRI	3	2	1			

Legend: AN=anorexia nervosa, BN=bulimia nervosa, BED=binge eating disorder, EDNOS=eating disorder not otherwise specified, SSRI=selective serotonin reuptake inhibitor.

etiology and risk does not produce iatrogenic effects [41], these programs are minimally effective in producing behaviour change, outside of increasing knowledge [40]. There are suggestions that programs utilising active prevention components may produce larger effects and many opportunities exist [39,42].

Cognitive dissonance or dissonance induction is one such active prevention approach which involves engaging in counter-attitudinal exercises that target potential risk factors for eating pathology (e.g., body dissatisfaction and internalisation of the 'thin-ideal') [61]. Research to date indicates these interventions show promise in changing attitudes associated with eating pathology over the short term [40-42], however further trials involving long term follow-up are need to determine if lasting effects on standardised eating pathology outcomes are possible. Media literacy programs have also shown promise and incorporating active dissonance exercises and simple CBT techniques has the potential to boost preventative effects.

Interestingly, our map failed to identify any controlled trials investigating prevention strategies involving families. This is curious given eating disorders often develop in adolescence; a time for many when the family structure is critical to functioning. Potential prevention components may involve education and skills-training for parents around talking about and identifying risk factors. Such components may assist in creating awareness, identifying the early stages of disordered eating or other symptomatology, ensuring parents have some control over their child's eating (particularly in those identified as at-risk) and importantly encouraging early help-seeking.

Research opportunities for those with established eating disorders

Systematic reviews

The evidence map revealed a paucity of systematic reviews summarising a range of treatment options for young people across the eating disorders. For example, many trials have now been conducted investigated interventions for BN such as CBT (22 trials) and SSRIs (9 trials) yet systematic reviews of these intervention modalities are absent. Results from individual trials are mixed regarding the effectiveness of either intervention, suggesting that submitting the trials to systematic review and meta-analysis may provide a summary answer to the effectiveness question. While both CBT and SSRIs have received attention in the adult literature, with systematic reviews demonstrating the clinical effectiveness of these approaches [21,62], the comprehensive synthesis of adolescent and young adult trial data would provide important clinical guidance about the appropriateness and effectiveness of these interventions in this younger population.

Stepped-care models of intervention

Stepped care for the management of mental disorders is not a new concept (e.g., [63-65]) yet these intervention models have received limited empirical attention in the field of eating disorders. Our map identified two trials investigating stepped-care models for the treatment of BN in young people [66,67]. Both trials compared a self-help manual with standard CBT in the initial phase, with those failing to respond being offered modified CBT in one trial [67] and fluoxetine plus CBT (if still unresponsive) in the second trial [66]. Both trials indicated that a stepped-care model was as effective as the main CBT intervention delivered, indicating a potentially lower cost/less resource intensive intervention model can produce similar effects.

Stepped care approaches typically commence with low-intensity treatment components and step up, depending on response and stage of illness, to more intensive, individualised, clinician delivered strategies. These are considered advantageous as they can be cost effective in a resource limited field, reduce delay-to-treat time by offering low-intensity components such as self-help as an initial step, and can be tailored to individual treatment plans according to illness severity and treatment response [65,68,69].

While these models do show promise, little can be definitively concluded about the effectiveness and appropriateness of stepped care interventions for young people with eating disorders. Significant questions remain regarding how decisions are made about progressing through intervention 'steps' (e.g., using response and/or stage of illness); appropriateness in younger age groups; how those who do not respond should be managed; and whether these models are appropriate for high severity disorders like AN which typically require intensive, sustained intervention [69]. Given these remaining questions and the potential benefits associated with these models, further research attention is warranted.

Binge eating disorder

Intervention research for BED among the adolescent and young adult population is lacking. Reviews of the adult literature point to CBT as a promising intervention in reducing binge frequency and other associated body image concerns, however changes in BMI are yet to be noted [70,71]. The map identified only two small trials of CBT in the adolescent and young adult population and while some positive effects on bingeing behaviour were noted [72,73], it remains difficult to draw conclusions about its appropriateness and effectiveness.

The promising nature of CBT warrants further investigation in the context of a much greater research effort directed towards BED given it is a stable and chronic syndrome, with serious physical and psychological ramifications including a heightened risk for obesity [74-76]. Despite a marginally later onset than other eating disorders, BED does occur in the younger population [1,2] highlighting the importance of developing effective interventions, particularly as adolescence represents a critical period for the development and maintenance of positive health behaviours [77].

While we acknowledge that the lack of intervention studies likely reflects BED's previous status as a research category according to DSM-IV-TR [78], it is anticipated that its inclusion as a diagnostic category in DSM-5 [79] will provide impetus for further intervention specific research in this area.

Family based therapy

Intervention research is dominated by trials of family based therapy, particularly for AN in the adolescent bracket. Even with the widespread implementation of FBTs due to clinical practice guideline recommendations (e.g., [20,80]), further well-conducted trials are still required, not only to provide a stronger evidence base for clinical recommendations, but to address significant clinical questions that remain. For example, is FBT the most effective psychological intervention for AN? Head to head trials with other validated psychological interventions adapted for the eating disorders are required. CBT is a potential candidate given its success in BN and the evidence base generated across other adolescent/young adult onset disorders. Interpersonal therapy also presents an interesting comparison as its relationship framework may have overlapping features with FBT. Important work is also needed to determine the effectiveness of FBT in populations other than adolescents. A recent review described developments of an adapted version of FBT for young adults (18+) [47]. The main adaptation being the definition of family where a pragmatic approach is used to define a 'family of choice' which may include partners, close friends, room mates etc. This approach has the potential to make an effective intervention available to a wider population.

Eating disorder not otherwise specified

The evidence map highlights the absence of intervention studies investigating EDNOS treatments in adolescents and young adults. This is concerning given that data suggest more than 50% of those diagnosed with an eating disorder have EDNOS [81,82] and it being the most common diagnosis reported in clinical and community populations with eating disorders [83,84]. Additionally, those with EDNOS follow a similar course to those diagnosed with AN and BN in terms of the nature, symptom severity, eating pathology and outcome of disorder [85-87].

Due to the similarities EDNOS shares with AN and BN, and problems recruiting sufficient sample sizes in eating disorder research [88], it can be common for researchers to include participants with EDNOS within trials investigating interventions for AN or BN, either by including EDNOS diagnosis or by using relaxed AN/BN inclusion criteria which facilitates entry of EDNOS participants. This may explain the lack of trials specifically targeting those with EDNOS, potentially masking the evidence base for effective EDNOS intervention. However, only a small number of trials explicitly reported doing so and those that did failed to provide the adequate sub-group analysis required to determine intervention effects according to eating disorder diagnosis.

Given the similarities between EDNOS and AN/BN categories and in line with guideline recommendations indicating treatment of EDNOS follow the disorder-symptom profile most closely resembled (either AN or BN [20]), those treatments which have previously shown promise in the AN and BN area (e.g., FBT, CBT) should be prioritised in future EDNOS intervention research.

Research opportunities for relapse prevention

While rates of relapse have yet to be systematically investigated, longitudinal cohort and treatment follow up studies estimate 20% to 50% of those with eating disorders will relapse [89-94]. Given these high relapse rates and the burden associated with a relapsing and chronic long-term condition, as is common among those with eating disorders, effective relapse prevention strategies are vital. The lack of trials investigating relapse prevention in adolescents and young adults with eating disorders is one of the most salient findings of this evidence map.

Three small trials were identified utilising CBT as a relapse prevention strategy with post-hospitalised, weight restored AN participants, showing positive preliminary results [95-97]. SSRIs were also investigated in another two trials using similar weight restored samples, however no effects above placebo were noted [98,99]. Of concern is that large proportions of intervention arm participants across these trials still experienced relapse.

CBT-based relapse prevention strategies appear promising, as noted in the above trials and highlighted in the adult AN literature [100], but require further investigation. Newer 'third wave' strategies like mindfulness, which has shown some degree of success in adults with depression [101,102], are now beginning to receive attention in the eating disorders literature (e.g., [103-105]) and similarly require investigation in younger populations. Given the age of onset of most eating disorders [1,2], it is interesting that family-based relapse prevention strategies have not yet been developed. Such strategies are noted in other high severity disorders affecting young people, for example first episode psychosis [106] and bipolar disorder [107]. Once a young person leaves primary treatment, they return to an environment that is potentially unchanged, where significant risk factors remain [108]. The family, and thus family-based interventions, may be well positioned to address factors associated with relapse and assert an important influence in maintaining behaviour change and preventing or minimising relapse.

Limitations

Syntheses of intervention effects were not undertaken, restricting us from drawing conclusions on intervention efficacy. Additionally, study quality appraisal was not conducted; therefore studies with methodological flaws may still be included. Furthermore, included studies were restricted to 'gold standard' research, which neglects important information available from studies utilising designs other than controlled trials and systematic reviews. For example, research areas where it may be unethical to randomise patients to particular conditions (e.g., those with chronic and severe disorders) would be absent from the evidence map. Nonetheless, this evidence map has systematically demonstrated what prevention and treatment interventions exist and has exposed important gaps in the current literature.

Conclusions

The onset of eating disorders frequently occurs in adolescence and young adulthood and is associated with significant psychological and physical burden. While promising interventions for this population have been identified, gaps exist and the body of evidence has not firmly established which interventions are most effective. Systematic reviews are required in some areas where the evidence base has yet to be summarised in a meaningful way (e.g., the use of CBT and antidepressants for diagnosed BN). Interventions which require further investigation in well conducted controlled trials include prevention programs for those at risk of developing eating disorders, focusing on intervention components other than passive psychoeducation; head-to-head trials of FBTs and other validated psychotherapies for AN; investigation of stepped-care intervention models; psychological interventions for BED and EDNOS; and interventions designed to prevent relapse or maintain treatment response. By systematically identifying existing interventions for young people with eating disorders and exposing gaps in the current evidence base, this evidence map can inform researchers, funding bodies and policy makers as to the opportunities for future research.

Abbreviations

AN: Anorexia nervosa; BN: Bulimia nervosa; EDNOS: Eating disorder not otherwise specified; BED: Binge eating disorder; FBT: Family based therapy; CBT: Cognitive behavioural therapy; PE: Psychoeducation; SSRI: Selective serotonin reuptake inhibitor.

Competing interests

The authors declare that they have no competing interests.

Authors' contributions

APB contributed to screening and coding of included articles and drafted the manuscript, AGP participated in the design of the study and helped draft the manuscript, LAC participated in screening and coding of included studies and helped draft the manuscript, LMH provided advice and helped draft the manuscript, PL participated in screening and coding of included studies and helped draft the manuscript, SEH conceived the study, participated in its design and helped draft the manuscript. All authors read and approved the final manuscript.

Acknowledgements

Headspace, National Youth Mental Health Foundation Ltd. is funded by the Australian Government Department of Health and Ageing under the Youth Mental Health Initiative Program. Orygen Youth Health Research Centre is affiliated with Melbourne Health and the University of Melbourne and receives funding from the Colonial Foundation. SEH is on a National Health and Medical Research Council Early Career Fellowship. The authors would like to thank Stefanie De Silva, Penelope Lucas, Patrick Callahan and Heidi Strickland for assisting with the early stages of study screening.

Author details

[1]Orygen Youth Health Research Centre, Centre for Youth Mental Health, The University of Melbourne, Locked Bag 10, Parkville, Melbourne, Victoria 3052, Australia. [2]Centre of Excellence in Youth Mental Health, headspace National Youth Mental Health Foundation Ltd, Level 2, South Tower, 485 La Trobe Street, Melbourne, Victoria 3000, Australia. [3]Melbourne School of Population Health, The University of Melbourne, Level 3, 207 Bouverie Street, Melbourne, Victoria 3010, Australia.

References

1. Hudson JI, Hiripi E, Pope HG, Kessler RC: **The prevalence and correlates of eating disorders in the national comorbidity survey replication.** *Biol Psychiatry* 2007, **61**(3):348–358.
2. Oakley-Browne MA, Wells JE, Scott KM, McGee MA: **Lifetime prevalence and projected lifetime risk of DSM-IV disorders in Te Rau Hinengaro: the New Zealand mental health survey.** *Aust N Z J Psychiatry* 2006, **40**(10):865–874.
3. Mathews R, Hall WD, Vos T, Patton GC, Degenhardt L: **What are the major drivers of prevalent disability burden in young Australians.** *Med J Aust* 2011, **194**(5):232–235.
4. Mond J, Rodgers B, Hay P, Korten A, Owen C, Beumont P: **Disability associated with community cases of commonly occurring eating disorders.** *Aust N Z J Public Health* 2004, **28**(3):246–251.

5. Madden S, Morris A, Zurynski YA, Kohn M, Elliot EJ: **Burden of eating disorders in 5-13-year-old children in Australia.** *Med J Aust* 2009, **190**(8):410–414.
6. Arcelus J, Mitchell AJ, Wales J, Nielsen S: **Mortality rates in patients with anorexia nervosa and other eating disorders: a meta-analysis of 36 studies.** *Arch Gen Psychiatry* 2011, **68**(7):724–731.
7. Berkman ND, Lohr KN, Bulik CM: **Outcomes of eating disorders: a systematic review of the literature.** *Int J Eat Disord* 2007, **40**(4):293–309.
8. Franko DL, Keel PK: **Suicidality in eating disorders: occurrence, correlates, and clinical implications.** *Clin Psychol Rev* 2006, **26**(6):769–782.
9. Preti A, Rocchi M, Sisti D, Camboni M, Miotto P: **A comprehensive meta-analysis of the risk of suicide in eating disorders.** *Acta Psychiatr Scand* 2011, **124**(1):6–17.
10. Braun DL, Sunday S, Halmi K: **Psychiatric comorbidity in patients with eating disorders.** *Psychol Med* 1994, **24**(4):859–867.
11. Calero-Elvira A, Krug I, Davis K, Lopez C, Fernandez-Aranda F, Treasure J: **Meta-analysis on drugs in people with eating disorders.** *Eur Eat Disord Rev* 2009, **17**(4):243–259.
12. Godart NT, Flament MF, Curt F, Perdereau F, Lang FO, Venisse JL, Halfon O, Bizouard P, Loas G, Corcos M: **Anxiety disorders in subjects seeking treatment for eating disorders: a DSM-IV controlled study.** *Psychiatry Res* 2003, **117**(3):245–258.
13. Kaye WH, Bulik CM, Thornton L, Barbarich N, Masters K: **Comorbidity of anxiety disorders with anorexia and bulimia nervosa.** *Am J Psychiatry* 2004, **161**(12):2215–2221.
14. Deloitte Access Economics: *Paying the price: the economic and social impact of eating disorders in Australia.* NSW, Australia: The Butterfly Foundation; 2012.
15. Barlow DH, Levitt JT, Bufka LF: **The dissemination of empirically supported treatments: a view to the future.** *Behav Res Ther* 1999, **37**(Suppl 1):147–162.
16. Wilson GT, Grilo CM, Vitousek KM: **Psychological treatment of eating disorders.** *Am Psychol* 2007, **62**(3):199–216.
17. Von Ranson KM, Robinson KE: **Who is providing what type of psychotherapy to eating disorder clients? a survey.** *Int J Eat Disord* 2006, **39**(1):27–34.
18. Simmons AM, Milnes SM, Anderson DA: **Factors influencing the utilization of empirically supported treatments for eating disorders.** *Eat Disord* 2008, **16**(4):342–354.
19. Haas HL, Clopton JR: **Comparing clinical and research treatments for eating disorders.** *Int J Eat Disord* 2003, **33**(4):412–420.
20. National Institute for Health and Clinical Excellence: *Eating disorders: core interventions in the treatment and management of anorexia nervosa, bulimia nervosa and related eating disorders.* London, UK: Author, CG9; 2004.
21. Hay P, Bacaltchuk J, Stefano S, Kashyap P: **Psychotherapy for bulimia nervosa and binging.** *Cochrane Database Syst Rev* 2009, **4**:CD000562.
22. Shapiro JR, Berkman ND, Brownley KA, Sedway JA, Lohr KN, Bulik CM: **Bulimia nervosa treatment: a systematic review of randomized controlled trials.** *Int J Eat Disord* 2007, **40**(4):321–336.
23. Pederson-Mussell M, Crosby RD, Crow SJ, Knopke AJ, Peterson CB, Wonderlich SA, Mitchell JE: **Utilization of empirically supported psychotherapy treatments for individuals with eating disorders: a survey of psychologists.** *Int J Eat Disord* 2000, **27**(2):230–237.
24. Crow S, Pederson Mussell M, Peterson C, Knopke A, Mitchell J: **Prior treatment received by patients with bulimia nervosa.** *Int J Eat Disord* 1999, **25**(1):39–44.
25. Cabana MD, Rand CS, Powe NR, Wu AW, Wilson MH, Abboud PAC, Rubin HR: **Why don't physicians follow clinical practice guidelines?** *JAMA* 1999, **282**(15):1458–1465.
26. Callahan P, Liu P, Purcell R, Parker AG, Hetrick SE: **Evidence map of prevention and treatment interventions for depression in young people.** *Depress Res Treat* 2012, **2012:**820735.
27. Liu P, Parker AG, Hetrick SE, Callahan P, De Silva S, Purcell R: **An evidence map of interventions across premorbid, ultra-high risk and first episode phases of psychosis.** *Schizophr Res* 2010, **123**(1):37–44.
28. De Silva S, Parker AG, Purcell R, Callahan P, Liu P, Hetrick SE: **Mapping the evidence of prevention and intervention studies for suicidal and self-harming behaviors in young people.** *Crisis* 2013, **34**(4):223–232.
29. Arksey H, O'Malley L: **Scoping studies: towards a methodological framework.** *Int J Soc Res Methodol* 2005, **8**(1):19–32.
30. Bragge P, Clavisi O, Turner T, Tavender E, Collie A, Gruen RL: **The global evidence mapping initiative: scoping research in broad topic areas.** *BMC Med Res Methodol* 2011, **11**:92.
31. Hetrick SE, Parker AG, Callahan P, Purcell R: **Evidence mapping: illustrating an emerging methodology to improve evidence-based practice in youth mental health.** *J Eval Clin Pract* 2010, **16**(6):1025–1030.
32. Katz DL, Williams A-I, Girard C, Goodman J, Comerford B, Behrman A, Bracken MB: **The evidence base for complementary and alternative medicine: methods of evidence mapping with application to cam.** *Altern Ther Health Med* 2003, **9**(4):22–30.
33. Mrazek PJ, Haggerty RJ: *Reducing risks for mental disorders: frontiers for preventive intervention research.* Washington, DC: National Academies Press; 1994.
34. American Psychiatric Association: *Diagnostic and statistical manual of mental disorders.* 4th edition. Washington, DC: Author: Text rev; 2000.
35. World Health Organisation: *ICD-10: International statistical classification of diseases and related health problems.* 10th edition. New York, NY: Author; 2008.
36. National Health and Medical Research Council: *NHMRC additional levels of evidence and grades for recommendations for developers of guidelines.* Canberra, Australia: Author; 2009.
37. Centre of Excellence in Youth Mental Health: *Evidence Maps.* Orygen Youth Health Research Centre and headspace, National Youth Mental Health Foundation. http://www.headspace.org.au/what-works/evidence-maps.
38. Siemer CP, Fogel J, Van Voorhees BW: **Telemental health and web-based applications in children and adolescents.** *Child Adolesc Psychiatr Clin N Am* 2011, **20**(1):135–153.
39. Stice E, Shaw H: **Eating disorder prevention programs: a meta-analytic review.** *Psychol Bull* 2004, **130**(2):206–227.
40. Yager Z, O'Dea JA: **Prevention programs for body image and eating disorders on university campuses: a review of large, controlled interventions.** *Health Promot Int* 2008, **23**(2):173–189.
41. Cororve-Fingeret M, Warren CS, Cepeda-Benito A, Gleaves DH: **Eating disorder prevention research: a meta-analysis.** *Eat Disord* 2006, **14**(3):191–213.
42. Stice E, Shaw H, Marti CN: **A meta-analytic review of eating disorder prevention programs: encouraging findings.** *Annu Rev Clin Psychol* 2007, **3**(1):207–231.
43. Beintner I, Jacobi C, Taylor CB: **Effects of an Internet-based prevention programme for eating disorders in the USA and Germany–a meta-analytic review.** *Eur Eat Disord Rev* 2012, **20**(1):1–8.
44. Rutherford L, Couturier J: **A review of psychotherapeutic interventions for children and adolescents with eating disorders.** *Can Child Adolesc Psychiatry Rev* 2007, **16**(4):153–157.
45. Tierney SWK: **What works for adolescents with AN? A systematic review of psychosocial interventions.** *Eat Weight Disord* 2005, **10**(2):66–75.
46. Kaslow NJ, Broth MR, Smith CO, Collins MH: **Family-based interventions for child and adolescent disorders.** *J Marital Fam Ther* 2012, **38**(1):82–100.
47. Stiles-Shields C, Hoste RR, Doyle PM, Le Grange D: **A review of family-based treatment for adolescents with eating disorders.** *Rev Recent Clin Trials* 2012, **7**(2):133–140.
48. Fisher CA, Hetrick SE, Rushford N: **Family therapy for anorexia nervosa.** *Cochrane Database Syst Rev* 2010, **4**, CD004780.
49. Gardner J, Wilkinson P: **Is family therapy the most effective treatment for anorexia nervosa?** *Psychiatr Danub* 2011, **23**(Suppl. 1):S175–S177.
50. Smith A, Cook-Cottone C: **A review of family therapy as an effective intervention for anorexia nervosa in adolescents.** *J Clin Psychol Med Settings* 2011, **18**(4):323–334.
51. Lock J, Le Grange D, Argas W, Dare C: *Treatment manual for anorexia nervosa. A family-based approach.* New York: The Guildford Press; 2001.
52. Robin ALSPT, Koepke T, Moye AW, Tice S: **Family therapy versus individual therapy for adolescent females with anorexia nervosa.** *J Dev Behav Pediatr* 1994, **15**(2):111–116.
53. Le Grange DC, Ross D, Rathouz Paul J, Leventhal Bennett L: **A randomized controlled comparison of family-based treatment and supportive psychotherapy for adolescent bulimia nervosa.** *Arch Gen Psychiatry* 2007, **64**(9):1049–1056.
54. Schmidt UL S, Beecham J, Perkins S, Treasure J, Yi I, Winn S, Robinson P, Murphy R, Keville S, Johnson-Sabine E, Jenkins M, Frost S, Dodge L, Berelowitz M, Eisler I: **A randomized controlled trial of family therapy and cognitive behavior therapy guided self-care for adolescents with bulimia nervosa and related disorders.** *Am J Psychiatry* 2007, **164**(4):591–598.
55. Court A, Mulder C, Hetrick SE, Purcell R, McGorry PD: **What is the scientific evidence for the use of antipsychotic medication in Anorexia Nervosa.** *Eat Disord: J Treat Prev* 2008, **16**(3):217–223.

56. Kishi T, Kafantaris V, Sunday S, Sheridan EM, Correll CU: **Are antipsychotics effective for the treatment of anorexia nervosa? Results from a systematic review and meta-analysis.** *J Clin Psychiatry* 2012, **73**(6):e757–e766.
57. McKnight RF, Park RJ: **Atypical antipsychotics and anorexia nervosa: a review.** *Eur Eat Disord Rev* 2010, **18**(1):10–21.
58. Flament MF, Bissada H, Spettigue W: **Evidence-based pharmacotherapy of eating disorders.** *Int J Neuropsychopharmacol* 2012, **15**(2):189–207.
59. Couturier JLJ: **Psychopharmacology update: a review of medication use for children and adolescents with eating disorders.** *J Can Acad Child Adolesc Psychiatry* 2007, **16**(4):173–176.
60. Hetrick S, McKenzie J, Merry S: **The use of SSRIs in children and adolescents.** *Curr Opin Psychiatry* 2010, **23**(1):53–57.
61. Stice E: **Risk and maintenance factors for eating pathology: a meta-analytic review.** *Psychol Bull* 2002, **128**(5):825–848.
62. Bacaltchuk J, Hay P: **Antidepressants versus placebo for people with bulimia nervosa.** *Cochrane Database Syst Rev* 2003, **4**:CD003391.
63. National Institute for Health and Clinical Excellence: *Depression in children and young people: identification and management in primary, community and secondary care. CG28.* London, UK: Author; 2005.
64. Van Straten A, Seekles W, Van't Veer-Tazelaar NJ, Beekman AT, Cuijpers P: **Stepped care for depression in primary care: what should be offered and how?** *Med J Aust* 2010, **192**(Suppl 11):36–39.
65. Bower P, Gilbody S: **Stepped care in psychological therapies: access, effectiveness and efficiency Narrative literature review.** *Br J Psychiatry* 2005, **186**(1):11–17.
66. Treasure J, Schmidt U, Troop N, Tiller J, Todd G, Turnbull S: **Sequential treatment for bulimia nervosa incorporating a self-care manual.** *Br J Psychiatry* 1996, **168**(JAN):94–98.
67. Mitchell JE, Agras S, Crow S, Halmi K, Fairburn CG, Bryson S, Kraemer H: **Stepped care and cognitive-behavioural therapy for bulimia nervosa: randomised trial.** *Br J Psychiatry* 2011, **198**(5):391–397.
68. Dunn E, Neighbors C, Larimer M: **Motivational enhancement therapy and self-help treatment for binge eaters.** *Psychol Addict Behav* 2006, **20**(1):44–52.
69. Wilson GT, Vitousek KM, Loeb KL: **Stepped care treatment for eating disorders.** *J Consult Clin Psychol* 2000, **68**(4):564–572.
70. Brownley KA, Berkman ND, Sedway JA, Lohr KN, Bulik CM: **Binge eating disorder treatment: a systematic review of randomized controlled trials.** *Int J Eat Disord* 2007, **40**(4):337–348.
71. Vocks S, Tuschen-Caffier B, Pietrowsky R, Rustenbach SJ, Kersting A, Herpertz S: **Meta-analysis of the effectiveness of psychological and pharmacological treatments for binge eating disorder.** *Int J Eat Disord* 2010, **43**(3):205–217.
72. Allen H, Craighead L: **Appetite monitoring in the treatment of binge eating disorder.** *Behav Ther* 1999, **30**(2):253–272.
73. Ricca V, Mannucci E, Mezzani B, Moretti S, Di Bernardo M, Bertelli M, Rotella C, Faravelli C: **Fluoxetine and fluvoxamine combined with individual cognitive-behaviour therapy in binge eating disorder: a one-year follow-up study.** *Psychother Psychosom* 2001, **70**(6):298–306.
74. Pope H, Lalonde J, Pindyck L, Walsh T, Bulik C, Crow S, McElroy S, Rosenthal N, Hudson J: **Binge eating disorder: a stable syndrome.** *Am J Psychiatry* 2006, **163**(12):2181–2183.
75. Hudson JI, Lalonde JK, Berry JM, Pindyck LJ, Bulik CM, Crow SJ, McElroy SL, Laird NM, Tsuang MT, Walsh BT: **Binge-eating disorder as a distinct familial phenotype in obese individuals.** *Arch Gen Psychiatry* 2006, **63**(3):313–319.
76. Dingemans A, Bruna M, Van Furth E: **Binge eating disorder: a review.** *Int J Obes* 2002, **26**(3):299–307.
77. Ortega F, Ruiz J, Castillo M, Sjostrom M: **Physical fitness in childhood and adolescence: a powerful marker of health.** *Int J Obes* 2007, **32**(1):1–11.
78. Striegel-Moore RH, Franko DL: **Should binge eating disorder be included in the DSM-V? A critical review of the state of the evidence.** *Annu Rev Clin Psychol* 2008, **4**(1):305–324.
79. American Psychiatric Association: *Diagnostic and statistical manual of mental disorders.* 5th edition. Arlington, VA: Author; 2013.
80. Royal Australian and New Zealand College of Psychiatrists: **Australian and New Zealand clinical practice guidelines for the treatment of anorexia nervosa.** *Aust N Z J Psychiatry* 2004, **38**:659–670.
81. Fairburn CG, Cooper Z: **Thinking afresh about the classification of eating disorders.** *Int J Eat Disord* 2007, **40**(Suppl 3):107–110.
82. Fairburn CG, Harrison PJ: **Eating disorders.** *Lancet* 2003, **361**(9355):407–416.
83. Dalle-Grave R, Calugi S: **Eating disorder not otherwise specified in an inpatient unit: the impact of altering the DSM-IV criteria for anorexia and bulimia nervosa.** *Eur Eat Disord Rev* 2007, **15**(5):340–349.
84. Rockert W, Kaplan AS, Olmsted MP: **Eating disorder not otherwise specified: the view from a tertiary care treatment center.** *Int J Eat Disord* 2007, **40**(Suppl 3):99–103.
85. Crow SJ, Peterson CB, Swanson SA, Raymond NC, Specker S, Eckert ED, Mitchell JE: **Increased mortality in bulimia nervosa and other eating disorders.** *Am J Psychiatry* 2009, **166**(12):1342–1346.
86. Fairburn CG, Cooper Z, Bohn K, O'Connor ME, Doll HA, Palmer RL: **The severity and status of eating disorder NOS: implications for DSM-V.** *Behav Res Ther* 2007, **45**(8):1705–1715.
87. Thomas JJ, Vartanian LR, Brownell KD: **The relationship between eating disorder not otherwise specified (EDNOS) and officially recognized eating disorders: meta-analysis and implications for DSM.** *Psychol Bull* 2009, **135**(3):407–433.
88. Agras WS, Brandt HA, Bulik CM, Dolan-Sewell R, Fairburn CG, Halmi KA, Herzog DB, Jimerson DC, Kaplan AS, Kaye WH: **Report of the national institutes of health workshop on overcoming barriers to treatment research in anorexia nervosa.** *Int J Eat Disord* 2004, **35**(4):509–521.
89. Carter JC, Blackmore E, Sutandar-Pinnock K, Woodside DB: **Relapse in anorexia nervosa: a survival analysis.** *Psychol Med* 2004, **34**(4):671–679.
90. Eckert ED, Halmi KA, Marchi P, Grove W, Crosby R: **Ten-year follow-up of anorexia nervosa: clinical course and outcome.** *Psychol Med* 1995, **25**(1):143–156.
91. Herzog DB, Dorer DJ, Keel PK, Selwyn SE, Ekeblad ER, Flores AT, Greenwood DN, Burwell RA, Keller MB: **Recovery and relapse in anorexia and bulimia nervosa: a 7.5-year follow-up study.** *J Am Acad Child Adolesc Psychiatry* 1999, **38**(7):829–837.
92. Keel PK, Dorer DJ, Franko DL, Jackson SC, Herzog DB: **Postremission predictors of relapse in women with eating disorders.** *Am J Psychiatry* 2005, **162**(12):2263–2268.
93. Pike KM: **Long-term course of anorexia nervosa: response, relapse, remission, and recovery.** *Clin Psychol Rev* 1998, **18**(4):447–475.
94. Strober M, Freeman R, Morrell W: **The long-term course of severe anorexia nervosa in adolescents: survival analysis of recovery, relapse, and outcome predictors over 10–15 years in a prospective study.** *Int J Eat Disord* 1997, **22**(4):339–360.
95. Pike M, Walsh B, Vitousek K, Wilson G, Bauer J: **Cognitive behavior therapy in the posthospitalization treatment of anorexia nervosa.** *Am J Psychiatry* 2003, **160**(11):2046–2049.
96. Carter J, McFarlane T, Bewell C, Olmsted M, Woodside D, Kaplan A, Crosby R: **Maintenance treatment for anorexia nervosa: a comparison of cognitive behavior therapy and treatment as usual.** *Int J Eat Disord* 2009, **42**(3):202–207.
97. Fichter MM, Quadflieg N, Nisslmüller K, Lindner S, Osen B, Huber T, Wünsch-Leiteritz W: **Does internet-based prevention reduce the risk of relapse for anorexia nervosa?** *Behav Res Ther* 2012, **50**(3):180–190.
98. Walsh B, Kaplan A, Attia E, Olmsted M, Parides M, Carter J, Pike K, Devlin M, Woodside B, Roberto C, Rockert W: **Fluoxetine after weight restoration in anorexia nervosa: a randomized controlled trial.** *JAMA* 2006, **295**(22):2605–2612.
99. Kaye W, Nagata T, Weltzin T, Hsu L, Sokol M, McConaha C, Plotnicov K, Weise J, Deep D: **Double-blind placebo-controlled administration of fluoxetine in restricting- and restricting-purging-type anorexia nervosa.** *Biol Psychiatry* 2001, **49**(7):644–652.
100. Bulik CM, Berkman ND, Brownley KA, Sedway JA, Lohr KN: **Anorexia nervosa treatment: a systematic review of randomized controlled trials.** *Int J Eat Disord* 2007, **40**(4):310–320.
101. Teasdale JD, Segal ZV, Williams JMG, Ridgeway VA, Soulsby JM, Lau MA: **Prevention of relapse/recurrence in major depression by mindfulness-based cognitive therapy.** *J Consult Clin Psychol* 2000, **68**(4):615–623.
102. Ma SH, Teasdale JD: **Mindfulness-based cognitive therapy for depression: replication and exploration of differential relapse prevention effects.** *J Consult Clin Psychol* 2004, **72**(1):31–40.
103. Wanden-Berghe RG, Sanz-Valero J, Wanden-Berghe C: **The application of mindfulness to eating disorders treatment: a systematic review.** *Eat Disord* 2011, **19**(1):34–48.
104. Merwin RM, Timko CA, Moskovich AA, Ingle KK, Bulik CM, Zucker NL: **Psychological inflexibility and symptom expression in anorexia nervosa.** *Eat Disord* 2011, **19**(1):62–82.

105. Baer RA, Fischer S, Huss DB: **Mindfulness and acceptance in the treatment of disordered eating.** *J Ration Emot Cogn Behav Ther* 2005, **23**(4):281–300.
106. Bird V, Premkumar P, Kendall T, Whittington C, Mitchell J, Kuipers E: **Early intervention services, cognitive-behavioural therapy and family intervention in early psychosis: systematic review.** *Br J Psychiatry* 2010, **197**(5):350–356.
107. Rea MM, Tompson MC, Miklowitz DJ, Goldstein MJ, Hwang S, Mintz J: **Family-focused treatment versus individual treatment for bipolar disorder: results of a randomized clinical trial.** *J Consult Clin Psychol* 2003, **71**(3):482–492.
108. Wilfley DE, Kolko RP, Kass AE: **Cognitive-behavioral therapy for weight management and eating disorders in children and adolescents.** *Child Adolesc Psychiatr Clin N Am* 2011, **20**(2):271–285.

Assessment of anorexia nervosa: an overview of universal issues and contextual challenges

Lois J Surgenor[1*] and Sarah Maguire[2]

Abstract

Aim: Anorexia Nervosa (AN) is a complex and clinically challenging syndrome. Intended for specialist audiences, this narrative review aims to summarise the available literature related to assessment in the adult patient context, synthesising both research evidence and clinical consensus guidelines.

Method: We provide a review of the available literature on specialist assessment of AN focusing on common trajectories into assessment, obstacles accessing assessment, common presenting issues and barriers to the assessment process, the necessary scope of assessment, and tools and techniques. It describes the further step of synthesising assessment information in ways that can inform resultant care plans.

Results: In addition to assessment of core behaviours and diagnostic skills, considerations for the expert assessor include the functions of primary care, systemic and personal barriers, knowledge of current assessment tools and research pertaining to comorbid pathology in AN, assessing severity of illness, role of family at assessment, as well as medical, nutritional and compulsory elements of assessment.

Conclusion: Comprehensive assessment of AN in the current healthcare context still remains largely the remit of the specialist ED clinician. Assessment should remain an on-going process, paying particular attention to available empirical evidence, thereby reducing the gap between research and practice.

Keywords: Anorexia nervosa, Assessment, Eating disorders

Introduction

Most health workers recognise that anorexia nervosa (AN) is a serious disorder that results in significant disability and impaired quality of life. Unfortunately for some, this disorder becomes a chronic or life-shortening illness. It is well-established that AN has the highest mortality rate of all psychiatric disorders [1]; compared with their peers without the illness the risk of premature death is approximately ten-fold in a person with AN [2]. Health consequences are widespread, both in terms of direct physical and mental health effects and economic costs to society overall; a recent Australian analysis placed the total yearly direct health system costs of AN at $59.8 million [3]. This means that although AN and AN-like conditions are relatively rare, severe and enduring forms of AN have impairment outcomes comparable to people with moderately severe depression and schizophrenia [3].

* Correspondence: lois.surgenor@otago.ac.nz
[1]Department of Psychological Medicine, University of Otago at Christchurch, 4 Oxford Terrace, Christchurch 8140, New Zealand
Full list of author information is available at the end of the article

Assessment and a resulting early diagnosis become a vital task for the health system and current research continues to suggest that, although primary care is the context of most presentation [4] areas with specialist services have more than double the number of diagnosable eating disorder (ED) cases, suggesting a sizeable proportion of diagnoses do not occur until the specialist service level [5]. What this means for both settings is worth discussion, but regardless, assessment skills and knowledge of the evidence base pertaining to diagnoses remain an important part of the skill set of the specialist clinician.

Regardless of the setting and complexity, there are descriptions of 'ideal practice' in the assessment of the disorder and associated health difficulties. However, assessment approaches do vary, along with models of service delivery, admission thresholds and the resources available in specialist settings [5]. Such factors will influence the composition of a multidisciplinary assessment team. There are suggestions about what constitutes an 'ideal' assessment team, but rarely will services have all recommended components, and multiple tasks may fall to 'mini teams' [6]. There is however areas of general consensus about many necessary and desirable tasks of assessment and given the above constraints it often falls to the specialist clinician working in relative isolation to be well versed in all factors pertinent to a comprehensive assessment. Focusing primarily on adult populations, this paper aims to reduce the gap between research and practice (as it relates to assessment of AN) by firstly providing a comprehensive review of the current literature relating to assessment pathways, barriers to assessment, diagnostic issues, instruments for assessment of illness and severity, role of the family at assessment, comorbid presentations relevant to assessment, medical, nutritional and compulsory assessment practises. Secondly, it discusses the process of synthesising information gathered at assessment for the purposes of formulation and ultimately to direct treatment.

Pathways to assessment

Links with primary care providers

Given the scarcity of specialist ED services, most people with AN will not be seen by a specialist service in the first instance, and for a significant number, specialist assessment may not occur at any stage. Half of those with an ED are first diagnosed by their primary care physician, although of concern a sizeable minority may go through life without any help whether this is for AN or other emotional problems [4]. General practitioners (GPs) and other primary health care providers are best placed to be the health practitioners first involved in conducting preliminary assessments, providing initial triage, and thereafter sharing case management with other clinicians [7]. This is partly because people with eating disorders attend GPs and other medical speciality services more frequently than their peer group, albeit often for conditions seemingly unrelated to the disorder. The presence of an ED also increases the rate of presentations to Emergency Departments [4]. In terms of accuracy of diagnosis, AN is the ED most often accurately diagnosed by primary care physicians [8]. Atypical cases, or those who do not present with all diagnostic criteria, can be misdiagnosed [9] or considered 'less serious' despite clearly having a clinically significant disorder that squarely sits within the AN spectrum.

A number of obstacles arise for primary care health professionals in their attempt to detect AN and refer on to ED services. Setting obstacles include the limited consultation time available and relatively limited exposure to AN. Clinical obstacles include patient minimisation of behavioural and psychological symptoms, the diversity of symptom expression, and well-hidden symptoms [7]. Further, there may be difficulty in determining which symptoms are most important in assessing medical acuity or how severe the condition has become.

Systemic issues also contribute to rates of diagnosis and their accuracy. GP education about risk factors and early warning signs as well as screening instruments like the SCOFF [10] can assist detection and management, particularly where GPs are expected to coordinate and manage concurrent medical and psychiatric conditions. Close and regular liaison with ED specialists may encourage more regular enquiry about eating difficulties in those who frequently present with emotional and/or physical problems. GPs are referral "gatekeepers" (whether intended or otherwise), and ED clinicians have a role in supporting and educating their colleagues about frontline assessment practices and referral thresholds. In the regions where there are specialist services, GPs are likely to have greater awareness of eating disorders and in turn refer to specialist services more frequently [6]. In any event, presentation to primary care or emergency services should always be used as an opportunity to introduce, or re-engage with an ED clinician or ED service if one is available.

Facilitating assessment following referral

Early identification and treatment of AN is consistently argued as a means to reduce the duration of AN [11,12]. A systematic review of treatment seeking has recently estimated that the median delay from onset to treatment for AN is 15 years [13]. Identifying the barriers between these two time points becomes pivotal, and will likely vary. A significant minority of people referred for ED problems fail to attend an initial assessment [14], and further significant attrition occurs between assessment and providing and/or completing treatment. The following sections discuss common obstacles and possible solutions.

System and resource barriers

There are extensive system factors contributing to delays in accessing assessment. The shortage of services often results in prolonged waiting lists for assessment, meaning that by the time of assessment, patients may be demotivated or otherwise less likely to engage in what is offered. Tatham et al. [15] trialled an active 'opt in' waitlist management strategy for an ED clinic, whereby following initial assessment patients were required to actively select to remain on the waitlist for treatment. While 'opting in' letters may reduce the waiting time for an assessment [16], this triage approach is not without significant risk. Specifically, those most in need of assessment may be the least able or willing to 'opt in'.

Long assessment waiting lists are likely to pose a barrier to engaging in any subsequent assessment - just as these do in many other health settings. It has been reported by patients that this can send a distorted message that the disorder is not serious enough. World-wide, services are caught in the ethical dilemma of setting priorities for how scarce resources should be allocated and prioritised. As these decisions have major clinical implications, resource priority-setting should be reviewed at regular intervals. Suggested strategies that have been shown to increase the likelihood of a valid referral resulting in an assessment include direct phone contact with the patient [14] accurate written knowledge services and, where appropriate, steps to engage significant others (for example, family) in the assessment process [11].

Barriers of ambivalence and motivation

There are multiple psychological reasons why people with AN may be reluctant to present for assessment or are guarded during an assessment. The disorder itself, at best, presents genuine ambiguity for many who suffer from it. As one woman described it, "I want to get rid of the disorder but not the body shape (of AN)...I want the best of both worlds" [17], page 29. AN has been demonstrated to serve more pivotal functions of affect numbing or identity and the individual may see no reason to alter it at all or, as is most common, the patient may move between wanting to address it and not seeing it as a problem. This ambivalence is complex and may shift even in the preliminary assessment interview. The interview may be infused with 'bargaining points' or requests for 'conditional' or no treatment at all. With these dynamics at play, careful clinical skills are required. It is important that such bargaining is not seen as 'manipulation' with the negative connotations of that concept. Rather, it represents a genuine struggle with symptoms that are both controlling and out of control, and at times deeply confusing for the person. It can be very validating to the client, and move the process of assessment along smoothly, to express understanding for the two seemingly opposite positions that can be held within the one person, and to not dismiss or invalidate the part of the client that wants to retain the illness. Family and carers may be equally conflicted about the need for treatment, with parents sometimes caught between loyalty for their offspring and wanting to heed professional advice. Assessment of family functioning is discussed later in this paper.

Although overlapping with ambivalence, motivation is a wider construct involving cognitive, behavioural, and biological systems. Appraising motivation for treatment and ability to change is an important component of any initial assessment: it often contributes to case formulation, decisions made at the conclusion of assessment, and subsequent treatment planning. Yet assessment of this is far from straight forward. Motivation may be symptom-specific: there may be high engagement in strategies to control physical side effects, but minimal engagement in behaviours directed towards weight gain. Engaging in conversations that highlight this variability at the beginning of a therapeutic interaction is likely to build alliance. As noted by [18], assessing what makes people want to recover, and what recovery represents to them, is important, and this is something highly valued by patients themselves.

Of note, there is controversy regarding the ability of clinicians to accurately assess motivation, and whether this predicts anything about the likelihood of engagement or even treatment outcome. Waller [19] provides a compelling overview of the complexities involved, including clinician overreliance on verbal expressions of change. Interestingly, similar critical analyses are now being extended to motivational enhancement techniques, noting that in regard to AN, the evidence is mixed at best [20]. Rieger et al. [21] specifically suggests motivation is not only required to alter the behavioural aspects of the illness (namely how much weight are patients are prepared to gain each week until they reach a healthy weight, and how motivated they feel to be at a normal weight) but also feeling of self-efficacy about achieving this. Some patients will state that they are very motivated to be at a normal weight and would be prepared to gain up to a kilo a week to do so, but when asked how confident they are that they can actually do this, the answer is quite different.

Clinicians as barriers

People presenting for assessment are often fearful of being judged or criticised. These fears are not unfounded as it has been repeatedly demonstrated that attitudes of health professionals, including mental health specialists towards EDs, are not always positive [22], and are no more empathic than those of non-professionals [23]. Negative professional attitudes may arise through lack of training or experience [24], inadequate resources and work pressure, and genuinely held stereotypes about AN being a personal choice. These factors can contribute to AN being seen as a disorder with relatively low prestige by health care professionals [25]. Training and support strategies may go some way to counter these effects. As clinical experience decreases the likelihood of negative reactions, services significantly benefit from retaining highly skilled staff.

Early drop-out

Failure to engage, or drop out once treatment begins has a negative association with prognosis [26,27] and increases the likelihood of intensive treatment utilisation in later stages of illness [28]. Specialist services have lower treatment drop out and allow greater continuity of care with the same service, yet studies suggest that amongst those with EDs who actually attend assessment, approximately one-in-five drop out before treatment can start [29]. Reliable predictors (clinical or otherwise) of drop-out from services are scarce [17,26,30], meaning that future assessment interviews should be seen as an opportunity to explore the factors involved from the patient's perspective. Hudson et al. [31] found life-time treatment for AN to be 33.8%, and thus much lower than other DSM-IV eating disorders (BN 43.2%; BED 43.6). Reducing drop-out before and after assessment is an obvious means to increase treatment take-up.

Diagnostic issues at assessment

AN is a syndrome involving considerable symptom variability between and within cases over time. Cross-over between AN subtypes is common, suggesting that those with AN-Restricting Type and AN-Binge-Eating/Purging Type may be phases of the same condition rather than distinct groups [32]. Diagnostic weight cut-offs are debated [9] and the severity of psychological versus physical symptomatology may not always highly correlate, albeit these will be highly intertwined at extremely low weights due to the behavioural, psychological, and cognitive effects of starvation [33]. The following sections discuss key issues regarding diagnostic variability.

Revised diagnostic criteria

The American Psychiatric Association diagnostic criteria (DSM-5) [34] have recently been reviewed. Hebebrand et al. [9] comprehensively discusses the rationale behind revised criteria, highlighting the reframing of psychological symptoms so that some pejorative attitudes are removed and other criteria are redefined to reflect the evidence. For example, eliminating the term 'refusal' (to maintain body weight), and replacing this with more objective terms describing food restriction. The removal of the diagnostic criteria of amenorrhea in post-menarcheal females is well overdue given the mounting evidence that this is of questionable utility. Similar changes are proposed for ICD-11 [35]. Clinicians involved in the assessment of AN should become familiar with current and future diagnostic debates in order to reduce the risk of adopting a rigid or outdated approach to formulating core psychopathology of AN and the expressions of this.

Effect of symptoms

Some features of AN can be difficult to assess meaningfully in that they decrease in 'severity' as illness severity increases. For example, fear of fatness can decrease as the individual's weight drops and they are no longer confronted with fat on their own body. Similarly, drive for thinness and body image dissatisfaction can also decrease as weight decreases. To generalist clinicians, this could result in a failure to diagnose individuals with potentially severe AN, as they appear to lack either one or both of the essential symptoms. Other clinicians may misconstrue this as 'denial' and engage in confrontational discussions with patients, which may be unhelpful.

At very low weights, the effects of starvation will always distort the expression of distress, and patients in general are not necessarily aware of why they behave in certain ways or why they may pursue certain goals. It may be useful to assess certain symptoms from the perspective of what it would be like not to have them. For example, assessing body dissatisfaction/drive for thinness not from the standpoint of how the person with AN feels about their body at its current weight, but rather how they would feel about their body, and how intense their drive to lose weight would be if they imagined their weight being within a normal weight range, holds some utility [36].

Culture and ethnicity

AN may present differently in people with a non-Western background (see Soh et al. [37] for a review), and there are significant body composition differences across ethnicities. For example, Asian women show higher levels of body fat for the same BMI than their Western peers [38]. There is more mixed evidence that cultural issues influence psychological symptom variability. While a commonly cited difference is that fear of fatness is less evident in patients from a non-Western background, many studies do not show this [39]. Likewise, levels of body image disturbance amongst clinical groups from different cultures have been found to be largely identical despite genuine cultural differences in body image concern in those who do not have an ED [40]. Studies that have historically highlighted symptom variability across cultures have commonly examined ethnic minorities residing in Western countries: when an ethnic group is studied in their country of origin, many of the proposed differences in clinical presentation cannot be found. Likewise, struggles with psychological control reported in AN appear universal, but importantly it is deviation from the cultural norm (whatever the culture) that seems to distinguish women with EDs from their peer group [41]. In short, rather than ethnicity explaining any noted symptom variations, the pertinent assessment issues may relate to understanding the current cultural norms and their dissonance with the culture of their ethnic background.

Gender

Although representing around one in ten people with AN [42], males with this condition are much less likely to be recognised. Amongst those who do present for assessment, medical complications are more likely apparent than with their female counterparts [43]. There are mixed views about whether males present for assessment much earlier (see Carlat et al. [44]) or later (see Siegel et al. [43])

than their female counterparts. Psychological symptoms are largely identical, although there is some limited evidence that males may have less severe scores on diagnostic tools and symptom rating scales [45] and are more likely present with particular weight control strategies (for example, excessive exercise [46]) and dissatisfaction with muscle size and shape. Too few studies have been conducted to examine whether the natural course of the illness differs by gender. Some studies report a more benign outcome in men at one year (e.g. Strober et al. [47]), while a recent long term follow-up study found no gender differences in 10-year survival rates [48]. Causal models particularly relevant to males are still largely speculative, although sexual orientation issues feature prominently in males [49]. However it may be that gay men may be more willing to seek help for psychological problems. At this stage therefore, the assessment of males presenting with AN largely should follow the same assessment considerations as females.

Assessment screening and severity tools

Screening tools

A large number of standardised self-report and interview-based measures are available to clinicians. There is long-standing debate about the superiority of interviews as opposed to self-report measures (whether paper and pencil or computerised), and ultimately the selection of any measure will depend on the purpose and context of assessment, along with constraints on time, availability of training and clinical factors. These issues are now discussed.

Self-report questionnaires are easy and quick to administer, although they differ in their utility. Shorter measures such as the Eating Attitudes Test (EAT-12; EAT-26) [50] and SCOFF [10] are useful in primary care situations where an ED may be suspected (NICE Guidelines; Allen et al., 2011), and identifying the need for second screening steps is a focus. However these are less useful in specialist settings where the more relevant task is to gather systematic information about severity and the extent of psychopathology. Here, longer self-report measures (for example, Eating Disorder Inventory (EDI-3) [51], Eating Disorder Examination Questionnaire (EDE-Q) [52], and Yale-Brown-Cornell Eating Disorders Scale (YBC-EDS, [53]) tend to assess two factors - a combination of risk factors and psychological disturbances associated with AN [54]. Detailed information about psychological symptoms can be elicited from these, which in turn adds to any clinical formulations. As standardised measures, they can be useful in assessing symptom change.

Semi-structured or structured clinical interviews such as the Structured Clinical Interview for DSM-IV Axis I Disorders Clinical Version (SCID-CV) [55], and Eating Disorder Examination (EDE) [56] are often referred to as *"gold standards"* (APA, 2006, p.46). These are more time-consuming, involve training and are more likely suitable for research purposes rather than clinical settings, although they do possess the advantage of being validated to render an ED diagnosis.

Irrespective of the measure used, scores are affected by a number of clinical, demographic and psychometric issues. Denial may occur in interviews due to embarrassment and reluctance to disclose, whereas the risk with self-report measures is that patients may inaccurately estimate the seriousness of core symptoms [57,58], or simply disagree that symptoms are problematic [59]. In very severe cases, administration of psychometric tests (AN-related or otherwise) is clearly inappropriate. Wider psychometric limitations arise from differences in international norms and few national clinical norms [54], and the utility of measures differ between adults and adolescents [60]. Furthermore, different formats of the same measure (e.g. EDE and EDE-Q) have only modest agreement ratings, with rates of agreement being dependent on the type of symptom being assessed [58]. In terms of AN, no measure reliably distinguishes between AN and EDNOS-AN [61].

A positive diagnosis can be made in most cases without the need for a battery of psychometric tests. The more useful place of standardised psychometric tools is to screen, assess symptom change and research. In the end, standardised psychometric tools cannot replace the advantages of a thorough clinical interview. As noted by Nordbø et al. [62], *"an assessment tool should never be regarded as a substitute for treating the patients individually or replace the need for an individual exploration in each single patient"* (page 660). This is further discussed in the final section of this paper.

What constitutes severity?

The use of the concept of illness severity is common in ED settings, and there are solid grounds for this. For example, severity markers can help aid treatment decisions, potentially aid prognosis, and promote more uniform international understandings about clinical presentations [63]. However, empirically supported definitions of severity are largely lacking. Clinicians commonly default to one or more symptom markers or treatment intensity markers such as BMI [64] or multiple severity indices based on different symptoms (not all of which are AN symptoms [65]), hospitalisation [66] or length of illness [67]. In an attempt to address problems with all of the above strategies, a more recent approach has been the development of empirically derived tools to stage AN severity [36,68]. Early indicators suggest that such measures involve multiple symptom dimensions, and neatly capture both clinical reality and patient subjective reality [36]. One of these instruments [67], the CASIAN, largely assess the behavioural features of the ED so as to minimise the factors of denial and the often perverse reduction in psychological distress discussed above, as the illness progresses (i.e. drive for thinness and body dissatisfaction can decrease with severity). Longitudinal data is still needed to determine how staging instruments could usefully aid assessment, treatment pathway decisions and the prediction of prognosis.

Family involvement and family assessment

Where possible, it is highly desirable to have carers or family involved in the assessment process given they provide much of the on-going care and share the extensive burden of the disorder. For younger patients still living at home, family members may need to be directly involved as treatment agents [69] as long as they are appropriately supported and advised, noting that family members can become entangled with behaviours that maintain the disorder [70]. For adolescents, the assessment phase may more directly involve assessment of family functioning. The inevitable distress about having a family member with AN may need addressing in its own right and assessment of family functioning is core where family therapy treatment models are to be employed. There is no clearly superior way to assess family functioning: approaches are likely to reflect the model of family therapy employed and there are several variants of this. Family therapy models have been met with enthusiasm although a recent Cochrane Collaboration review suggests a need to temper this enthusiasm due to a range of methodological shortcomings in the small number of published treatment trials [71]. Such moderation should equally apply to assessment processes meaning that rigid approaches to assess families should be avoided.

Co-morbidity

Given psychiatric co-morbidity is common in people with AN, consideration of these associated problems should be routine. Those presenting for assessment may have higher rates of co-morbidity than AN community samples due to the additional burden and distress of these comorbid conditions. Indeed, these conditions may be the precipitant for presentation rather than AN itself. If psychiatric co-morbidity is recognised, conclusions about the actual presence of a primary anxiety (or mood disorder) is often best delayed until the symptom contribution of AN can be clarified, especially in the case of severe AN. Co-morbidity may impact on treatment engagement, in both directions, with co-morbidity prompting assessment or in other circumstances reducing engagement. The following sections discuss common forms of co-morbidity and implications for assessment.

Mood disorders

While major depression features prominently, depressive symptoms may also result from severe malnutrition, which almost certainly elevate these rates. Generally, however, there is robust evidence for elevated rates of major depression in all AN populations, irrespective of whether these are clinic or community samples. Godart et al. [72] found life-time prevalence rates ranging from 9.5% - 71.3%, with the variability in findings likely due to methodological differences across studies. The overall lifetime prevalence for eating disorders patients is estimated at 40%. There is debate about the most common sequencing of these comorbidities with some suggesting that the mood disorder more often precedes the ED (Cooper et al., 2002) and others highlighting past problems of over-diagnosing depression when instead symptoms may be secondary to malnutrition [57]. The consensus is that the relationship is complex. Scores on depression screening measures can be significantly elevated by an ED [73] resulting in a need to set higher cut-off scores in order to be meaningful. Vigilance for mood symptoms should also be ongoing given that improvements in AN can be experienced as depressogenic, with some sufferers construing the relinquishing of symptoms as a sign of losing control or giving in (to treatment) [74].

Bipolar disorder co-morbidity in AN is rare [75]. Affective disorders along this spectrum are more likely to be associated with forms of disordered eating involving bingeing or over-eating. How EDs and bipolar disorders overlap requires further study.

Assessment of self-harm and suicide risk

A recent meta-analysis observed a decreased risk of completed suicide in AN [76] over recent decades, with a standardised mortality ratio (SMR) of 31. This SMR still represents an elevated risk when compared with other EDs and the general population. The extent to which AN directly contributes to this risk as opposed to the combined effects of AN and co-morbidity to this risk is still debated [77].

Information gathering about risk comprises a two stepped approach. First, standard suicide self-harm risk assessment considerations apply. Thus, just with non-ED populations, the presence of depression increases the risk of suicidal behaviours and completed suicide and a sizeable proportion of these people will have had contact with their GP in the week or months before death. Other risk factors include a history of mental disorder, more severe psychopathology overall, Axis 2 psychopathology, history of self-harm/suicide attempts, and substance misuse (see Hawton et al. [78]). It follows that assessment of these standard risk factors should always occur when engaging with a person presenting with AN.

Second, the presence of particular AN symptoms or a history of AN may produce additional risks. These include the presence of binge-purge patterns [79], markers of chronicity including illness duration and very low weight [80], and high anxiety in AN-R [79]. Rates of completed suicides in people with AN are debated [2], with one study reporting suicide as the second most frequent cause of death in a retrospective study of those treated in an ED service [81]. The most consistent finding is approximately 20% of deaths in AN are attributable to suicide [82]. It is self-evident that assessment of suicidal ideation and behaviours is important, especially in those presenting with co-morbidity.

Unusual forms of self-harm have been reported that are directly linked with efforts to maintain AN. For example, ingesting large quantities of salt [83], scratching [84] and blood-letting [85]. How these phenomena fall under the umbrella of wider deliberate self-harm (DSH) phenomena is unclear as DSH has multiple intended functions [86]. If present, such behaviours are unlikely to come to light in outpatient assessment settings. Although the conscientious clinician will assess for them, these may only be revealed following close monitoring, as occurs in inpatient settings.

Anxiety disorders

There is extensive overlap between anxiety and AN symptoms, with AN exacerbating concurrent anxiety disorders in addition to extensive anxiety symptoms forming part of the AN syndrome [87]. This makes assessment of anxiety a necessary component of any formulation, irrespective of any suspected Axis 1 anxiety disorder. This is because common anxiety treatment techniques inevitably will be part of treatment. Assessment questions include the extent of pre-morbid anxiety, the presence of genuine co-morbidity and the degree to which anxiety symptoms are actually part of AN. These issues are addressed in turn.

Reported lifetime prevalence rates of anxiety disorders vary considerably ranging from 23%-75% (see Swinbourne and Touyz [88] for a review). Generally the anxiety disorder is more likely to precede the onset of AN rather than the other way around [89], although this may depend on the anxiety disorder in question [90]. Of the anxiety disorders, obsessive-compulsive disorder (OCD) is the most researched condition [91], although social phobia, other phobic states and Generalised Anxiety Disorder (GAD) and anxiety-based problems such as clinical perfectionism [92] have all received attention.

Teasing out the functional relationship between wider anxiety phenomena and/or the presence of a primary anxiety disorder can be challenging, and even after weight-restoration anxiety symptoms tend to persist [93]. Detailed functional analysis of behavioural and cognitive rituals, the scope of intrusive thoughts, the scope of avoidance, and any other symptoms of fear may help clarify how these features are directly part of AN or more correctly attributed to another primary anxiety disorder. Importantly, anxiety symptoms may not be reported due to the success of avoidance or engaging in subtle "safety behaviours" that keep symptoms at bay. In such cases, anxiety symptoms may only emerge once there are treatment demands for change. As a result, the absence of anxiety symptoms on initial assessment should not be taken as evidence of the absence of anxiety.

Obsessions and compulsions particularly increase with starvation, and sometimes to an intensity that is comparable to people with OCD. Conclusions about the presence of a primary anxiety disorder should wait until the effects of starvation have abated.

Substance abuse and dependence

Reported rates of substance abuse in AN vary widely and are significantly associated with AN subtype (binge/purge), with rates as high as 35% in those who cross over to Bulimia Nervosa (BN) after weight restoration [94]. In general, the presence of any bulimic symptomatology significantly increases the likelihood of co-morbidity involving a variety of substances, both illicit and legal [95,96]. The sequencing of co-morbid alcohol problems and AN shows no distinctive pattern [97]. However the concurrent presence of alcohol misuse and AN should prompt enquiry into wider psychopathology given the increased odds of this in this subpopulation [98] and the known increased mortality [2].

Other substance abuse and dependence problems include the use of diet pills, laxatives, diuretics and other illicit stimulants for appetite suppression and increased metabolic effects [99]. Opioid and sedative use is also significantly elevated. In short, the assessment of substance misuse should cast a wide net, seeking information about illicit and over-the-counter drugs, including common substances containing high levels of caffeine. The assessment should also include patient understandings about how these substances maintain AN symptoms (for example, warding off normal signals of hunger) or manage other psychological symptoms or distress.

Nutritional, weight, and eating behaviour assessment

Obtaining a weight and nutritional history is a critical component of assessment, although this can be far from straight-forward. Being asked to be weighed is one of the most anxiety-provoking demands for someone with AN, even when many know their weight due to excessive self-monitoring. In the situation of outright refusal to be weighed, this can be a temporary impasse if the anxiety about this is explored. Clinicians who allow the continued avoidance of assessing weight may find themselves inadvertently colluding with the disorder.

Body mass index (BMI) is the most common metric used, with extreme levels (BMI ≤ 13) consistently showing a risk of a poorer outcome and elevated medical risks [81,100]. Centile charts are recommended for patients who are younger than 18 years of age [101]. Percentage of body fat is another useful indicator of risk as this also has been associated with outcome [102].

Apart from ascertaining current weight, there are several aspects of weight history that are clinically important. These include obtaining information about highest and lowest-ever weight (BMI), means of weight control, and if amenorrhea is present, weight at which menses were lost or in the case of primary amenorrhea consideration of the effect of delayed puberty. A history of a very low BMI at any point in the illness trajectory is a risk factor for premature death [2]. BMI alone is problematic in younger populations for whom BMI-for-age is argued as more appropriate [103]. Patient perception of their 'ideal' weight, and how they determined this, can provide useful clinical information about maintaining factors, and how AN is serving to manage psychological difficulties. Commonly, a particular weight may be fixated upon with an expectation that achieving this will bring a sense of well-being and success. Inevitably such rewards are not forthcoming often resulting in a decision to work towards a lower weight - as if the original goal was miscalculated.

A food and fluid diary may help assess aspects of nutritional pathology, or at least start the discussion about nutritional intake. Shame, embarrassment, and anxiety about increasing nutritional intake, are amongst the factors that affect the accuracy of food diaries and other forms of self-recording. Additional enquiry should be made about avoided foods, behaviours and rituals around eating, evidence of self-imposed caloric limits, and the full repertoire of compensatory behaviours.

Medical assessment

The main causes of increased mortality in AN are those directly related to the disease [82]. Fortunately advances in assessment and careful treatment of AN-related medical abnormalities have helped reduce the rates of mortality [104] compared with earlier practices. Multiple organ systems should be reviewed at assessment and abnormal medical findings can provide compelling objective evidence to ambivalent attendees who may contest the need for treatment. The types of medical complications presenting are influenced by age, clinical history, and weight history. The extent of medical and physical investigations undertaken will depend on these factors although there is some consensus on commonly recommended laboratory investigations. These include a full blood count, urea and electrolytes, biochemistry including calcium, magnesium, and phosphate, and glucose and liver functioning [105]. Assessment and monitoring for phosphate depletion is particularly important. Hypophosphatemia is well known to be associated with catastrophic consequences in the context of refeeding particularly for the severely underweight person.

Of concern, complications that are not reversible can occur in those who have yet to develop a chronic problem, and these include altered linear growth, osteoporosis, and structural or functional brain changes [106]. It is important to recognise that patients may initially appear asymptomatic due to slow adaptation to starvation over time. More detailed medical assessments may be indicated for those presenting with severe AN, as it is a mistake to consider mild AN as a benign condition. Even those with mild AN may experience prolonged periods of debilitating symptoms [11].

A full medical history and physical examination is essential to highlight immediate medical problems such as hypotension, hypothermia, bradycardia, skin conditions, and intercellular changes such as dehydration. Enquiry should extend to other gastrointestinal problems such as diarrhoea, constipation and abdominal cramping. A small number of patients may have had extensive previous medical work-up in an attempt to locate a medical condition that could explain symptoms that are more correctly caused by AN. Likewise, although rare, other non-psychiatric causes of significant weight loss (for example, medical conditions resulting in mal-absorbing consequences) should be considered early in the assessment process.

A medical review should include considering the presence of other conditions that may have serious consequences while occurring in the context of AN (e.g. diabetes) or other causes of weight loss unrelated to AN (e.g. primary gastrointestinal disorders), along with a review of medications that may compromise or contribute to medical risks occurring (for example, medications that prolong QT intervals). Since cardiac abnormalities have been estimated to occur in up to 86% of patients [107], and cardiovascular causes are a major cause of death [108], cardiac investigations (ECG) should check for a range of cardiomyopathies, of which there are many [109]. Studies suggest that is unclear when QT prolongation first occurs in the natural history of AN and when the period of greatest risk of cardiac abnormalities may occur [107]. Endocrine screens are useful, particularly checking thyroid functions and other hormonal disturbances.

Other checks may need to include bone density scans assessing for osteoporosis and spontaneous or low impact fractures, particularly if pain is a presenting complaint. When symptoms of self-induced vomiting are present, the risk of dental complications is high even after a relatively short history of vomiting [110] and dental reviews are recommended. Common gastrointestinal disturbances include gastric pain, prolonged gastric emptying and constipation [108], all of which can perpetuate the desire to continue restricting.

The presence of medical complications may or may not lead to hospital admission. As noted earlier, significant contextual factors, availability and regional treatment philosophies influence admission decisions [111] both within and between countries. When acute medical presentations occur, particular care is needed to avoid the refeeding syndrome and other treatment-related complications. Medical symptoms may be alarming and prompt consideration of urgent steps, but cautious use of otherwise considered routine interventions (for example, intravenous fluids) is required in order to avoid catastrophic consequences [112]. A small number of patients will require an explicit medical admission.

Compulsory assessments

On occasions, preliminary assessments occur under duress after formal steps have been taken to initiate the assessment. Engagement of a reluctant patient who may require persuasion, formal or otherwise, to accept urgent investigations or treatment requires skill and tact. The legal options and legislative pathways for compulsory assessment vary across countries, but the principles are relatively universal and well discussed in the literature [113,114]. Legal coercion is required relatively infrequently [115]. Importantly, patient perceptions of coercion, with or without the use of formal compulsion, occur along a continuum [116] with many later describing formal treatment orders as helpful. Much can be done to mitigate distress when a compassionate and trusting approach is taken [117]. Decision-making must consider patient capacity to make decisions, the urgency of presenting symptoms and the outcomes where compulsory steps have been previously utilised to detain the patient.

Synthesis and formulation of assessment information

A comprehensive assessment interview is likely to take several hours, and where clinically indicated, may require several appointments. Once sufficient and necessary information has been gathered, the next step is to synthesise this with other findings from other standard assessment steps such as history taking and mental status examination.

A case formulation approach is recommended to develop *"a more complete picture of the patient than can be associated with a diagnosis"* [[118], page 1] incorporating all presenting issues, past treatment outcomes and patient perspectives. It involves assimilating information from multiple sources and using clinical judgement to weigh up both converging and conflicting data. A case formulation approach is also conducive to building a therapeutic alliance which is vital in psychotherapeutic treatments both generally and specifically in regarding to AN [119].

The formulation may include tentative hypotheses about predisposing, precipitating and maintaining factors. Families commonly ask about causal factors fearing that assessment findings will implicate them in some way. Pressed for answers from distressed families (and patients themselves), clinicians may be tempted to be drawn on predisposing factors. However causes of AN are far from understood. Tentative hypotheses are best, and better framed as general risk factors in the interim. Given the typically prolonged time between onset and assessment combined with difficulties establishing age of onset, articulating more immediate precipitating factors is equally fraught. It will be more possible to draw conclusions about maintaining factors due to the extensive knowledge about reinforcement schedules and behavioural traps in the lived experience of AN.

In a large multidisciplinary team, varying perspectives and formulations may emerge and this can be clinically useful. However such differences should never divert from the importance of all team members uniting behind any arising triage or treatment plan. The end result of the case formulation should be a set of working hypotheses articulated into a coordinated care plan followed by all team members. This care plan should be both detailed and broad covering immediate treatment needs and priorities for further investigation.

Conclusion

This overview in limited in its ability to fully discuss all relevant factors in assessment; a decision was made to include issues that would be pertinent to a wide audience. Likewise, the scope of this overview precludes discussion of the steps instigating treatment following from assessment, although it follows that management of acute physical and psychiatric problems naturally take priority.

Experienced clinicians know that the process of assessment is an on-going one, encompassing a need to repeat and monitor medical investigations and revise psychological formulations as more information comes to light, symptoms worsen or improve and priorities shift. A preliminary assessment should never attempt to reach firm opinions about cause although formulations relating to factors maintaining the disorder may be more apparent.

In conclusion, assessments require a systematic, rigorous, and empathic approach that strikes an important balance between carefully listening to patient needs and dilemmas, while remaining firm and focused about the need for treatment. Even difficult assessment interviews conducted under duress should leave the patient with a sense of dignity and that they have been heard. The assessment interaction should be seen as an important therapeutic interaction to begin building a therapeutic alliance, balancing both an atmosphere of acceptance [120] yet firmness without being over-confident or paternalistic. The most important assessment tool is the clinician and the knowledge and stance they take into the interpersonal interaction. An assessment will always be a deeply complex interpersonal interaction requiring a careful clinical interview, and one based on a sound understanding of the symptoms and issues faced by the patient.

On-going efforts are required to address substantive knowledge gaps and to encourage the uptake of evidenced-based approaches where such evidence is assessed as strong. As noted recently, "*the bond that tethers our patient to our treatment is a fragile one*" [[121], page 178]. At times this could be rephrased to say that the bond that tethers assessing clinicians to the evidence is equally fragile. There is a universal problem transferring research evidence into clinical practice, and this overview aims to reduce that 'leakage' [122] between research and practice.

While not above criticism themselves, a number of practice guidelines are available that outline in some detail the required and desired assessment investigations, and at least draw clinicians' attention to the quality and limitations of evidence. These include the Australasian [123] (currently undergoing review), North American [124], and the British [101] guidelines. The latter of these (and the most recently published) appeared just under a decade ago, but a recent review of the literature indicates that these guidelines are as relevant today as they were in 2004, (http://www.nice.org.uk/nicemedia/live/10932/55781/55781.pdf, downloaded 17 Sept 2012).

Competing interests
Both authors declare that they have no competing interest.

Authors' contributions
LS carried out the literature review and drafted the early version. SM revised initial manuscript drafts and critically commented on the intellectual content. Both authors read and approved the final manuscript.

Author details
[1]Department of Psychological Medicine, University of Otago at Christchurch, 4 Oxford Terrace, Christchurch 8140, New Zealand. [2]Centre for Eating and Dieting Disorders, University of Sydney, 92-94 Parramatta Road, Camberdown, New South Wales 2050, Australia.

References
1. Harris EC, Barraclough B: **Excess mortality of mental disorder.** *Br J Psychiatry* 1998, **173**:11–53.
2. Button EJ, Chadalavada B, Palmer RL: **Mortality and predictors of death in a cohort of patients presenting to an eating disorders service.** *Int J Eat Disord* 2010, **43**:387–392.
3. Butterfly Foundation: *Paying the Price: The economic and social impact of eating disorders.* Butterfly Foundation: Melbourne; 2012. Available from: www.thebutterflyfoundation.org.au.
4. Dooley-Hash S, Lipson SK, Walton MA, Cunningham RM: **Increased emergency department use by adolescents and young adults with eating disorders.** *Int J Eat Disord* 2012, **45**:883–890.
5. Simon J, Schmidt U, Pilling S: **The health service use and cost of eating disorders.** *Psychol Med* 2005, **35**:1543–1551.
6. House J, Schmidt U, Craig M, Landau S, Simic M, Nicholls D, Hugo P, Berelowitz M, Eisler I: **Comparison of specialist and nonspecialist care pathways for adolescents with anorexia nervosa and related eating disorders.** *In J Eat Disord* 2012, **45**:949–956.
7. Marks P, Beumont P, Birmingham CL: **GPs managing patients with eating disorders. a tiered approach.** *Aust Fam Physician* 2003, **32**:509–514.
8. Allen KL, Fursland A, Watson H, Byrne SM: **Eating disorder diagnoses in general practice settings: comparison with structured clinical interview and self-report questionnaires.** *J Ment Health* 2011, **20**:270–280.
9. Hebebrand J, Bulik CM: **Critical appraisal of the provisional DSM-5 criteria for anorexia nervosa and an alternative proposal.** *Int J Eat Disord* 2011, **44**:665–678.
10. Hill LS, Reid F, Morgan JF, Lacey JH: **SCOFF, the development of an eating disorder screening questionnaire.** *Int J Eat Disord* 2010, **43**:344–351.
11. Treasure J, Russell G: **The case for early intervention in anorexia nervosa: theoretical exploration of maintaining factors.** *Br J Psychiatry* 2011, **199**:5–7.
12. Von Holle A, Pinheiro AP, Thornton LM, Klump KL, Berrettini WH, Brandt H, Crawford S, Crow S, Fichter MM, Halmi KA, Johnson C, Kaplan AS, Keel P, La Via M, Mitchell J, Strober M, Woodside DB, Kaye WH, Bulik CM: **Temporal patterns of recovery across eating disorder subtypes.** *Aust NZ J Psychiatry* 2008, **42**:108–117.
13. Hart LM, Granillo MT, Jorm AF, Paxton SJ: **Unmet need for treatment in the eating disorders: a systematic review of eating disorder specific treatment seeking among community cases.** *Clin Psychol Rev* 2011, **31**:727–735.
14. Waller G, Schmidt U, Treasure J, Murray K, Aleyna J, Emanuelli F, Crockett J, Yeomans M: **Problems across care pathways in specialist adult eating disorder services.** *Psychiatr Bull* 2009, **33**:26–29.
15. Tatham M, Stringer H, Perera S, Waller G: **"Do you still want to be seen?": the pros and cons of active waiting list management.** *Int J Eat Disord* 2012, **45**:57–62.
16. Carmen D, Shah S, Gilbert S, Russell F: **Improving attendance at an eating disorder clinic by means of an "opt in" letter.** *Clin Psych Forum* 2007, **173**:22–25.
17. Surgenor LJ, Plumridge EW, Horn J: **'Knowing one's self' anorexic: implications for therapeutic practice.** *Int J Eat Disord* 2003, **33**:22–32.
18. Nordbo RH, Gulliksen KS, Espeset EM, Skarderud F, Geller J, Holte A: **Expanding the concept of motivation to change: the content of patients' wish to recover from anorexia nervosa.** *Int J Eat Disord* 2008, **41**:635–642.
19. Waller G: **The myths of motivation: time for a fresh look at some received wisdom in the eating disorders?** *Int J Eat Disord* 2012, **45**:1–16.
20. Knowles L, Anokhina A, Serpell L: **Motivational interventions in the eating disorders: What is the evidence?** *Int J Eat Disord* 2012, **46**:97–107.
21. Rieger E, Touyz SW, Beumont PJV: **The anorexia nervosa stages of change questionnaire (ANSOCQ): Information regarding its psychometric properties.** *Int J Eat Disord* 2002, **32**:24–38.
22. Morgan JF, Jones WR, Saeidi S: **Knowledge and attitudes of psychiatrists towards eating disorders.** *Eur Eat Disord Rev* 2012, **21**:84–88.
23. Stewart MC, Schiavo RS, Herzog DB, Franko DL: **Stereotypes, prejudice and discrimination of women with anorexia nervosa.** *Eur Eat Disord Rev* 2008, **16**:311–318.
24. Reid M, Williams S, Burr J: **Perspectives on eating disorders and service provision: A qualitative study of healthcare professionals.** *Eur Eat Disord Rev* 2010, **18**:390–398.
25. Album D, Westin S: **Do diseases have a prestige hierarchy? A survey among physicians and medical students.** *Soc Sci Med* 2008, **66**:182–188.
26. Sly R: **What's in a name? Classifying 'the dropout' from treatment for anorexia nervosa.** *Eur Eat Disord Rev* 2009, **17**:405–407.
27. Strober M, Freeman R, Morrell W: **The long-term course of severe anorexia nervosa in adolescents: survival analysis of recovery, relapse, and outcome predictors over 10–15 years in a prospective study.** *Int J Eat Disord* 1997, **22**:339–360.
28. Baran SA, Weltzin TE, Kaye WH: **Low discharge weight and outcome in anorexia nervosa.** *Am J Psychiatry* 1995, **152**:1070–1072.

29. Watkins CE Jr: **The supervision of psychotherapy supervisor trainees.** *Am J Psychother* 1994, **48:**417–431.
30. Wallier J, Vibert S, Berthoz S, Huas C, Hubert T, Godart N: **Dropout from inpatient treatment for anorexia nervosa: critical review of the literature.** *Int J Eat Disord* 2009, **42:**636–647.
31. Hudson JI, Hiripi E, Pope HG Jr, Kessler RC: **The prevalence and correlates of eating disorders in the National Comorbidity Survey Replication.** *Biol Psychiatry* 2007, **61:**348–358.
32. Eddy KT, Dorer DJ, Franko DL, Tahilani K, Thompson-Brenner H, Herzog DB: **Diagnostic crossover in anorexia nervosa and bulimia nervosa: implications for DSM-V.** *Am J Psychiatry* 2008, **165:**245–250.
33. Keys A, Brozek J, Henschel A, Mickelsen O, Taylor HL: *The biology of human starvation.* Minneapolis: University of Minnesota Press; 1950.
34. American Psychiatric Association: *Diagnostic and Statistical Manual of Mental Disorders (DSM-5).* American Psychiatric Publishing: Washington, DC; 2013. ISBN 5.
35. Uher R, Rutter M: **Classification of feeding and eating disorders: review of evidence and proposals for ICD-11.** *World Psychiatry* 2012, **11:**80–92.
36. Maguire S, Touyz S, Surgenor L, Crosby RD, Engel SG, Lacey H, Heywood-Everett S, Grange DL: **The clinician administered staging instrument for anorexia nervosa: development and psychometric properties.** *Int J Eat Disord* 2012, **45:**390–399.
37. Soh N, Touyz S, Surgenor LJ: **Eating and body image disturbances across cultures.** *Eur Eat Disord Rev* 2006, **14:**54–65.
38. Wang J, Thornton JC, Russell M, Burastero S, Heymsfield S, Pierson RN Jr: **Asians have lower body mass index (BMI) but higher percent body fat than do whites: comparisons of anthropometric measurements.** *Am J Clin Nutr* 1994, **60:**23–28.
39. Ung EK, Lee S, Kua EH: **Anorexia nervosa and bulimia–a Singapore perspective.** *Singapore Med J* 1997, **38:**332–335.
40. Soh NL, Touyz S, Dobbins T, Surgenor L, Clarke S, Kohn M, Lee EL, Leow V, Rieger E, Ung KE, Walter G: **Body image disturbance in young North European and East Asian women with and without eating disorders in Australia and in Singapore.** *Eur Eat Disord Rev* 2008, **16:**287–296.
41. Soh N, Surgenor LJ, Touyz S, Walter G: **Eating disorders across two cultures: does the expression of psychological control vary?** *Aust NZ J Psychiatry* 2007, **41:**351–358.
42. Rhys Jones W, Morgan JF: **Eating disorders in men: a review of the literature.** *J Public Ment Health* 2010, **9:**23–31.
43. Siegel JH, Hardoff D, Golden NH, Shenker IR: **Medical complications in male adolescents with anorexia nervosa.** *J Adolesc Health* 1995, **16:**448–453.
44. Carlat DJ, Camargo CA Jr, Herzog DB: **Eating disorders in males: a report on 135 patients.** *Am J Psychiatry* 1997, **154:**1127–1132.
45. Nunez-Navarro A, Aguera Z, Krug I, Jimenez-Murcia S, Sanchez I, Araguz N, Gorwood P, Granero R, Penelo E, Karwautz A, Moragas L, Saldana S, Treasure J, Menchon JM, Fernandez-Aranda F: **Do men with eating disorders differ from women in clinics, psychopathology and personality?** *Eur Eat Disord Rev* 2012, **20:**23–31.
46. Marks LI: **Deconstructing locus of control: Implications for practitioners.** *J Counsel Devel* 1998, **76:**251–260.
47. Strober M, Freeman R, Lampert C, Diamond J, Teplinsky C, DeAntonio M: **Are there gender differences in core symptoms, temperament, and short-term prospective outcome in anorexia nervosa?** *Int J Eat Disord* 2006, **39:**570–575.
48. Gueguen J, Godart N, Chambry J, Brun-Eberentz A, Foulon C, Divac Phd SM, Guelfi JD, Rouillon F, Falissard B, Huas C: **Severe anorexia nervosa in men: comparison with severe AN in women and analysis of mortality.** *Int J Eat Disord* 2012, **45:**537–545.
49. Keel PK, Brown TA: **The impact of relationships on the association between sexual orientation and disordered eating in men.** *Int J Eat Disord* 2012, **45:**792–799.
50. Garner DM, Olmsted MP, Bohr Y, Garfinkel PE: **The eating attitudes test: Psychometric features and clinical correlates.** *Psychol Med* 1982, **12:**871–878.
51. Garner DM: *Eating disorder inventory-3.* Lutz, Florida: Psychological Assessment Resources, Inc.; 2004.
52. Beglin S, Fairburn CG: **Eating Disorder Examination Questionnaire (EDQ-Q 6.0).** In *Cognitive behaviour therapy and eating disorders.* Edited by Fairburn CG. New York: Guildford Press; 2008:265–308.
53. Sunday SR, Halmi KA, Einhorn A: **The Yale-Brown-Cornell Eating Disorder Scale: a new scale to assess eating disorder symptomatology.** *Int J Eat Disord* 1995, **18:**237–245.
54. Clausen L, Rosenvinge JH, Friborg O, Rokkedal K: **Validating the Eating Disorder Inventory-3 (EDI-3): A Comparison Between 561 Female Eating Disorders Patients and 878 Females from the General Population.** *J Psychopath Behav Assess* 2011, **33:**101–110.
55. First MB, Spitzer RL, Gibbon M, Williams JBW: *Structured Clinical Interview for DSM-IV Axis I Disorders, Clinical Version (SCID-CV).* Washington, DC: American Psychiatric Press Inc.; 1996.
56. Fairburn CG, Cooper Z: **The eating disorders examination.** In *Binge Eating: Nature, Assessment and Treatment.* Edited by Fairburn CG, Wilson GT. New York: Guildford Press; 1993:317–360.
57. Mattar L, Huas C, Duclos J, Apfel A, Godart N: **Relationship between malnutrition and depression or anxiety in Anorexia Nervosa: a critical review of the literature.** *J Affect Disord* 2011, **132:**311–318.
58. Wolk SL, Loeb KL, Walsh BT: **Assessment of patients with anorexia nervosa: interview versus self-report.** *Int J Eat Disord* 2005, **37:**92–99.
59. Allen S, Dalton WT: **Treatment of eating disorders in primary care: a systematic review.** *J Health Psychol* 2011, **16:**1165–1176.
60. Binford RB, Le Grange D, Jellar CC: **Eating Disorders Examination versus Eating Disorders Examination-Questionnaire in adolescents with full and partial-syndrome bulimia nervosa and anorexia nervosa.** *Int J Eat Disord* 2005, **37:**44–49.
61. Le Grange D, Crosby RD, Engel SG, Cao L, Ndungu A, Crow SJ, Peterson CB, Mitchell JE, Wonderlich SA: **DSM-IV-defined anorexia nervosa versus subthreshold anorexia nervosa (EDNOS-AN).** *Eur Eat Disord Rev* 2013, **21:**1–7.
62. Nordbo RH, Espeset EM, Gulliksen KS, Skarderud F, Geller J, Holte A: **Reluctance to recover in anorexia nervosa.** *Eur Eat Disord Rev* 2012, **20:**60–67.
63. Maguire S, Le Grange D, Surgenor LJ, Marks P, Lacey H, Touyz S: **Staging anorexia nervosa: conceptualising illness severity.** *Early Intervent Psych* 2008, **2:**3–10.
64. Touyz S, Thornton C, Rieger E, George L, Beumont P: **The incorporation of the stage of change model in the day hospital treatment of patients with anorexia nervosa.** *Eur Child Adolesc Psychiatry* 2003, **12**(Suppl 1):I65–I71.
65. Loeb KL, Jones J, Roberto CA, Sonia Gugga S, Marcus SM, Attia E, Timothy Walsh B: **Adolescent-adult discrepancies on the eating disorder examination: a function of developmental stage or severity of illness?** *Int J Eat Disord* 2011, **44:**567–572.
66. Milos G, Spindler A, Schnyder U, Martz J, Hoek HW, Willi J: **Incidence of severe anorexia nervosa in Switzerland: 40 years of development.** *Int J Eat Disord* 2004, **35:**250–258.
67. Treasure J, Tchanturia K, Harrison A, Davies H, Roberts M, Oldershaw A, Stahl D, Morris R, Schmidt U: **Cognitive flexibility and clinical severity in eating disorders.** *Plos One (Electronic Resource)* 2001, **6:**e20462.
68. Bauer S, Winn S, Schmidt U, Kordy H: **Construction, scoring, and validation of the short evaluation of eating disorders (SEED).** *Eur Eat Disord Rev* 2005, **13:**191–200.
69. Treasure J, Sepulveda AR, MacDonald P, Whitaker W, Lopez C, Zabala M, Kyriacou O, Todd G: **The assessment of the family of people with eating disorders.** *Eur Eat Disord Rev* 2008, **16:**247–255.
70. Schmidt U, Treasure J: **Anorexia nervosa: valued and visible. A cognitive-interpersonal maintenance model and its implications for research and practice.** *Br J Clin Psychol* 2006, **45:**343–366.
71. Fisher CA, Hetrick SE, Rushford N: **Family therapy for anorexia nervosa.** *Cochrane Database Syst Rev* 2010:. Issue 4: Art. No: CD004780.
72. Godart NT, Perdereau F, Rein Z, Berthoz S, Wallier J, Jeammet P, Flament MF: **Comorbidity studies of eating disorders and mood disorders. Critical review of the literature.** *J Affect Disord* 2007, **97:**37–49.
73. Kennedy SH, Kaplan AS, Garfinkel PE, Rockert W, Toner B, Abbey SE: **Depression in anorexia nervosa and bulimia nervosa: discriminating depressive symptoms and episodes.** *J Psychosom Res* 1994, **38:**773–782.
74. Mischoulon D, Eddy KT, Keshaviah A, Dinescu D, Ross SL, Kass AE, Franko DL, Herzog DB: **Depression and Eating Disorders.** *J Affect Disord* 2011, **130:**470–477.
75. McElroy SL, Frye MA, Hellemann G, Altshuler L, Leverich GS, Suppes T, Keck PE, Nolen WA, Kupka R, Post RM: **Prevalence and correlates of eating disorders in 875 patients with bipolar disorder.** *J Affect Disord* 2011, **128:**191–198.
76. Preti A, Rocchi MB, Sisti D, Camboni MV, Miotto P: **A comprehensive meta-analysis of the risk of suicide in eating disorders.** *Acta Psychiatr Scand* 2011, **124:**6–17.
77. Bodell LP, Joiner TE, Keel PK: **Comorbidity-independent risk for suicidality increases with bulimia nervosa but not with anorexia nervosa.** *J Psychiatr Res* 2013, **47:**617–621.

78. Hawton K, Casanas ICC, Haw C, Saunders K: **Risk factors for suicide in individuals with depression: A systematic review.** *J Affect Disord* 2013, **147**:17–28.
79. Forcano L, Alvarez E, Santamaria JJ, Jimenez-Murcia S, Granero R, Penelo E, Alonso P, Sanchez I, Menchon JM, Ulman F, Bulik CM, Fernandez-Aranda F: **Suicide attempts in anorexia nervosa subtypes.** *Compr Psychiatry* 2011, **52**:352–358.
80. Favaro A, Santonastaso P: **Suicidality in eating disorders: clinical and psychological correlates.** *Acta Psychiatr Scand* 1997, **95**:508–514.
81. Rosling AM, Sparen P, Norring C, von Knorring AL: **Mortality of eating disorders: a follow-up study of treatment in a specialist unit 1974–2000.** *Int J Eat Disord* 2011, **44**:304–310.
82. Papadopoulos FC, Ekbom A, Brandt L, Ekselius L: **Excess mortality, causes of death and prognostic factors in anorexia nervosa.** *Br J Psychiatry* 2009, **194**:10–17.
83. Morgan JF, Ahene P, Lacey JH: **Salinophagia in anorexia nervosa: case reports.** *Int J Eat Disord* 2010, **43**:190–192.
84. Morgan JF, Lacey JH: **Scratching and fasting: a study of pruritus and anorexia nervosa.** *Br J Dermatol* 1999, **140**:453–456.
85. Morgan JF, Lacey JH: **Blood-letting in anorexia nervosa: a case study.** *Int J Eat Disord* 2000, **27**:483–485.
86. Skegg K: **Self-harm.** *Lancet* 2005, **366**:1471–1483.
87. Steinglass JE, Sysko R, Glasofer D, Albano AM, Simpson HB, Walsh BT: **Rationale for the application of exposure and response prevention to the treatment of anorexia nervosa.** *Int J Eat Disord* 2011, **44**:134–141.
88. Swinbourne JM, Touyz SW: **The co-morbidity of eating disorders and anxiety disorders: a review.** *Eur Eat Disord Rev* 2007, **15**:253–274.
89. Touyz S, Swinbourne J, Hunt C, Abbott M, Russell J, St Clare T: **The comorbidity between eating disorders and anxiety disorders: prevalence in an eating disorder sample and anxiety disorder sample.** *Aust NZ J Psychiatry* 2012, **46**:118–131.
90. Pallister E, Waller G: **Anxiety in the eating disorders: understanding the overlap.** *Clin Psychol Rev* 2008, **28**:366–386.
91. Godart NT, Flament MF, Perdereau F, Jeammet P: **Comorbidity between eating disorders and anxiety disorders: a review.** *Int J Eat Disord* 2002, **32**:253–270.
92. Fairburn CG, Cooper Z, Shafran R: **Cognitive behaviour therapy for eating disorders: a "transdiagnostic" theory and treatment.** *Behav Res Ther* 2003, **41**:509–528.
93. Yackobovitch-Gavan M, Golan M, Valevski A, Kreitler S, Bachar E, Lieblich A, Mitrani E, Weizman A, Stein D: **An integrative quantitative model of factors influencing the course of anorexia nervosa over time.** *Int J Eat Disord* 2009, **42**:306–317.
94. Krug I, Pinheiro AP, Bulik C, Jimenez-Murcia S, Granero R, Penelo E, Masuet C, Aguera Z, Fernandez-Aranda F: **Lifetime substance abuse, family history of alcohol abuse/dependence and novelty seeking in eating disorders: comparison study of eating disorder subgroups.** *Psychiatry Clin Neurosci* 2009, **63**:82–87.
95. Herzog DB, Franko DL, Dorer DJ, Keel PK, Jackson S, Manzo MP: **Drug abuse in women with eating disorders.** *Int J Eat Disord* 2006, **39**:364–368.
96. O'Brien KM, Vincent NK: **Psychiatric comorbidity in anorexia and bulimia nervosa: nature, prevalence, and causal relationships.** *Clin Psychol Rev* 2003, **23**:57–74.
97. Baker JH, Thornton LM, Strober M, Brandt H, Crawford S, Fichter MM, Halmi KA, Johnson C, Jones I, Kaplan AS, Klump KL, Mitchell JE, Treasure J, Woodside DB, Berrettini WH, Kaye WH, Bulik CM: **Temporal sequence of comorbid alcohol use disorder and anorexia nervosa.** *Addict Behav* 2013, **38**:1704–1709.
98. Bulik CM, Klump KL, Thornton L, Kaplan AS, Devlin B, Fichter MM, Halmi KA, Strober M, Woodside DB, Crow S, Mitchell JE, Rotondo A, Mauri M, Cassano GB, Keel PK, Berrettini WH, Kaye WH: **Alcohol use disorder comorbidity in eating disorders: a multicenter study.** *J Clin Psychiatry* 2004, **65**:1000–1006.
99. Root TL, Pisetsky EM, Thornton L, Lichtenstein P, Pedersen NL, Bulik CM: **Patterns of co-morbidity of eating disorders and substance use in Swedish females.** *Psychol Med* 2010, **40**:105–115.
100. Pinter O, Probst M, Vandereycken W, Pieters G, Goris M: **The predictive value of body mass index for the weight evolution in anorexia nervosa.** *Eat Weight Disord* 2004, **9**:232–235.
101. National Institute for Clinical Excellence: *Eating disorders: Core interventions in the treatment and management of anorexia nervosa, bulimia nervosa, and related eating disorders.* London: National Institute for Clinical Excellence; 2004.
102. Bodell LP, Mayer LE: **Percent body fat is a risk factor for relapse in anorexia nervosa: a replication study.** *Int J Eat Disord* 2011, **44**:118–123.
103. Flegal KM, Wei R, Ogden C: **Weight-for-stature compared with body mass index-for-age growth charts for the United States from the Centers for Disease Control and Prevention.** *Am J Clin Nutr* 2002, **75**:761–766.
104. Lindblad F, Lindberg L, Hjern A: **Improved survival in adolescent patients with anorexia nervosa: a comparison of two Swedish national cohorts of female inpatients.** *Am J Psychiatry* 2006, **163**:1433–1435.
105. Nicholls D, Hudson L, Mahomed F: **Managing anorexia nervosa.** *Arch Dis Child* 2011, **96**:977–982.
106. Katzman DK: **Medical complications in adolescents with anorexia nervosa: a review of the literature.** *Int J Eat Disord* 2005, **37**(Suppl):S52–S59. discussion S87-9.
107. Lesinskiene S, Barkus A, Ranceva N, Dembinskas A: **A meta-analysis of heart rate and QT interval alteration in anorexia nervosa.** *World J Biol Psychia* 2008, **9**:86–91.
108. Zipfel S, Sammet I, Rapps N, Herzog W, Herpertz S, Martens U: **Gastrointestinal disturbances in eating disorders: clinical and neurobiological aspects.** *Auton Neurosci* 2006, **129**:99–106.
109. Casiero D, Frishman WH: **Cardiovascular complications of eating disorders.** *Cardiol Rev* 2006, **14**:227–231.
110. Montecchi PP, Custureri V, Polimeni A, Cordaro M, Costa L, Marinucci S, Montecchi F: **Oral manifestations in a group of young patients with anorexia nervosa.** *Eat Weight Disord* 2003, **8**:164–167.
111. Sylvester CJ, Forman SF: **Clinical practice guidelines for treating restrictive eating disorder patients during medical hospitalization.** *Curr Opin Pediatr* 2008, **20**:390–397.
112. Mascolo M, Trent S, Colwell C, Mehler PS: **What the emergency department needs to know when caring for your patients with eating disorders.** *Int J Eat Disord* 2012, **45**:977–981. Early view - Online Only.
113. Ayton A, Keen C, Lask B: **Pros and cons of using the Mental Health Act for severe eating disorders in adolescents.** *Eur Eat Disord Rev* 2009, **17**:14–23.
114. Carney T, Tait D, Touyz S, Ingvarson M, Saunders D, Wakefield A: *Managing anorexia nervosa: Clinical, legal, and social perspectives on involuntary treatment.* New York: Nova; 2006.
115. Carney T, Tait D, Touyz S: **Coercion is coercion? Reflections on trends in the use of compulsion in treating anorexia nervosa.** *Australas Psychiatry* 2007, **15**:390–395.
116. Guarda AS, Pinto AM, Coughlin JW, Hussain S, Haug NA, Heinberg LJ: **Perceived coercion and change in perceived need for admission in patients hospitalized for eating disorders.** *Am J Psychiatry* 2007, **164**:108–114.
117. Tan JO, Stewart A, Fitzpatrick R, Hope T: **Attitudes of patients with anorexia nervosa to compulsory treatment and coercion.** *Int J Law Psychiatry* 2010, **33**:13–19.
118. Gody A, Haynes SN: **Clinical case formulation: Introduction to a special section.** *Eur J Psychol Assess* 2011, **27**:1–3.
119. Swain-Campbell NR, Surgenor LJ, Snell DL: **An analysis of consumer perspectives following contact with an eating-disorders service.** *Aust NZ J Psychiatry* 2001, **35**:99–103.
120. Holte A, Gulliksen KS, Espeset EM, Nordbo RH, Skarderud F, Geller J: **Preferred therapist characteristics in treatment of anorexia nervosa: The patient's perspective.** *Int J Eat Disord* 2012, **45**:932–941. Early View.
121. Strober M, Johnson C: **The need for complex ideas in anorexia nervosa: why biology, environment, and psyche all matter, why therapists make mistakes, and why clinical benchmarks are needed for managing weight correction.** *Int J Eat Disord* 2012, **45**:155–178.
122. Mickan S, Burls A, Glasziou P: **Patterns of 'leakage' in the utilisation of clinical guidelines: a systematic review.** *Postgrad Med J* 2011, **87**:670–679.
123. Royal Australian and New Zealand College of Psychiatrists Clinical Practice Guidelines Team for Anorexia Nervosa: **Australian and New Zealand clinical practice guidelines for the treatment of anorexia nervosa.** *Aust NZ J Psychiatry* 2004, **38**:659–670.
124. American Psychiatric Association: **Practice guidelines for the treatment of patients.** *Am J Psychiatry* 2000, **157**:1–39.

Changing the course of comorbid eating disorders and depression: what is the role of public health interventions in targeting shared risk factors?

Carolyn Black Becker[1*], Maribel Plasencia[1], Lisa Smith Kilpela[1], Morgan Briggs[1] and Tiffany Stewart[2]

Abstract

Public health has a productive history of improving global health due to its focus on reaching large populations using effective and scalable interventions. Yet, the marriage between evidence-based science and the implementation of community/public health interventions within mental illness remains underdeveloped. Research suggests that major depression is the most commonly cited comorbidity for eating disorders (EDs). Thus, identification of public health strategies that jointly impact depression and EDs, including shared risk factors, has the potential to significantly impact mental health suffering. The primary aim of this paper is to examine and discuss such public health approaches as well as explore cues taken from public health efforts to inform future directions in research and clinical practice. As a comprehensive review of all public health initiatives that address EDs and depression is beyond the scope of this paper, this paper reviews a series of programs/approaches that either are of large scale and/or have received empirical support. In particular, public health related interventions that aim to reduce variable risk factors associated with EDs and depression, as well as interventions that aim to reduce continuous measures of ED and depression symptoms are reviewed. To date, despite significant progress in modifying risk factors for EDs and depression, the field still lacks a public health study that has been appropriately designed and/or adequately powered to assess true ED/depression prevention effects. Further, although several programs show promise, many widely disseminated approaches lack empirical support, raising concerns about the potential for waste of limited resources. In summary, although the combination of prevention and public health based approaches appear to have merit when trying to move the needle on risk factors and symptoms associated with EDs and/or depression, further research is needed to investigate the reach and effectiveness of large scale dissemination efforts of such endeavors.

Keywords: Eating disorders, Depression, Prevention, Public health interventions, Risk factors, Obesity

Introduction

Despite significant advances within the mental health field in the development and testing of treatments for mental illness, the distance between scientific findings and community-based implementation of evidence-based interventions remains sizeable [1-3]. Moreover, Kazdin and colleagues have convincingly argued that the dominant delivery mode of intervening with mental illness (i.e., face-to-face psychotherapy provided by a highly trained masters or doctoral level therapist) will never be sufficient to meet the needs of those suffering from mental illness due to a variety of factors (e.g., insufficient number of trained therapists, cost, geographical challenges) [1,4]. As such, they called on the mental health field broadly to increase the range of models for delivering mental health services. One proposed strategy involves increased collaboration with other disciplines in moving beyond a focus on standard one-on-one psychotherapy [1]. The aim of this paper is to investigate to what degree current research supports the adoption of strategies drawn from public health with the aim of impacting the course of comorbid eating disorders (EDs) and depression through the targeting of shared risk factors and to make suggestions for future directions,

* Correspondence: cbecker@trinity.edu
[1]Department of Psychology, Trinity University, San Antonio, TX 78212, USA
Full list of author information is available at the end of the article

both clinically and empirically. We focus on EDs and depression because public health initiatives that can address these dual issues are likely to have greater effect in reducing mental health suffering.

Public health appears to offer a tremendous resource to the ED and depression fields in our efforts to reduce mental illness suffering [5]. More specifically, public health interventions have a longstanding history of contributing to health on a national and international scale. For example, throughout the 20th century, the field of public health improved the United States' population health, adding 25 years to the nation's average life expectancy [6]. Important public health achievements, which were not limited to the United States, during this time included: immunizations, motor-vehicle safety, control of infectious diseases, food safety, prenatal care, fluoridation of drinking water, and identification of tobacco use as a hazardous health behavior [6]. Of note, these public health initiatives evidenced high scalability (i.e., interventions could be "scaled up" and delivered to large populations without losing effectiveness); thus the impact of such initiatives was far-reaching and change observable across the population.

Furthermore, as illustrated by the aforementioned examples, the field of public health provides a myriad of strategies and perspectives for widespread impact regarding health behaviors and illness prevention. Although a variety of definitions exist, most public health approaches to behavior change include four main concepts: 1) a focus on population health and public policy; 2) emphasizing promotion and prevention; 3) addressing determinants of health (i.e., risk factors); and 4) engaging in a three-step action plan (i.e., gathering data, creating policies, and ensuring policies are implemented and enforced) [7]. These concepts are evident in an array of existing public health initiatives targeting mental illness.

Written from the perspective of the eating disorder field, the aim of this paper is to address public health efforts that could impact comorbid EDs and depression. We first briefly review the literature on comorbidity. We then discuss shared variable risk factors (i.e., risk factors that have the potential to be changeable [8]) for EDs and depression given that, to our knowledge, no public health program/intervention exists that targets both clinical ED and depression diagnoses. As such, we focus on a variety of public health related interventions that aim to reduce variable risk factors associated with EDs and depression, as well as interventions that seek to reduce continuous measures of ED and depression symptomatology.

Review

Eating disorders and depression: comorbidity

The term comorbidity describes the situation in which a given individual meets criteria for more than one disorder. Thus, in the case of EDs and depression, comorbidity rates describe the percentage of a given population that meets criteria for both disorders. Research suggests that EDs and depression are highly comorbid [9-11]. For instance, Green and colleagues found that lifetime prevalence rates of major depression in patients diagnosed with EDs ranged from 36% to 86% [9]. It is important to note, however, that other disorders also are highly comorbid with EDs. For instance, although studies generally reveal higher rates of depression as compared with anxiety disorders in anorexia nervosa [12-15], researchers have used the high rates of anxiety disorders in EDs to argue against a specific relationship between EDs and depression [12]. Further, Schwalberg and colleagues [16] found no significant difference between the lifetime prevalence rates of depression between individuals with bulimia nervosa, social phobia, or panic disorder, suggesting that the connection between depression and EDs may be nonspecific.

It also can be helpful to examine the association of continuous measures of depressive and ED symptoms (versus rates of comorbid full syndrome disorders), particularly in younger populations given that they are often a primary target for public health prevention approaches. Research here again supports a link. For instance, in a sample of 241 male and female high school students Santos, Richards, and Bleckley [17] found disordered eating attitudes and depressive symptoms to be positively correlated such that as disordered eating attitudes increased, depressive symptoms also increased. Moreover, results indicated that disordered eating attitudes accounted for significant variance in self-reported depressive symptoms even when statistically controlling for the effects of body dissatisfaction, social support and self-esteem [17]. In summary, significant research supports the comorbid relationship between EDs and depression at both clinical and sub-threshold levels.

Shared variable risk factors

As noted above, one of the common components of public health approaches is a focus on determinants of health, or risk factors for illness. The risk factor approach identifies an antecedent condition and its association to a subsequent outcome. This approach aims to identify factors that increase the probability of a negative outcome compared to the rate of a control population. Additionally, researchers may identify protective factors that increase the probability of a positive outcome or decrease the probability of a negative outcome. Although it is beyond the scope of this paper to conduct a comprehensive review of shared risk factors for depression and EDs, we provide an overview of some major commonalities in this area. Notably, we focus on potentially modifiable risk factors, or what have been referred to as variable risk factors versus fixed markers [8]. Fixed markers are risk factors that cannot be changed. For instance, being female is a very potent risk factor for both EDs and depression. Yet, because one cannot truly alter gender (i.e., we can only alter appearance of gender with surgery and hormones), it is not a useful risk factor when it comes to intervening with EDs or depression except with respect to identifying higher risk populations.

Described by Jacobi and Fittig [18] as one of the most potent and best confirmed ED risk factors, body dissatisfaction (including weight concerns/shape concerns) also increases risk for depression. Indeed, research indicates that body dissatisfaction prospectively predicts a host of negative outcomes including increases in low self-esteem, depression, binge eating, emotional eating, use of unhealthy weight control behaviors, decreased physical activity, and, among overweight girls, increased weight gain between 1–5 years later [19-21]. One model that accounts for the association between body dissatisfaction, EDs and depression has been mapped out by Stice, Nemeroff, and Shaw [22]. The dual pathway model posits that internalization of the thin-ideal standard of female beauty increases risk for body dissatisfaction which in turn increases risk for both dietary restraint and negative affect (i.e., depressed mood), both of which in turn increase risk for ED symptomatology. Research also suggests that the relationship between dieting and depressed mood may interact to increase risk for EDs. For instance, Isomaa, Isomaa, Marttunen, Kaltiala-Heino, and Björkqvist [23] found that dieters who were also depressed and dieters who endorsed "feeling fat" had a 15-fold increased risk of developing a lifetime ED as compared to "vanity" (i.e., dieting to achieve the thin-ideal) or "overweight" (i.e., dieting to reduce negative health outcomes associated with being overweight) dieters.

As described below, the dual pathway model and associated research linking cultural pressures to achieve the thin-ideal standard of beauty, thin-ideal internalization, body dissatisfaction, negative affect, dieting, and ED symptoms have driven many public health-based attempts to target the course of EDs and depressed mood. It is important to note that additional research by Stice and colleagues supports a more complex multidirectional relationship between these variables, rather than a one-way relationship in which depressed mood always precedes ED symptoms. For instance, longitudinal research with over 1000 adolescent girls revealed that body dissatisfaction, dietary restraint, and bulimic symptoms predicted later onset of depression even after controlling for baseline negative mood in initially non-depressed participants [24]. Other studies also have yielded similar results suggesting that eating- and weight-related disturbances increase risk for subsequent depression [25,26]. Adding further complexity, a study conducted by Abrantes and colleagues [27] found that dieters at an adolescent inpatient psychiatric program were more likely to meet criteria for an ED, reported greater levels of distress, and had higher rates of major depression in the previous year compared to non-dieters.

Research also has implicated a role for low self-esteem in both EDs and depression. For instance, in a large-scale prospective study examining the relation between eating and weight-related disturbances, Rawana [25] found that self-esteem moderated the prospective relationship between trying to lose weight and depression. In addition, low self-esteem has been identified as a risk factor for bulimia nervosa [18], and high self-esteem was found to be protective in the development of later EDs in a large-scale study of Spanish adolescents [28]. Isomaa and colleagues [23] also found that their high-risk dieting group (i.e., feeling fat dieters and depressed dieters) reported lower self-esteem and more depressed mood than lower risk dieters.

Another potential target for public health initiatives is bullying, including weight-related teasing. Research supports the influence of bullying both in the development of EDs and depression. For instance, using a retrospective design, Striegel-Moore, Dohm, Pike, Wilfley, and Fairburn [29] found that bullying was significantly more common among both black and white women with binge ED compared to healthy controls. Importantly, the rate of bullying was not elevated relative to a psychiatric control group, of which 50% were diagnosed with a mood disorder. This provides evidence that bullying is a nonspecific risk factor for the development of eating pathology and that it also increases risk for other forms of mental illness.

With regards to prospective research on bullying and teasing, Haines, Neumark-Sztainer, Einsenberg, and Hannan [30] used a longitudinal design and found that weight related teasing at baseline significantly increased risk for binge eating with loss of control in boys as well as use of unhealthy weight control behaviors. Among girls, weight-related teasing significantly increased risk for becoming a frequent dieter. Although the literature on bullying and later onset of depression is somewhat mixed [31], recent longitudinal research indicates that among youth at risk for later suicide (e.g., due to baseline suicidal ideation or elevated depression) bullying was associated with increased suicidal ideation and functional impairment at 2-year follow-up [31].

As noted above, a comprehensive review of all shared variable risk factors is beyond the scope of this article. It is worth noting that a variety of risk factors may increase risk for many forms of psychopathology, including EDs and depression. For instance, both childhood sexual abuse and pregnancy complications (including pre-term birth/low birth weight) may increase risk for a number of psychiatric disorders including EDs [18,29] and depression in some individuals [32-38]. Such risk factors may be considered potential future targets for changing the course of

EDs and depression. Because we are not aware of public health initiatives to influence these risk factors with the intention of reducing EDs/depression, we do not focus on them in this article.

Public health approaches: programs and campaigns

Although we are not aware of any public health initiatives aimed at EDs and depression on the scale of some of the public health campaigns described above (e.g., immunizations), there are a number programs/campaigns in which one can recognize key the elements of standard public health approaches. Below, we review a series of approaches that are either particularly noteworthy because of their scale or empirical support. We also examine approaches that are simply very common. We do not claim that this is a comprehensive review of all programs in existence as there are many (likely hundreds) of regional initiatives across many countries that use approaches similar to what is described a below.

All of the programs below aim at some level to reduce risk factors for EDs, if not EDs per se. Moreover, because all of the programs below target nonspecific risk factors that are shared with depression, theoretically they should improve the course of depression *if* they sufficiently impact the targeted risk factor. It is important to note that changing risk factors for EDs and depression has proven more challenging than many expected and one problem that will be highlighted in this review is the lack of adequate evidence for the effectiveness of many approaches. Moreover, successful alteration of a risk factor may or may not alter the course of the end point disorder of interest (i.e., EDs, depression). Thus, ultimately risk factor reduction studies will need to be followed by rigorous research aimed at determining whether or not the courses of EDs and depression are in fact altered. As can be seen from the review below, this final step has yet to be taken in virtually all of the public health approaches.

Lastly, in some cases, researchers, clinicians or organizations may not be highly motivated to determine whether or not the course of endpoint disorders (i.e., EDs and depression) is in fact changed if the risk factor itself holds sufficient interest. For instance, below we describe a public health initiative by Dove and the World Association of Girl Guides and Girl Scouts (WAGGGS). The primary aim of this initiative is to increase body confidence and self-esteem. Changes in depression or EDs would, of course, be appreciated, but they are not a primary goal of this program. Such initiatives seek to simply reduce risk factors for the sake of reducing distress associated with the risk factors.

The Institute of Medicine (IOM) differentiates three types of prevention approaches: universal, selective, and indicated programs [39]. Universal programs target all individuals in a population regardless of risk status. Universal programs are distinct from selective prevention programs, which target individuals believed to be at high risk for developing a particular mental disorder based on the presence of identified risk factors. Indicated prevention programs target individuals with symptoms of a mental disorder but who do not meet the full criteria for a disorder. Note that this categorical organization of prevention programs is imperfect given that risk is a continuous variable and because many populations that are broadly considered high risk still consist of a mix of both higher- and lower-risk individuals. For instance, one can argue that any program that targets females could be categorized as selective given that female gender is a significant risk factor for both depression and EDs. Such labeling, however, may obfuscate significant differences between programs that aim to reach all females (i.e., program is universally delivered to both low and high body dissatisfied females) versus programs that are designed only to reach the higher risk females (e.g., only those with high body dissatisfaction).

As noted above, public health initiatives typically seek to focus on the health of an entire population versus focus on a small subset. For this reason, in this paper we only focus on initiatives that have been implemented on a universal/selective basis (e.g., to all women in a given population) versus selective/indicated basis (e.g., self-selected women with elevated body dissatisfaction or women showing early symptoms of EDs). To date no universal/selective study has been adequately powered or appropriately designed to assess true prevention effects, in large part because these studies were generally conducted with less grant support. We define true "prevention effects" as demonstrating that a given program reduces the onset of clinically significant EDs and depression (e.g., cases of DSM-IV bulimia nervosa and major depressive disorder) relative to a control condition. In the absence of true prevention effects, most studies are designed to reduce variable risk factors and continuous measures of ED and depressive symptomatology. Presently, despite decades of research, only three programs (*Student Bodies*, the *Body Project*, and a *Healthy Weight Intervention*) have yielded what could be referred to as true prevention effects with respect to EDs. To our knowledge, no studies have examined whether or not onset of clinical depression was also changed, although reductions in continuous measures of negative affect have been found. The two studies that demonstrated the above three EDs prevention programs could produce true prevention effects were both selective/indicated studies [40,41], and thus are not reviewed here. Instead, we review public health approaches and campaigns that have targeted shared risk factors for EDs and depression.

Public health approaches targeting body dissatisfaction

Programs focusing on body dissatisfaction are appealing for a number of reasons from a public health perspective. First, body dissatisfaction is exceedingly common particularly among females [42], and as noted above it is a variable risk factor for an array of negative outcomes, including EDs and depression. Thus, at least theoretically, wide scale and clinically significant improvement in body dissatisfaction should improve the mental health (e.g., eating disorders and depression), and potentially the physical health, of a large percentage of the population. As noted above, however, this assumption has yet to be to be adequately tested. Below we review a number of different public health related approaches to improving body dissatisfaction.

The body project

Developed by Stice and colleagues, the *Body Project* is based on the dual pathway model of EDs described above, and utilizes a cognitive dissonance-based approach. A well-known psychological phenomenon [43], dissonance is the uncomfortable psychological state that occurs when an individual's beliefs and actions are misaligned. To reduce psychological tension, individuals typically alter beliefs to align with behavior. In the *Body Project*, participants voluntarily speak and act against the thin-ideal, a behavior which is inconsistent with any previously held pro-thin-ideal beliefs. Theoretically, this leads participants to reduce thin-ideal internalization, which decreases body dissatisfaction and subsequently dietary restraint, depressed mood and ED symptomatology. This intervention has been branded under a variety of names (e.g., *Sorority Body Image Program, Reflections: Body Image Program®; Succeed Body Image Programme*); to avoid confusion and because it was originally published under the title of the *Body Project* [44,45], we use this label.

The *Body Project* is supported by significant high quality research when implemented in a selective/indicated fashion [40,46-49]. From a public health perspective, however, what distinguishes the *Body Project* from *Student Bodies* and the *Healthy Weight Intervention* has been the relatively extensive testing, dissemination and implementation of the *Body Project* on a more universal/selective basis using community providers. The use of low cost community providers is often critical for public health approaches given problems with scaling interventions to reach larger populations if interventions must be implemented by highly trained (i.e., expensive) providers. Thus, task shifting to less trained and less expensive providers fits a public health perspective [50]. Community providers also can spread the message of a program within the community even when a program is not formally being run.

In a series of studies, Becker and colleagues [51-53] investigated if the *Body Project* remained effective when it was delivered universally to members of a university sub-community (i.e., local sororities) by peers on a mandatory basis. These studies had the potential to identify key weaknesses in the *Body Project* from a public health perspective. For instance, if the *Body Project* only worked when implemented on a voluntary basis, by more highly educated providers, and with only higher risk participants this would have undermined the likely scalability of the intervention.

Results from three randomized controlled trials (RCTs [51-53]) indicated that the *Body Project* could be implemented on a mandatory basis by peer-leaders with significant changes in thin-ideal internalization, body dissatisfaction, dietary restraint, and ED pathology. Moreover, the *Body Project* yielded benefits for both lower- and higher-risk participants whereas an alternative intervention only benefitted higher-risk participants [52]. Lastly, results indicated that at 14-months, the magnitude of effects was similar for this delivery mode of the *Body Project* as compared to selective/indicated, voluntary delivery with more highly educated providers; the *Body Project* in this format also reduced negative affect, which included depressed mood [53]. No other public health approach has amassed this level of scientific support.

The Becker et al. studies were not only RCTs, but also relied on research methodology known as community-based participatory research (CBPR). CBPR is commonly used in public health approaches, with the goal of ensuring that interventions designed to address the health needs of communities are implemented in partnership with community leaders and/or members [54]. In CBPR, researchers engage community partners in an egalitarian manner that truly shares power and decision making with the aim of integrating knowledge about health problems [54]. CBPR also aims to improve problems solving, build on community strengths, and facilitate the creation of sustainable programs [54]. For instance, in the above studies, with the exception of Becker, the research team consisted of community members. In addition, sorority leaders and members played a key role in determining how the *Body Project* should be implemented.

CBPR methods also played a significant role in a 7-year *Body Project* dissemination effort throughout North America [55]. In 2005, having learned of the partnership between Becker and the local sororities at her university, the Delta Delta Delta fraternity (Tri Delta) began piloting the *Body Project* on a national scale. For readers outside North America, sororities are largely North American institutions created by early female pioneers in academia with the aim of providing community and a sense of belonging.

Between 2005 and 2012, Tri Delta and Becker disseminated the *Body Project* to over 100 campuses within the

United States and Canada [55]. The primary vehicle for dissemination involved the creation of a *"Body Image Academy,"* a 2-day training workshop. University professionals were trained as peer-leaders trainers in a "train-the-trainer" model that allowed for greater scalability at their home institutions. Although *Body Image Academy* is no longer active, many of the universities that sent professionals continue to implement the *Body Project* on an annual basis. The *Body Image Academy* model also was adopted by the Succeed Foundation in its efforts to disseminate the *Body Project* throughout the United Kingdom via universities.

To date, the *Body Project* has been tested almost exclusively with secondary school and university-aged participants. Recent evidence, however, suggests that the dissonance approach may work with younger ages when appropriately adapted. For instance, Halliwell & Diedrichs [56] found that a dissonance-based approach reduced thin-ideal internalization, body dissatisfaction and increased resilience to negative media in 12–13 year old girls. This is an important study from a public health perspective as schools are often considered prime settings for implementing public health programming.

Most recently, Dove and WAGGGS used the *Body Project* as the foundation for a new initiative which aims to either directly or indirectly reach 3.5 million girls, ages 7–14, within the WAGGGS global network. In consultation with Becker, Stice and Diedrichs (who collaborated with the Succeed Foundation and their *Body Project* efforts) WAGGGS and Dove developed the dissonance-based program, *"Free Being Me,"* as part of Dove's global campaign to improve body confidence in girls and women [57]. This represents a very important step for Dove in that their previous public health initiatives were less evidence-based (see below). The Dove/WAGGGS effort also builds off the Tri Delta/Succeed Foundation train-the-trainers model as part of their global dissemination effort [58]. To our knowledge, *Free Being Me* represents the largest organized effort to disseminate evidence-based body image programming worldwide and as such will be an important program to watch. Still, we must sound two cautionary notes with regards to this effort. First, as noted above, limited research has investigated the effects of a dissonance program in younger girls. Importantly, however, limited research currently exists supporting *any* program in this age group. As such, Dove/WAGGGS are acting in the spirit of an evidence-based approach in seeking to adapt the program with the greatest volume of support in reducing body dissatisfaction in females. In addition, the extensive scale of the project will undoubtedly raise new logistical challenges and it will be interesting to see how these are addressed by Dove/WAGGGS over time.

Media literacy programs

Media smart

Australian program Media literacy programs such as *Media Smart*, like several other programs described below, seek to influence a risk factor for body dissatisfaction with the aim of thereby reducing body dissatisfaction and creating a cascading effect that impacts EDs and depression. Media both influences and reinforces prevailing social norms, beliefs, and attitudes about appearance, and the effects of media exposure on body image have been well documented [59-61]. More specifically, findings from meta-analyses indicate that even brief exposure to media that portrays the thin-ideal of beauty [61] increases body dissatisfaction, which, as noted above, is a potent a risk factor for EDs and depression.

Several recent studies [62-65] employed a universal approach to evaluate if *Media Smart* was effective in reducing ED risk factors in a young-adolescent, mixed sex audience. For instance, *Media Smart* was evaluated in a controlled efficacy trial with assessment of ED risk factors at baseline, post-intervention, 6 month, and 2.5 year follow up time points ($N = 540$ girls and boys in the 8th grade). The authors concluded that media literacy reduced shape and weight concern, body dissatisfaction, ineffectiveness, and depression in a universal, young adolescent population of girls and boys. It should be noted, however, that reductions in shape and weight concern among girls were only present at 2.5 year follow up when attrition had reached approximately 46%. Also, a preliminary controlled efficacy trial of *Media Smart* with adolescent girls 15 years of age demonstrated that *Media Smart* was comparable to a control group and less effective than a perfectionism-focused prevention intervention [65]. In this trial, *Media Smart* did not improve weight and shape concern or any other ED risk factors in this population. These results suggest that replication trials are needed to fully ascertain the effectiveness of *Media Smart* with adolescents.

Recently, depression was examined as a moderator of the impact of the *Media Smart* program [66]. Results indicated a reduction in ED risk factors (shape and weight concern, media internalization, dieting) for participants with high depression, and a reduced rate in development of ED risk factors (shape and weight concern) for participants with low depression. In sum, *Media Smart* is supported by research that suggests that it can be useful for a universal audience that is under the age of 15 who is at both low- and high-risk of developing an ED. That said, replication trials, particularly independent replication trials, in this line of research are needed with young individuals, as it has been suggested that ED risk factor constructs may be less stable in young adolescents, as opposed to older adolescents [67].

Media smart

United Kingdom (UK) program *Media Smart UK* [68] is a UK based media literacy initiative that consists of one lesson aimed at improving body image. Some other components of this program also are known as *Be Adwise. Media Smart UK*, which was launched in 2002 and provides free educational materials, targets primary school children (children aged 7–11) and aims to aid children in understanding and interpreting advertising. This non-profit initiative was funded by the for-profit advertising industry, which collaborated with media literacy specialists. The body image lesson, which targets 10–11 year olds and was launched in 2011, was created to align with the UK government *Body Confidence Campaign* (see below). Since its inception, the *Media Smart UK* body image lesson has been downloaded over 1500 times [69].

To our knowledge, only one study has evaluated the effectiveness of the *Media Smart UK* body image lesson. Diedrichs and colleagues randomly assigned 204 boys and girls to either the body image lesson or a waitlist control [69]. Results indicated no benefit of the *Media Smart UK* body image lesson over the wait list control condition for all body image variables; in fact the control group outperformed *Media Smart UK* in weight esteem for boys. In summary, *Media Smart UK* not only lacks evidence for its benefits, but one study provides support for the interpretation that the program simply does not work at altering body image. Although well-intentioned, *Media Smart UK* provides a cautionary example of the problem with distributing public health type approaches prior to rigorous testing.

Labeling/banning of photo retouching or very underweight models

Recently, significant attention has been focused on the effects of photo retouching in popular media (e.g. magazines and online media) to "correct" flaws in the appearance (e.g. imperfections in eyes, wrinkles, skin tone, hair) and/or body shape and size of individuals featured in the media [70]. Concerns generally focus on the notion that the result of "retouching" presents an extremely unattainable image for individuals to achieve, thus increasing body dissatisfaction. Thus, like media literacy programs, efforts targeting photo retouching aim to modify a risk factor of an ED/depression risk factor (i.e., body dissatisfaction) with the aim of altering body dissatisfaction and associated negative outcomes.

Several countries, including France, Australia, and the United Kingdom [71-73] have proposed or are currently initiating efforts to add disclaimers or warning labels to media images retouched using Photoshop. The most far reaching example of this occurred in Israel in 2012 when the Adatto Photoshop bill became law. This law bans the use of models with a Body Mass Index (BMI) of less than 18.5 and requires labeling of photoshopped images [74]. These actions fit with policy approaches in public health. Parallel initiatives from other areas include putting warning labels on items/substances that are harmful (e.g., cigarettes) or to simply ban said stimuli (e.g., USA Food and Drug Administration effort to potentially remove artificial trans fats in processed foods) in an effort to reduce consumption of those items [75,76].

Research on the likely benefit of these efforts has yielded mixed outcomes [77,78]. In a study conducted by Slater and colleagues [77] participants who viewed images with a warning label reported lower levels of body dissatisfaction than participants who viewed the images without a warning label, irrespective of the degree of the internalization of the thin-ideal. In contrast, Alta, Thompson, & Small [78] found no benefit on body dissatisfaction or intent to diet with either a disclaimer label ("Retouched photograph aimed at changing a person's physical appearance.") or a warning label ("Warning: Trying to look as thin as this model may be dangerous to your health.") relative to control conditions. In sum, research examining the effects of labeling media images on female's body dissatisfaction and mood is mixed. Further, at this time it is unclear if such labeling will significantly impact body dissatisfaction on a population level, let alone EDs and depression. However, we should note that to date studies have been small, investigating the effects of short term exposure to such stimuli. To our knowledge no research has investigated longer term effects of a markedly changed media environment such as might result from the Israeli government's efforts; indeed we are not sure how such research could be conducted in a controlled, experimental design. Thus, the mental health benefits of environmental changes resulting from government-based policy with respect to media images likely will have to be studied longitudinally as country-wide social experiments.

Campaigns promoting positive messaging aimed at body image and/or sexism

Body image and gender activists have designed and implemented numerous "campaigns" aimed at promoting positive body image and/or addressing sexism. Typically, not unlike other public health awareness campaigns, these efforts are largely not classified as "interventions" or "programs" but simply as campaigns to increase awareness around certain topics (e.g. body acceptance, body appreciation, building body confidence, reducing sexism in the media). In some cases, activists may develop interventions or workshops aimed at promoting their causes in schools as sub-elements of their campaign. In many cases, such campaigns and associated curricula are highly adopted by the general public (e.g., *The Representation Project*), despite lacking empirical support for their effects on the targeted issue. We outline several of these efforts below.

We note that campaigns vary in the degree to which they are explicit about the intended effects of their efforts on body image as well as the degree to which they state or imply that their campaign will ultimately affect variables such as EDs and depression. For instance, although neither *The Representation Project* nor the *Campaign for Body Confidence* explicitly state they will alter body image or the course of eating disorders, both do explicitly describe negative mood and eating disorders as potential results of sexism/objectification and pressure to conform to unrealistic images (see *Miss Representation* movie; and http://campaignforbodyconfidence.wordpress.com/about/). Thus, there is an implication that correcting said forces will reduce onset of EDs and depression. Other campaigns (e.g., *Love your Body Campaign* by the National Organization for Women) describe predicted effects of improved body image as an outcome (e.g., "feeling less stressed about appearance" at http://loveyourbody.nowfoundation.org/whatsitallabout.html). Lastly, as noted above with regards to regulating models and photoshopped images, some elements of campaigns may be very difficult to test whereas others (e.g., associated curricula) would be easier.

FAT TALK FREE WEEK

In 2008, Tri Delta launched a worldwide advocacy campaign called *Fat Talk Free Week* (FTFW). Coined by Nichter and Vuckovic [79,80] fat talk is a term that refers to gendered dialogue between females that reinforces the thin-ideal standard of female beauty. Research indicates that as little as 3–5 minutes of fat talk can significantly increase body dissatisfaction [81].

FTFW was designed as a social marketing campaign aimed at increasing awareness of fat talk and its harmful effects. FTFW also promoted Tri Delta's *Body Project* dissemination effort. Since its launch, FTFW has been implemented in dance studios, fitness studios, primary and secondary schools, retail stores, and universities throughout the United States and internationally.

To date, only one study has examined the effectiveness of FTFW. Garnett, Buelow, Franko, Becker, Rodgers, and Austin [82] investigated the effects of FTFW on a sample of university women. Some participants in the study attended FTFW events, whereas others did not. Results indicated that both samples showed significant reductions in self-fat talk, in body comparison, and on a measure of body dissatisfaction post-FTFW, possibly suggesting diffusion effects. Campaign saliency emerged as the strongest predictor of decreased fat talk, suggesting that the message worked best for individuals who found the message resonated with them. In summary, one very preliminary study provides some support for FTFW in reducing fat talk and impacting body dissatisfaction, but more research is needed before concluding the campaign achieves its aims. Further, there is no evidence that FTFW impacts the course of EDs or depression. To be fair, however, the campaign was originally designed as a marketing platform for the *Body Project* and was not expected to be sufficiently potent to impact EDs or depression.

THE REPRESENTATION PROJECT

The Representation Project (formerly *Miss Representation*) is classified by its developers as "a movement that uses media and film content to expose injustices created by gender stereotypes and to shift peoples' consciousness towards change" [83]. This effort began in 2011 with the release and promotion of the film, *Miss Representation*, a film aimed at highlighting sexist depictions of women in the media and the consequent effects on women's ability to reach their potential (e.g. reduced upward mobility in the workplace; body dissatisfaction; lack of desire for leadership as girls age). This effort also includes a curriculum that is designed to boost media literacy in children in K-12th grade. Although the curriculum does not explicitly target body image in its learning objectives, body dissatisfaction is a theme that emerges throughout the original film, in *The Representation Project*'s partnerships (e.g., *Endangered Bodies*), and on their website (e.g., the statistics page which includes information about EDs and body dissatisfaction) [83]. As such, *The Representation Project* is commonly accepted as attempting to impact body image as well as broader goals.

The Representation Project has received significant exposure at schools, universities, and public forums across the country and has successfully improved discourse about the damaging effects of media. To our knowledge, however, efficacy studies have not examined the campaign and, perhaps more importantly, the media literacy curriculum. As highlighted in the case of the *Media Smart UK* program, even well-meaning media literacy programs like *The Representation Project* curriculum may fail to have the intended effect and thus waste valuable school time. As such, research is urgently needed to investigate whether or not the effects of the curriculum, which is being used in 17 countries [83], justify its widespread dissemination.

CAMPAIGN FOR BODY CONFIDENCE

The *Campaign for Body Confidence* is a positive body image advocacy initiative in the UK, led by a partnership between the UK government (i.e., the All Party Parliamentary Group on Body Image) and the Central YMCA [84,85]. The goal of this campaign is to promote greater body confidence in men and women, and to circulate psycho educational materials (digital and otherwise) about body dissatisfaction, dysregulated eating behaviors, unhealthy appearance-related behaviors (e.g., cosmetic surgery), and media literacy. Still in its beginning stages, the campaign provides facts and base rates about eating behaviors, societal appearance ideals, and the principles of body diversity and acceptance. Further, the campaign calls for body activists to organize and propagate further campaigns and events to tackle societal pressures for appearance ideals and for efforts to change policies regarding media messages. To our knowledge, no research has been published regarding the efficacy or effectiveness of participating in this campaign. One positive aspect of this campaign, however, is the collaboration and support of the UK government, which is unique to body image campaigns. Government involvement has been crucial in many other successful public health endeavors in other areas. Additionally, campaigns like the *Campaign for Body Confidence* and *The Representation Project* promote further activism and discussion related to body diversity and body acceptance. Lastly, the UK government has the capacity to push evidence-based programming for body image, though to date they have not aggressively done so as far as we can discern. In summary, although well-intentioned, without research investigating the effects of spreading positive messages via campaigns, the degree to which the *Campaign for Body Confidence* has the potential to impact the course of body dissatisfaction and ultimately EDs, or depression it is ambiguous at best.

NATIONAL ORGANIZATION OF WOMEN'S LOVE YOUR BODY CAMPAIGN

The United States National Organization for Women (NOW) focuses on an overarching goal of achieving equality for women through education and litigation. NOW concentrates on a wide range of women's rights issues including women's body image. Through NOW's *Love Your Body Campaign*, the organization challenges the message that society evaluates a woman's value according to her willingness and ability to manifest current beauty standards [86]. The *Love Your Body Campaign* utilizes mainstream media (e.g. websites, Facebook, and twitter) to provide information about EDs and body image and to promote body image activism. NOW's website offers a multiplicity of body image activism ideas that women can undertake in addition to projects that the organization develops such as "Let's Talk About It" [86]. Although body image activism is one component of the *Body Project* program described above, NOW's *Love Your Body Campaign* lacks empirical research supporting the efficacy of the campaign's ability to improve women's body image. In contrast to *The Representation Project* and *Media Smart UK*, however, we are not aware of any efforts by NOW to secure significant school time. Thus the potential cost of this program, even if ineffective, is substantially lower.

Public health approaches targeting self-esteem

Dove workshops

The Dove Self-Esteem Project (DSEP) [87], previously known as the Dove Self-Esteem Fund, is a program targeting girls aimed at improving body image and self-esteem, both of which targets are variable risk factors for EDs and depression. As part of the DSEP, Dove created the Dove Self Esteem ToolKit for girls [88]. The workshops are open to adolescent girls (ages 8–17 years) and their adult female mentors. The educational and interactive sessions focus on society's creation of ideal images of beauty and promote the initiation of positive dialogue about beauty and self-esteem. Several incarnations of these workshops exist, including *BodyThink* in Australia which targets media literacy, self-esteem, internalization of the media ideal, body comparison and appearance teasing in young men and women. This self-esteem initiative by Dove also received input from BEAT (the UK EDs association), the Butterfly Foundation (Australia), and the Girl Scouts of the USA. This program has been disseminated throughout the UK in schools using the title of *BodyTalk.* In Australia, the Butterfly Foundation provided training to over 900 professionals for the dissemination of this program. As of June 2008, 40,000 adolescents (ages 10–17 years) had participated in the program [89].

To our knowledge, only one study investigated the efficacy of this widely disseminated program. Richardson, Paxton, and Thomson [89] conducted a study of 277 grade 7 students from 4 secondary schools in Australia. The adolescents in the intervention group participated in *BodyThink* during four 50-minute class periods while the adolescents in the control condition attended class as usual. In both adolescent males and females Richardson et al. [90] found no significant differences between the groups on measures of body dissatisfaction or dietary restraint and bulimic symptoms. The results largely demonstrate *BodyThink*'s lack of impact on body image or ED symptoms (depression was not assessed), and once again raise concerns about organizations widely disseminating media literacy programs prior to investing in the rigorous testing needed to determine if they work. As noted above, however, Dove has recently adopted a more evidence-based philosophy in its partnership with WAGGGS which is very encouraging.

Full of ourselves

Yet another public health program targeting self-esteem, confidence, and self-acceptance is the wellness program "Full of Ourselves: Advancing Girl Power, Health, and Leadership" [90,91]. This program was designed as an

EDs and obesity prevention program with a strong feminist approach that focuses on esteem-building, building leadership skills, and providing opportunities for both leadership and receiving mentorship. Two expected outcomes are improvements in the depression/ED variable risk factors, body image and self-esteem.

The program includes two phases; during the first phase, small groups of 11–14 year-old girls receive the program, 8 units total, delivered by adult women. Phase one employs an interactive structure with discussions, role-plays, and out-of-session activities (e.g. daily self-proclamations, letter-writing to advertiser or magazine about problems with material related to body esteem). In phase two, participants from phase one become peer leaders for younger girls, ages 8–11 years-old.

In a strong effort to assess effectiveness of the program, Steiner-Adair and colleagues [90] evaluated an implementation of *Full of Ourselves* in a partially randomized controlled trial across 24 schools in the Northeast United States comparing the program to an assessment-only control group. Results indicated that participants in the *Full of Ourselves* program reported increased knowledge (regarding health, weightism/appearance, and media literacy), as well as improved weight-related body esteem as compared to control participants through 6 month follow-up. Results did not suggest a difference between participants and controls in self-reported dysregulated eating behaviors (e.g. skipping meals). Of note, although results indicated an increase in knowledge and body esteem, there were no significant program effects on measures of body dissatisfaction, a critical and established risk factor for EDs and depression. A notable strength of the *Full of Ourselves* program is the ability to implement in school systems on a large scale while maintaining modest effectiveness at reducing some risk factors. Additionally, research assessing outcomes of participating in the program exists, which is an aspect that we have argued in this paper as necessary prior to large-scale implementation efforts. Although results of this program suggested modest improvement in some target variables further research is needed to investigate whether or not this program has a true prophylactic effect for onset of EDs, obesity, or depression.

Public health approaches targeting bullying

Very important kids

Very Important Kids (V.I.K.) is a school-based program designed to reduce weight-related teasing and unhealthy weight control behaviors (e.g., skipping a meal, taking diet pills) in children in grades 4 through 6. This multi-component program is aimed at producing change at both the individual level and the greater school/community environment [92]. A study evaluating the effectiveness and feasibility of VIK [92] found that this program was effective in reducing weight-related teasing in those schools that received the intervention compared to those serving as assessment only controls. Specifically, after controlling for baseline measures of overall teasing, this study found students in the intervention condition reported significantly lower odds of being teased about their appearance. Overall, intervention schools reported a 10% decrease in teasing from pre to posttest. Additionally, students who received the intervention reported significantly greater self-efficacy to change or impact weight-related teasing (e.g. stand up for a peer who was being teased) and a decrease in negative weight-related norms (e.g. talking about a peer's weight). Somewhat less encouraging, V.I.K. largely failed to impact secondary outcomes such as body image concerns and unhealthy weight control behaviors. A major strength of V.I.K was the developers' use of a CBPR approach for implementation; students in V.I.K. actively contributed throughout the course of the program, ensuring ideas and concepts were culturally relevant. As with other programs that target risk factors for the development of EDs and depression, it remains unclear if V.I.K will impact the course of these endpoint disorders. However, in contrast to some programs reviewed here, V.I.K. has not been widely disseminated ahead of testing.

Public health approaches targeting eating disorder and obesity

Due to the overlap in risk factors for EDs and obesity (e.g., body dissatisfaction, depression, dieting, media consumption) researchers have called for programs that aim to prevent both EDs and obesity (e.g. Neumark-Sztainer et al. [93]). Given that obesity is considered a prominent public health target, we would be remiss in not touching on a few of these programs even though a more detailed review is beyond the scope of this paper. Two examples of this approach include *Planet Health* and *Life Smart.*

Planet health

Planet Health is a two-year obesity prevention program for girls and boys in grades 6–8 that was tested in a large-scale school-based cluster RCT. Ten schools were randomly assigned to receive *Planet Health* or a control condition. The primary aim of *Planet Health* was to create change in four primary areas: reduce television watching to less than 2 hours per day, increase moderate and vigorous physical activity, decrease consumption of high-fat foods, and increase consumption of fruits and vegetables. Although the primary aim of *Planet Health* was to impact obesity, later analyses investigated effects of Planet Health on ED related behavior. Results indicated that in addition to reducing rates of obesity [94], *Planet Health* also reduced onset of purging behaviors amongst girls in the intervention condition [95]. To our knowledge no data indicates whether or not *Planet*

Health impacted depressive symptoms. In summary, there is some limited evidence to suggest *Planet Health*, a public health program aimed at obesity, impacted one dimension of ED symptomatology, but it is unclear to what degree full syndrome EDs were impacted.

Life smart

Life Smart consists of an eight session school-based program aimed at reducing the risk of both EDs and obesity in young adolescent girls and boys [96]. In a recent pilot study conducted by Wilksch and Wade [96], grade 7 girls and boys ($N = 115$) were randomly assigned to *Life Smart* or a control group. Risk factors were measured at baseline and post-intervention, which occurred five weeks after the delivery of the intervention. Results indicated that participants enjoyed the program and perceived it as valuable. Further, *Life Smart* showed promising results in reducing such ED/depression risk factors as shape and weight concern, body dissatisfaction, peer-teasing, and media internalization in girls. Boys who participated in *Life Smart* experienced no significant benefits [96]. Further research will be needed to determine if this program is capable of yielding true prevention effects.

Conclusions

Public health approaches to disease prevention and health promotion have achieved many impressive outcomes in the area of physical health. Given the limitations of the expensive, expert treatment provider approach to reducing mental health suffering on a global scale [1,4], it is past time to investigate how public health approaches can further inform mental health programming. In this paper we focus on altering the course of EDs and depression.

The results of this review are both encouraging and discouraging in our opinion. On the encouraging side, research [51-53] increasingly supports the public health utility of one program (i.e., the *Body Project*) which has been found to actually reduce onset of EDs in selective/indicated research [40], and we are seeing increased efforts at dissemination of this program on increasingly larger scales. Further, more preliminary research supports several other programs in reducing at least one ED and depressive risk factor when delivered in a manner consistent with public health approaches (e.g., *Media Smart* (*Australia*), *V.I.K.*, *Planet Health*; *Life Smart*). Additionally, there is some evidence that at least some of these programs also reduce depressive symptoms/negative affect. We also are encouraged to see that some major players in this area (e.g., Dove) are increasingly disseminating evidence-based approaches (including with schools) instead of widely disseminating untested programs. Lastly, we think that it is encouraging that EDs and associated risk factors (e.g., body dissatisfaction) finally appear to be on the radars of policy makers in at least some national governments.

On the discouraging or concerning side, most public health efforts to impact the course of EDs and depression, or the course of risk factors for these disorders, lack empirical support at best (e.g., *The Representation Project*; *Media Smart* (*UK*)), and those discussed in this paper are just the large scale examples of the types of programs that regional organizations and advocates frequently deliver in our experience. Thus, the overall landscape of public health approaches consists of a vast amount of time, energy and in some cases money being spent on programs that either have no demonstrated efficacy or, in the worst instances, actually have been shown to not work. One might ask whether or not this is in fact a problem if well-meaning individuals and organizations are at least trying to have an impact. We argue it is a problem and turn to evidence from another public health intervention from another area, namely substance prevention in the United States, to support our case. The Drug Abuse Resistance Education (DARE) program is a widely distributed substance abuse prevention program that launched in the early 1980's without prior testing. In 1998 evidence emerged that the DARE program was ineffective at best [97]. Although DARE has since received funding to update its programming, one must ask what was the cost of those years when an ineffective program was being widely distributed. The General Accounting Office of the US Government placed the price tag at approximately 2 million dollars in the year 2000 alone [98]. Yet, an independent economist [99] estimated that the real cost of DARE was approximately one billion dollars per year when all costs (e.g., lost classroom space/time, law enforcement officer time etc.) were taken into account. We consider this history a warning for advocates and organizations seeking to impact risk factors for EDs and depression using public health approaches. There are real (yet often hidden) costs to ineffective programs, not the least of which is that when schools and other community settings invest in ineffective programs they are not using their resources to implement more effective programs or alternative educational initiatives that could work.

We consider attempts to label photographs and ban models of a certain size as potentially positive. Research clearly supports the negative impact of thin-ideal media images on body dissatisfaction, and body dissatisfaction is an ED/depression risk factor. Thus it is understandable that people want to see if reversing the trend in media images could be beneficial; indeed it may be that if governments can create sufficiently large scale change, there will be benefits. At the same time, this appears also to be yet one more instance when public health approaches are moving very far ahead of the empirical literature. It would seem to us that a more logical approach would be to invest further in appropriate research before changing policy.

Lastly, even with the most promising programs, we still need more research. For instance, it is unclear if public health type dissemination of the *Body Project* will yield true prevention effects, particularly when the program is delivered on a very large scale. We also need additional research investigating best practices for dissemination and implementation of efficacious programs. In addition, no program has been demonstrated to impact the onset of both clinically significant EDs and depression.

In summary, although public health approaches offer much promise in changing the course of EDs and depression, in our opinion we need significantly more research to determine a) which efficacious programs can be widely disseminated, b) which campaigns actually have an impact on behavior, risk factors and/or EDs and depression, and c) which programs and campaigns should be judged ineffective and eliminated to conserve and better deploy resources. In addition, we suggest that greater restraint is needed by organizations and advocates so that there is less dissemination of untested programs, which have the potential to waste significant resources. We appreciate the desire by many advocates, organizations and even governments to intervene so as to reduce the burden of EDs, depression and associated risk factors. Yet, it is critical in resource tight environments to be cognizant of costs and to not assume that a desire to do something positive will in fact have a positive outcome.

Abbreviations
ED: Eating disorder; FTFW: Fat talk free week; NOW: National Organization of Women; DSEP: Dove self-esteem project.

Competing interests
Carolyn Black Becker is co-director of the Body Project Collaborative, a social entrepreneurship company aimed at facilitating dissemination and implementation of the *Body Project* program that is described in this paper. She also sits on the scientific advisory board of Emerge (see below under Tiffany Stewart). As noted in this body of this paper, she consulted with Dove and WAGGGS on the development of the *Free Being Me* program. Lisa Smith Kilpela is a trainer for the Body Project Collaborative. Tiffany Stewart is co-founder and chief scientific officer for Emerge (www.emergebodyimage.com/), a body image technology development company, which is a listed partner for *The Representation Project*.

Authors' contributions
All authors contributed to conducting the literature review, writing and editing of this paper. No section of this paper was exclusively produced by one author. All authors read and approved the final version of this manuscript.

Acknowledgments
Publication of this article was facilitated by Beyondblue Australia. All content is independent of Beyondblue.

Author details
[1]Department of Psychology, Trinity University, San Antonio, TX 78212, USA. [2]Pennington Biomedical Research Center, 6400 Perkins Rd, Baton Rouge, LA 70808, USA.

References
1. Kazdin AE, Blase SL: **Rebooting psychotherapy research and practice to reduce the burden of mental illness.** *Perspect Psychol Sci* 2011, **6**(1):21–37.
2. Lilienfeld SO, Ritschel LA, Lynn SJ, Cautin RL, Latzman RD: **Why many clinical psychologists are resistant to evidence-based practice: Root causes and constructive remedies.** *Clin Psychol Rev* 2013, **33**(7):883–900.
3. Proctor EK, Landsverk J, Aarons G, Chambers D, Glisson C, Mittman B: **Implementation research in mental health services: An emerging science with conceptual, methodological, and training challenges.** *Adm Policy Ment Health* 2009, **36**(1):24–34.
4. Kazdin AE, Rabbitt SM: **Novel models for delivering mental health services and reducing the burdens of mental illness.** *Clin Psychol Sci* 2013, **1**(2):170–191.
5. Austin SB: **A public health approach to eating disorders prevention: It's time for public health professionals to take a seat at the table.** *BMC Public Health* 2012, **12**(1):854.
6. **Achievements in Public Health, 1900–1999: Changes in the Public Health System.** http://www.cdc.gov/mmwr/preview/mmwrhtml/mm4850a1.htm.
7. Miles J, Espiritu RC, Horen N, Sebian J, Waetzig E: *A public health approach to children's mental health: A conceptual framework.* Washington, DC: Georgetown University Center for Child and Human Development, National Technical Assistance Center for Children's Mental Health; 2010.
8. Jacobi C, Hayward C, De Zwaan M, Kraemer HC, Agras WS: **Coming to terms with risk factors for eating disorders: application or risk terminology and suggestions for a general taxonomy.** *Psychol Bull* 2004, **130**(1):19–64.
9. Green MA, Scott NA, Cross SE, Liao KYH, Hallengren JJ, Davids CM, Carter LP, Kugler DW, Read KE, Jepson AJ: **Eating disorder behaviors and depression: a minimal relationship beyond social comparison, self-esteem, and body dissatisfaction.** *J Clin Psychol* 2009, **65**(9):989–999.
10. Grilo CM, White MA, Masheb RM: **DSM-IV psychiatric disorder comorbidity and its correlates in binge eating disorder.** *Int J Eat Disord* 2009, **42**(3):228–234.
11. Wilfley DE, Friedman MA, Dounchis JZ, Stein RI, Welch RR, Ball SA: **Co-morbid psychopathology in binge eating disorder: Relation to eating disorder severity at baseline and following treatment.** *J Consult Clin Psychol* 2000, **68**(4):641–649.
12. Fornari V, Kaplan M, Sandberg DE, Matthews M, Skolnick N, Katz JL: **Depressive and anxiety disorders in anorexia nervosa and bulimia nervosa.** *Int J Eat Disord* 1992, **12**(1):21–29.
13. Halmi KA: **Psychological Comorbidity of Eating Disorders.** In *The Oxford Handbook of Eating Disorders.* Edited by Agras WS. USA: Oxford University Press; 2010:292–303.
14. Halmi KA, Eckert E, Marchi P, Sampugnaro V, Apple R, Cohen J: **Comorbidity of psychiatric diagnoses in anorexia nervosa.** *Arch Gen Psychiatry* 1991, **48**(8):712–718.
15. Herzog DB, Keller MB, Sacks NR, Yeh CJ, Lavori PW: **Psychiatric comorbidity in treatment-seeking anorexics and bulimics.** *J Am Acad Child Adolesc Psychiatry* 1992, **31**(5):810–818.
16. Schwalberg MD, Barlow DH, Alger SA, Howard LJ: **Comparison of bulimics, obese binge eaters, social phobics, and individuals with panic disorder on comorbidity across DSM-III-R anxiety disorders.** *J Abnorm Psychol* 1992, **101**(4):675–681.
17. Santos M, Richards CS, Bleckley MK: **Comorbidity between depression and disordered eating in adolescents.** *Eat Behav* 2007, **8**(4):440–449.
18. Jacobi C, Fittig E: **Psychosocial Risk Factors for Eating Disorders.** In *The Oxford Handbook of Eating Disorders.* Edited by Agras WS. USA: Oxford University Press; 2010:123–136.
19. Johnson F, Wardle J: **Dietary restraint, body dissatisfaction, and psychological distress: a prospective analysis.** *J of Abnorm Psychol* 2005, **114**:119–125.
20. Neumark-Sztainer D, Paxton SJ, Hannan PJ, Haines J, Story M: **Does body satisfaction matter? Five-year longitudinal associations between body**

satisfaction and health behaviors in adolescent females and males. *J of Adolesc Health* 2006, **39**:244–251.
21. Van den Berg P, Neumark-Stzainer D: **Fat 'n' happy 5 years later: is it bad for overweight girls to like their bodies.** *J of Adolesc Health* 2007, **41**:415–417.
22. Stice E, Nemeroff C, Shaw HE: **Test of the dual pathway model of bulimia nervosa: Evidence for dietary restraint and affect regulation mechanisms.** *J Soc Clin Psychol* 1996, **15**(3):340–363.
23. Isomaa R, Isomaa AL, Marttunen M, Kaltiala-Heino R, Björkqvist K: **Psychological distress and risk for eating disorders in subgroups of dieters.** *Eur Eat Disord Rev* 2010, **18**(4):296–303.
24. Stice E, Hayward C, Cameron RP, Killen JD, Taylor CB: **Body-image and eating disturbances predict onset of depression among female adolescents: a longitudinal study.** *J Abnorm Psychol* 2000, **109**(3):438–444.
25. Rawana JS: **The relative importance of body change strategies, weight perception, perceived social support, and self-esteem on adolescent depressive symptoms: Longitudinal findings from a national sample.** *J Psychosom Res* 2013, **75**(1):49–54.
26. Bearman SK, Presnell K, Martinez E, Stice E: **The skinny on body dissatisfaction: A longitudinal study of adolescent girls and boys.** *J Youth Adolesc* 2006, **35**(2):217–229.
27. Abrantes AM, Strong DR, Ramsey SE, Lewinsohn PM, Brown RA: **Characteristics of dieting and nondieting adolescents in a psychiatric inpatient setting.** *J Child Fam Stud* 2006, **15**(4):418–432.
28. Cervera S, Lahortiga F, Martínez-González MA, Gual P, Irala-Estévez JD, Alonso Y: **Neuroticism and low self-esteem as risk factors for incident eating disorders in a prospective cohort study.** *Int J Eat Disord* 2003, **33**(3):271–280.
29. Striegel-Moore RH, Dohm FA, Pike KM, Wilfley DE, Fairburn CG: **Abuse, bullying, and discrimination as risk factors for binge eating disorder.** *Am J Psychiatry* 2002, **159**(11):1902–1907.
30. Haines J, Neumark-Sztainer D, Eisenberg ME, Hannan PJ: **Weight teasing and disordered eating behaviors in adolescents: longitudinal findings from Project EAT (Eating Among Teens).** *Pediatrics* 2006, **117**(2):e209–e215.
31. Klomek AB, Kleinman M, Altschuler E, Marrocco F, Amakawa L, Gould MS: **Suicidal Adolescents' experiences with bullying perpetration and victimization during high school as risk factors for later depression and suicidality.** *J Adolesc Health* 2013, **53**(1):S37–S42.
32. Costello EJ, Worthman C, Erkanli A, Angold A: **Prediction from Low birth weight to female adolescent depression: a test of competing hypotheses.** *Arch Gen Psychiatry* 2007, **64**(3):338–344.
33. Jaffee SR, Moffitt TE, Caspi A, Fombonne E, Poulton R, Martin J: **Differences in early childhood risk factors for juvenile-onset and adult-onset depression.** *Arch Gen Psychiatry* 2002, **59**(3):215–222.
34. Nikulina V, Widom CS, Brzustowicz LM: **Child abuse and neglect, *MAOA*, and mental health outcomes: a prospective examination.** *Biol Psychiatry* 2012, **71**(4):350–357.
35. Widom CS, DuMont KA, Czaja SJ: **A prospective investigation of major depressive disorder and comorbidity in abused and neglected children grown up.** *Arch Gen Psychiatry* 2007, **64**:176–187.
36. Gibb BE, Butler AC, Beck JS: **Childhood abuse, depression, and anxiety in adult psychiatric outpatients.** *Depress Anxiety* 2003, **17**:226–228.
37. Brown GR, Anderson B: **Psychiatric morbidity in adult inpatients with childhood histories of sexual and physical abuse.** *Am J Psychiatry* 1991, **148**:55–61.
38. Kendler KS, Bulik CM, Silberg J, Hettema JM, Myers J, Prescott CA: **Childhood sexual abuse and adult psychiatric and substance use disorders in women: An epidemiological and cotwin control analysis.** *Arch Gen Psychiatry* 2000, **57**:953–959.
39. Mrazek P, Haggerty RJ: *Reducing Risks for Mental Disorders: Frontiers for Preventive Intervention Research.* Washington, DC: The National Academies Press; 1994.
40. Stice E, Marti CN, Spoor S, Presnell K, Shaw H: **Dissonance and healthy weight eating disorder prevention programs: Long-term effects from a randomized efficacy trial.** *J Consult Clin Psychol* 2008, **76**(2):329–340.
41. Taylor CB, Bryson S, Doyle AAC, Luce KH, Cunning D, Abascal LB, Rockwell R, Field AE, Striegel-Moore R, Winzelberg AJ, Wilfley DE: **The adverse effect of negative comments about weight and shape from family and siblings on women at high risk for eating disorders.** *Pediatrics* 2006, **118**(2):731–738.
42. Levine MP, Smolak L: **Body Image Development in Adolescence.** In *Body Image: A Handbook of Theory, Research, and Clinical Practice.* Edited by Cash TF, Pruzinsky T. New York: Guilford Press; 2004:74–82.
43. Festinger L: *A Theory of Cognitive Dissonance.* Stanford, CA: Stanford University Press; 1957.
44. Stice E, Presnell K: *The Body Project.* New York: Oxford University Press; 2007.
45. Stice E, Rohde P, Shaw H: *The Body Project: A Dissonance-Based Eating Disorder Prevention Intervention (Programs That Work).* New York: Oxford University Press; 2012.
46. Stice E, Mazotti L, Weibel D, Agras WS: **Dissonance prevention program decreases thin-ideal internalization, body dissatisfaction, dieting, negative affect, and bulimic symptoms: A preliminary experiment.** *Int J Eat Disord* 2000, **27**(2):206–217.
47. Stice E, Trost A, Chase A: **Healthy weight control and dissonance-based eating disorder prevention programs: Results from a controlled trial.** *Int J Eat Disord* 2003, **33**(1):10–21.
48. Stice E, Shaw H, Burton E, Wade E: **Dissonance and healthy weight eating disorder prevention programs: a randomized efficacy trial.** *J Consult Clin Psychol* 2006, **74**(2):263–275.
49. Stice E, Rohde P, Gau J, Shaw H: **An effectiveness trial of a dissonance-based eating disorder prevention program for high-risk adolescent girls.** *J Consult Clin Psychol* 2009, **77**(5):825–834.
50. Patel V, Chowdhary N, Rahman A, Verdeli H: **Improving access to psychological treatments: Lessons from developing countries.** *Behav Res Ther* 2011, **49**(9):523–528.
51. Becker CB, Smith LM, Ciao AC: **Peer-facilitated eating disorder prevention: A ramdomized effectiveness trial of cognitive dissonance and media advocacy.** *J Consult Clin Psychol* 2006, **53**(4):550–565.
52. Becker CB, Bull S, Schaumberg K, Cauble A, Franco A: **Effectiveness of peer-led eating disorders prevention: A replication trial.** *Consult Clin Psychol* 2008, **76**(2):347–354.
53. Becker CB, Wilson C, Williams A, Kelly M, McDaniel L, Elmquist J: **Peer-facilitated cognitive dissonance versus healthy weight eating disorders prevention: A randomized comparison.** *Body Image* 2010, **7**(4):280–288.
54. Israel BA, Eng E, Schulz AJ, Parker EA: **Methods in community-based participatory research for health.** In *Introduction to methods in community-based participatory research for health.* 2nd edition. Edited by Israel BA, Eng E, Shulz AJ, Parker EA. San Francisco: Jossey-Bass; 2005:3–26.
55. Becker CB, Stice E, Shaw H, Woda S: **Use of empirically-supported interventions for psychopathology: Can the participatory approach move us beyond the research-to-practice gap?** *Behav Res Ther* 2009, **47**(4):265–274.
56. Halliwell E, Diedrichs PC: **Testing a dissonance body image intervention among young girls.** *Health Psychol* 2014, **33**(2):201–204. doi: 10.1037/a0032585.
57. **Free Being Me.** http://www.free-being-me.com/.
58. **Free Being Me Global Training.** http://www.wagggs.org/en/news/22767.
59. Thompson JK, Herbozo S, Himes S, Yamamiya Y: **Effects of weight-related teasing in adults.** In *Weight bias: Nature, Consequences and Remedies.* 1st edition. Edited by Brownell KD, Puhl RM, Schwartz MB, Rudd L. New York: Guilford Press; 2005:137–149.
60. Grabe S, Ward LM, Hyde JS: **The role of the media in body image concerns among women: a meta-analysis of experimental and correlational studies.** *Psychol Bull* 2008, **134**(3):460–476.
61. Yamamiya Y, Cash TF, Melnyk SE, Posavac HD, Posavac SS: **Women's exposure to thin-and-beautiful media images: body image effects of media-ideal internalization and impact-reduction interventions.** *Body Image* 2005, **2**(1):74–80.
62. Wilksch SM, Tiggemann M, Wade TD: **Impact of interactive school-based media literacy lessons for reducing internalization of media ideals in young adolescent girls and boys.** *Int J Eat Disord* 2006, **39**(5):385–393.
63. Wilksch SM, Wade TD: **Reduction of shape and weight concern in young adolescents: A 30-month controlled evaluation of a media literacy program.** *J Am Acad Child Adolesc Psychiatry* 2009, **48**(6):652–661.
64. Wilksch SM: **Universal school-based eating disorder prevention: Benefits to both high-and low-risk participants on the core cognitive feature of eating disorders.** *Clin Psychol* 2010, **14**(2):62–69.
65. Wilksch SM, Durbridge MR, Wade TD: **A preliminary controlled comparison of programs designed to reduce risk of eating disorders targeting perfectionism and media literacy.** *J Am Acad Child Adolesc Psychiatry* 2008, **47**(8):939–947.
66. Wilksch SM, Wade TD: **Depression as a moderator of benefit from Media Smart: A school-based eating disorder prevention program.** *Behav Res Ther* 2014, **52**:64–71.

67. Wilksch SM, Wade TD: **Examination of the sociocultural attitudes towards appearance questionnaire-3 in a mixed-gender young-adolescent sample.** *Psychol Assess* 2012, **24**(2):352–364.
68. **Media Smart.** http://www.mediasmart.org.uk/.
69. Diedrich PC, Paraskeva N, Yager Z, Halliwell E: *Media Smart? Evaluating a Government Endorsed Body Image Program for pre-Adolescent Boys and Girls.* Montreal: Paper presented at the International Conference on Eating Disorders; 2013.
70. Metzmacher D: **70 Beauty-Retouching Photoshop Tutorials. Smashing Magazine, from.** http://www.smashingmagazine.com/2008/07/15/70-beauty-retouching-photoshop-tutorials/.
71. Erlanger S: **Point, Shoot, Retouch and Label?** http://www.nytimes.com/2009/12/03/fashion/03Boyer.html?pagewanted=all&_r=0.
72. National Advisory Group: *A proposed National Strategy on Body Image.* Australia: Commonwealth of Australia; 2009. http://www.youth.gov.au/sites/Youth/bodyImage/Documents/Proposed-National-Strategy-on-Body-Image.pdf.
73. Duffett H: **Jo Swinson: Ban airbrushing in children's adverts.** In *Liberal Democrat Voice.* 2009. http://www.libdemvoice.org/jo-swinson-ban-airbrushing-in-childrens-adverts-15807.html.
74. Ya'ar C: **Knesset Passes New Anorexia Law.** http://www.israelnationalnews.com/News/News.aspx/153937#.Uuk5jj1dXEY.
75. **Tobacco Products.** http://www.fda.gov/TobaccoProducts/GuidanceComplianceRegulatoryInformation/ucm276626.htm.
76. U.S. Food and Drug Administration: **FDA Targets Trans Fat in Processed Foods.** http://www.fda.gov/ForConsumers/ConsumerUpdates/ucm372915.htm.
77. Slater A, Tiggemann M, Firth B, Hawkins K: **Reality Check: An experimental investigation of the addition of warning labels to fashion magazine images on women's mood and body dissatisfaction.** *J Soc Clin Psychol* 2012, **31**:105–122.
78. Ata RN, Thompson JK, Small BJ: **Effects of exposure to thin-ideal media images on body dissatisfaction: testing the inclusion of a disclaimer versus warning label.** *Body Image* 2013, **10**(4):472–480.
79. Nichter M: *Fat talk: What girls and their parents say about dieting.* Cambridge: Harvard University Press; 2001.
80. Nichter M, Vuckovic N: **Fat Talk.** In *Many mirrors: Body image and social relations.* Edited by Sault N. New Brunswick: Rutgers University Press; 1994:109–132.
81. Stice E, Maxfield J, Wells T: **Adverse effects of social pressure to be thin on young women: an experimental investigation of the effects of "fat talk".** *Int J Eat Disord* 2003, **34**:108–117.
82. Garnett BR, Buelow R, Franko DL, Becker B, Rodgers RF, Austin SB: **The importance of campaign saliency as a predictor of attitude and behavior change: a pilot evaluation of social marketing campaign fat talk free week.** *Health Commun* 2013, **29**:1–12.
83. **Representation Project.** therepresentationproject.org.
84. **All Party Parliamentary Group on Body Image.** http://www.ymca.co.uk/bodyimage/.
85. All Party Parliamentary Group on Body Image: **Reflections on Body Image.** http://issuu.com/bodyimage/docs/reflections_on_body_image.
86. **National Organization for Women.** http://loveyourbody.nowfoundation.org/.
87. **Dove.** http://www.dove.us/social-mission/campaign-for-real-beauty.aspx.
88. **Dove Self-Esteem Toolkit and Resources.** http://www.dove.us/Our-Mission/Girls-Self-Esteem/Get-Involved/default.aspx.
89. Richardson SM, Paxton SJ, Thomson JS: **Is BodyThink an efficacious body image and self-esteem program? A controlled evaluation with adolescents.** *Body Image* 2009, **6**(2):75–82.
90. Steiner-Adair C, Sjostrum L, Franko DL, Pai S, Tucker R, Becker AE, Herzog DB: **Primary prevention of risk factors for eating disorders in adolescent girls: Learning from practice.** *Int J Eat Disord* 2002, **32**:401–411.
91. Sjostrom LA, Steiner-Adair C: **Full of ourselves: A wellness program to advance girl power, health, and leadership: An eating disorders prevention program that works.** *J Nutr Educ Behav* 2005, **37**:141–144.
92. Haines J, Neumark-Sztainer D, Perry CL, Hannan PJ, Levine MP: **VIK (Very Important Kids): a school-based program designed to reduce teasing and unhealthy weight-control behaviors.** *Health Educ Res* 2006, **21**(6):884–895.
93. Neumark-Sztainer D, Levine MP, Paxton SJ, Smolak L, Piran N, Wertheim EH: **Prevention of body dissatisfaction and disordered eating: What next?** *Ea Disord* 2006, **14**:265–285.
94. Gortmaker SL, Peterson K, Wiecha J, Sobol AM, Dixit S, Fox MK, Laird N: **Reducing obesity via a school-based interdisciplinary intervention among youth: planet health.** *Arch Pediatr Adolesc Med* 1999, **153**(4):409–418.
95. Austin SB, Field AE, Wiecha J, Peterson KE, Gortmaker SL: **The impact of school-based obesity prevention trial on disordered weight control behaviors in early adolescent girls.** *Arch Pediatr Adolesc Med* 2005, **159**:225–230.
96. Wilksch SM, Wade TD: **Life Smart: A Pilot Study of a School-Based Program to Reduce the Risk of Both Eating Disorders and Obesity in Young Adolescent Girls and Boys.** *J Pediatr Psychol* 2013, **38**(9):1044–1050.
97. Rosenbaum DP, Hanson GS: **Assessing the Effects of School-based Drug Education: A 6-year Multilevel Analysis of Project D.A.R.E.** *J Res Crime Delinq* 1998, **35**(4):381–412.
98. **U.S. Government Accountability Office.** http://www.gao.gov/new.items/d03172r.pdf.
99. Shepard EM: *The Economic Costs of D.A.R.E.* http://www.drugpolicy.org/docUploads/DAREfinalRP.pdf.

A preliminary study of motivational interviewing as a prelude to intensive treatment for an eating disorder

Carmen V Weiss[1], Jennifer S Mills[2*], Henny A Westra[2] and Jacqueline C Carter[3]

Abstract

Background: Engaging patients with an eating disorder in change is difficult and intensive treatment programs have high drop-out rates. The purpose of the study was to determine whether Motivational Interviewing (MI) in the form of a brief, pre-treatment intervention would be associated with higher completion rates in subsequent intensive treatment for an eating disorder.

Thirty-two participants diagnosed with an eating disorder participated in the study. All participants were on the waitlist for admission to an intensive, hospital-based treatment program. Sixteen participants were randomly assigned to four individual sessions of MI that began prior to entrance into the treatment program (MI condition) and 16 participants were assigned to treatment as usual (control condition). The main outcome was completion of the intensive treatment program. Participants also completed self-report measures of motivation to change.

Results: Participants in the MI condition were significantly more likely to complete intensive treatment (69% completion rate) than were those in the control condition (31%).

Conclusions: MI can be a useful intervention to engage individuals with severe eating disorders prior to participation in intensive treatment. MI as a brief prelude to hospital-based treatment for an eating disorder may help to improve completion rates in such programs. Further research is required to determine the precise therapeutic mechanisms of change in MI.

Keywords: Motivational interviewing, Eating disorders, Treatment

Background

Motivational Interviewing (MI) [1] is a treatment approach that was originally designed for use within the field of addictions to help enhance motivation to recover from substance abuse. In general, MI seeks to explore and resolve a client's ambivalence toward change by acknowledging both the pros and cons of changing behaviour, by normalizing the experience of ambivalence, and by helping the client situate his/her behaviour within the context of his/her values and goals [1]. Resistance to change in a therapeutic context is seen as an indication of a mismatch between the intervention and the client's readiness to change. Such resistance is considered to be a warning to the therapist to begin to validate the client's concerns about making changes, rather than pushing for behavioural change, which would likely be met with more resistance. In so doing, the therapist gives the client the opportunity to consider and then critically evaluate both the benefits and costs of change. MI facilitates a movement towards change by encouraging the client to put the pros and cons in the context of his/her values and goals. Originally developed for patients with substance abuse, MI is generally well suited for use as an intervention for conditions in which ambivalence is common.

There is agreement among clinicians that eating disorders, including anorexia nervosa (AN) and bulimia nervosa (BN) are very difficult disorders to treat. Treatment for these disorders is often marked by premature drop-out and relapse [2]. Intensive, hospital-based treatment programs for eating disorders have notoriously poor completion rates and high rates of recidivism. Ambivalence toward recovery and low motivation to change are

* Correspondence: jsmills@yorku.ca
[2]Department of Psychology, York University, Toronto, Ontario, Canada
Full list of author information is available at the end of the article

hallmarks of eating disorders [3]. Motivation to change has been found to be especially low in individuals with AN [4-6]. Other studies have reported no differences between these two groups on motivation to change [7,8].

Understanding ED patients' ambivalence toward recovery and increasing their motivation to change is critical to increasing treatment effectiveness for these disorders. Early research by Geller and colleagues was among the first of studies to show a link between readiness to change one's eating and outcome from treatment for an eating disorder [9]. A study by Bewell and Carter sought to determine whether a patient's ambivalence about recovery would predict completion of an intensive hospital-based treatment program for AN [10]. They found not only that readiness to change eating and weight, as measured after four weeks in the program, predicted intensive treatment completion, but also that readiness to change fully mediated the relationship between ED symptomatology at admission to the program and later treatment completion. Similar findings were demonstrated in an adolescent population treated in an intensive hospital-based treatment program [11]. Other research has shown than individuals with BN who are more motivated to change at baseline experience a greater reduction in binge eating during therapy than do those who are initially less motivated to change [12,13], and that motivation to change has been shown to be a predictor of relapse in individuals with BN [14,15]. In sum, there is strong evidence that readiness for change impacts the course of treatment for an eating disorder.

Because MI specifically targets ambivalence about change, it has been thought to be useful in the treatment of eating disorders. Some studies have shown that MI and MI-based treatments are useful as either a standalone treatment or as a pre-treatment in recovery from binge eating [16,17]. There has also been some evidence that MI-based treatments and assessment techniques have been associated with increases in motivation and readiness to change in individuals with AN [18,19]. On the other hand, recent reviews by Dray and Wade [20] as well as Knowles and colleagues [21] conclude that although MI approaches appear to increase motivation in participants, there is still no compelling scientific evidence that MI approaches actually enhance treatment outcomes for eating disorders. Better designed studies, including the use of randomized controlled trials and improved treatment integrity, are called for.

Individuals with an eating disorder who enter and then prematurely drop out of intensive treatment do so for various reasons, including inability and unwillingness to comply with program rules (e.g., abstention from symptoms) or distress from eating that is so significant as to interfere with treatment. Given the substantial financial cost of these programs and the paucity of admission spots that are available for eating disorders, research needs to uncover ways in which to make individuals more likely to successfully complete treatment. The extant literature on motivation to change eating disorder symptoms suggests that it may be important to consider (and foster) an individual's level of motivation to change before engaging the individual in intensive treatment for disordered eating. The present research evaluated the clinical efficacy of a brief MI intervention delivered to patients before admission to an intensive treatment program for an eating disorder. Based on the previous literature, it was hypothesized that individuals in the MI treatment condition would be more likely to complete the intensive treatment program than were those who did not receive the MI pre-treatment. Specifically, Gowers and Smyth [22] found that an MI pre-treatment led to improvements in self-reported motivation to change, which then predicted early treatment response. Therefore, it was further hypothesized that participants in the MI treatment condition would show a larger increase in their motivation to change (as measured by self-report questionnaires) across the 4-week pre-treatment interval than would those in the control condition.

Methods

Participants

The participants were recruited from the waiting lists for the Inpatient and Day Hospital Units of Toronto General Hospital's Eating Disorder Program between January 2008 and June 2009. The inpatient and ambulatory programs for eating disorders at this hospital have been described in detail elsewhere [23]. Briefly, they are both well-established intensive group therapy programs that treat adult patients (ages 17 and older) and are primarily directed towards symptom control, normalized eating, and body weight restoration to a minimum body mass index (BMI) of 20 (in the case of those who are initially underweight). The inpatient program is typically recommended for patients who are potentially medically unstable and is primarily comprised of patients with AN. Patients begin the program as inpatients and are granted outside privileges as they demonstrate symptom control and meet minimal standards of weight gain. Approximately two thirds of the way through their stay, if they are progressing well in their recovery, they are discharged as an inpatient, but continue to attend the program as a day-patient (i.e., attending all groups and eating two meals and a snack with the inpatient group). Once patients reach a BMI of 20, they typically are kept in the program for 2–3 additional weeks, to solidify their gains, and then they are discharged to the follow-up care program at the hospital. The ambulatory treatment program is comprised entirely of outpatients. However, the program is intensive, as patients typically attend the program from 10 am until 6 pm, Monday to Friday, and complete two staff-supervised meals and one supervised snack each day in hospital. The ambulatory program is comprised of individuals with clinical and subclinical levels of AN and BN. Patients who do not require weight gain are given a maximum admission of eight weeks, whereas those who have weight to gain are admitted until they reach a BMI of 20.

All participants in this study were female and met DSM-IV criteria for AN, BN, or Eating Disorder Not Otherwise Specified (EDNOS). These assessments were completed by psychologists, psychiatrists, and Master's level therapists in the Toronto General Hospital Eating Disorders program. Participants also were required to have a BMI greater than or equal to 13, as we were concerned that patients with a BMI of less than 13 would be too medically unstable to participate. It was decided that clients who were suicidal (i.e., those who expressed suicidal intent and plans for how they would hurt themselves) would be included in the study since suicidality is so common in eating disordered populations [24]. These patients were monitored closely throughout pre-treatment and intensive treatment. Only one patient demonstrated severe suicidal ideation, and she was admitted to an acute mental health unit after only one MI session, and was subsequently excluded from the analyses.

In total, 69 participants meeting the inclusion criteria agreed to be contacted about the study (see Figure 1). Of these individuals, 39 (56.5%) consented to participate and entered the trial. One participant in the MI condition was excluded because she attended a different hospital's treatment program after completing her MI sessions.[a] Two participants in the control condition were excluded; one had a disruption in her intensive treatment due to unrelated medical issues and one had significant missing questionnaire data.

Definition of treatment completion

Twenty-one participants were randomized to the MI condition. Four patients completed only one session, two completed three sessions, and 14 completed all four MI sessions. There are currently no guidelines for an appropriate "dose" of MI, but it was agreed by the authors that completion of three out of four sessions of MI could be considered treatment completion. It was noted by the first author that there was little new material introduced after the third session and that the fourth session served mainly to reiterate issues raised in previous sessions.

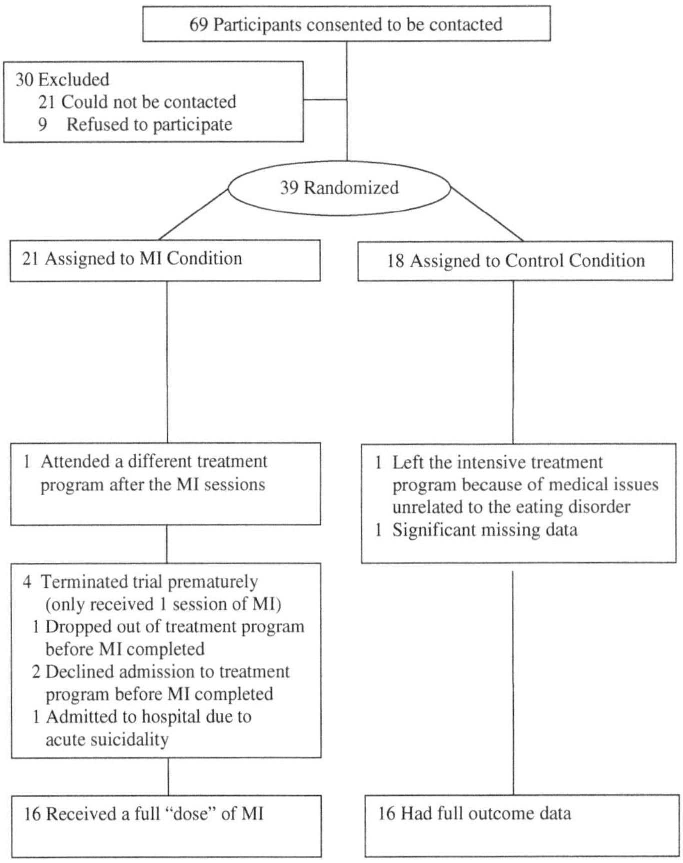

Figure 1 Flow of participants through the study.

Before excluding participants on the basis of MI non-completion, a series of t-tests were run to compare the groups on all the measures of motivation measured at pre-randomization. It was determined that there was only one difference between the "completers" and the "non-completers": the MI non-completers (i.e., the four participants who received only one out of four sessions) had lower baseline scores on confidence about changing weight and shape preoccupation (t (16) = 3.20, p = 0.01). There was no evidence that this variable predicted hospital treatment completion or introduced other confounds. Thus, it was decided that, with no other differences between the groups, the four participants who received only one session of MI would be excluded from further analysis.

The final sample consisted of 32 participants. Sixteen had been randomly assigned to the MI treatment condition (15 females, 1 male), and 16 to the waiting list control condition (15 females, 1 male) (see Figure 1).

Procedure

This study received ethical approval from the Research Ethics Boards of both York University and the hospital ethics board. Participants who consented to participate were asked to complete some self-report questionnaires. They also participated in a brief assessment interview inquiring about demographic information, diagnostic information and age of onset of their eating disorder, eating disorder treatment history, and information about the treatment they were receiving at the time of randomization. Finally, participants were randomized (through permuted block randomization) into either the treatment or control condition. Treatment staff in the subsequent intensive treatment program was kept blind to participants' group assignment.

Treatment condition

The MI condition received weekly 50-minute sessions of MI over four consecutive weeks. Treatment followed the principles and techniques outlined in Miller and Rollnick's MI manual. At the end of each session, participants completed a measure of therapeutic alliance. It should be noted that we considered our MI intervention to be "brief" only in comparison to the typical length of treatment for an eating disorder. MI as an adjunct to other treatments is usually done over 1–2 one hour sessions. However, we wanted our intervention to include all of the key components to Miller and Rollnick's MI manual. Participants in the MI condition were also able to continue to receive "treatment-as-usual," meaning they could carry on as they normally would (e.g., seeing a family doctor, taking medication, etc.). This treatment most often included regular medical monitoring by their physician or psychiatrist and the use of anti-depressant medication. Some participants were also receiving psychotherapy with psychologists and clinical social workers, and some were seeing dietitians, as is common.

Control condition

Participants assigned to the control condition did not receive any MI treatment over the four-week treatment period, but remained on the waiting list and received treatment as usual. Admission to intensive treatment was not delayed for any participant as a function of condition.

Approximately four weeks after randomization (and after the final therapy session for those in the MI condition), participants in both groups were asked to complete another copy of the original questionnaire packet. They also consented to allow the researcher to access their hospital chart to determine whether they completed the subsequent treatment program, and these charts were examined to determine whether the participant completed treatment or dropped out prematurely.

The length of time between randomization and the participant's admission to the intensive treatment program varied considerably (ranging from .43 to 30.5 weeks). This inconsistency was primarily accounted for by the varying nature of the waitlists for both of the hospital treatment programs. At the time of randomization, it wasn't known when the participant would be entering intensive treatment. When the waitlists were short, there was often not sufficient time to recruit participants and finish the four-week assessment period before the participant was admitted to the program. Thus, 24 (75%) of participants were attending the treatment program for some portion of time while they were receiving the MI treatment or waiting to complete the final questionnaire packet (if they were in the control group). In other words, for some participants in both conditions, "treatment as usual" included intensive treatment in the hospital eating disorder program. A Chi-square analysis indicated that there were no differences between the MI group and the control group in the proportions of participants who completed their second set of questionnaires while in the program, $X^2(1, 32) = 3.46, p = .06$.

Therapist and therapist training

This study formed part of the doctoral dissertation of the first author (CW) and all MI treatment was delivered by this author. Training consisted of attending a 2-day intensive workshop on MI led by Dr. William Miller (one of the founders of MI), readings, on-going supervision (including live observation and videotape review) with a highly experienced MI therapist (HW), and ongoing supervision with a highly experienced therapist specializing in eating disorders (JC).

Measures

Pros and Cons of Eating Disorders Scale (PCED) [25]. This self-report measure asks participants to identify the extent to which they agree with 70 statements addressing both the pros and cons of ED. The items have been shown to have good internal consistency and test-retest reliability (ranging from .72 to .92) [26].

Motivation to change scale - modified version (MTC)

Motivation rulers (motivation, confidence, readiness) were used in the current study. These measures have been used previously in other research and have shown good psychometric properties [27], but have not yet been validated for use with eating disorders. Our measure was based on a scale comprised of three questions aimed at addressing an individual's motivation to change his/her behaviour ("How important is it for you to eat normally and to gain weight?"), confidence ("If you decided to change your eating and weight, how confident are you that you would succeed?"), and feelings of readiness to change ("How ready are you to change your eating and weight?"). For clarity, the original questions were also changed by deleting any reference about gaining weight, because some of the patients had normal BMIs. In other words, "How important is it for you to eat normally and to gain weight?" became "How important is it for you to eat normally?" Each question is presented in a 10-point Likert-scale format. The current study also included questions re-worded for the symptoms of both Food Restriction and Weight/Shape Preoccupation.

MI treatment integrity

Twenty percent of the MI treatment sessions were randomly selected and a twenty-minute videotaped segment was randomly chosen from each. These segments were then coded by two independent raters according to the Motivational Interviewing Treatment Integrity coding system (MITI, 2.0) [28]. These raters had been trained in the MITI rating system, and participated as raters on a previous MI treatment trial [29]. The MITI coding system creates global rating scores based on two dimensions: Empathy/Understanding and Spirit. Treatment integrity in the present study was set as 5 on a 7-point scale, based on the cut-off used in previous research.

Results

Sample characteristics

Taking the 32 participants as a whole, participants had a mean age of 28.0 years ($SD = 8.8$), a mean age of ED onset of 17.3 years ($SD = 4.5$), and a mean duration of illness of 10.7 years ($SD = 8.9$). Ninety-four percent of the participants were female. Eighty-two percent were single, 13% were married or in common-law relationships, and 6% were divorced. In terms of ethnic background, all participants identified themselves as Caucasian. Twenty-one participants (65.6%) were diagnosed with AN (9 with AN restricting subtype and 12 with AN binge-purge subtypes), 10 (31.3%) with BN, and 1 (3.1%) with Eating Disorder Not Otherwise Specified (EDNOS). The BMI ranges at admission to intensive treatment are as follows: AN-R (13.4-19.0), AN-BP (13.3-17.7), BN (16–26.2), EDNOS (21.22). Ninety-four percent of participants were currently receiving some form of additional treatment at pre-randomization. The most common forms of treatment were medications (most often anti-depressants), psychotherapy (with psychologists, psychiatrists, psychological associates, or social workers) and medical monitoring (with psychiatrists or general practitioners). Many participants were currently engaging in all three of these forms of treatment when they were randomized. Sixteen participants (50.0%) completed the intensive treatment program, whereas 16 (50.0%) dropped out prematurely.

There were no differences between the groups in terms of subtype, age, age of onset of their ED, length of illness, admission BMI, or type of intensive treatment program (inpatient vs. ambulatory treatment). Table 1 presents the sample characteristics broken down by treatment group.

There also were no significant differences between the groups on any of the questionnaires measured at pre-randomization. Table 2 presents means and SDs for all measures across time by treatment group, as well as within group effect sizes.

MI treatment integrity

According to the treatment integrity ratings, the quality of the MI sessions was high, with no session being rated as lower than 5 on either global dimension, and many receiving ratings of 6 or 7. The overall mean for the global "Empathy/Understanding" score was 5.88/7 ($SD = .62$), and the overall mean for the global "Spirit" score was 5.81/7 ($SD = .75$).

The impact of MI on treatment completion rates

Intention to treat analysis, in which all participants are included regardless of whether they adhered to the treatment, was deemed to be inappropriate for the current study since it often underestimates the comparative effectiveness of a treatment [30]. The current study had several characteristics that contributed to that decision, including an emphasis on treatment integrity, a significant number of drop-outs and non-completers, and longer time between MI treatment and outcome. A logistic regression was run with condition (MI versus control) as the independent variable and treatment completion as the dependent variable. The overall model was significant ($X^2(1, 32) = 4.61$, $p = .032$, Nagelkerke $R^2 = .18$), and correctly predicted 69% of cases. Condition was found to

Table 1 Sample characteristics by treatment group

Measure	MI group (n = 16)	Control group (n = 16)
Gender	15 Female	15 Female
	1 Male	1 Male
Age	M =28.0 years (S.D. = 9.5)	M = 28.4 years (S.D. = 7.8)
Ethnicity	16 Caucasian	16 Caucasian
Marital status	13 Single	13 Single
	2 Married/Common-law	2 Married
	1 Divorced	1 Divorced
Employment status	8 Students	6 Students
	6 Employed	7 Employed
	2 Unemployed	3 Unemployed
Age of onset	M = 17.1 years (S.D. = 4.0)	M = 17.5 years (S.D. = 5.1)
Duration of illness	M = 11.0 years (S.D. = 10.0)	M = 10.9 years (S.D. = 7.8)
Subtype	4 AN-R	5 AN-R
	8 AN-BP	5 AN-BP
	4 BN	6 BN
Admission BMI	*M* = 17.7 (*SD* = 2.9)	*M* = 18.4 (*SD* = 4.8)
Type of intensive treatment program	8 Inpatient program	7 Inpatient program
	8 Day hospital program	9 Day hospital program

be a significant predictor of outcome ($B = 1.58$, Wald Statistic = 4.27, $p = .039$), and examination of the odds ratio indicated that participants in the MI condition were 4.8 times more likely than those in the control condition to complete the subsequent treatment program. In this analysis, 11 (68.8%) of participants in the MI group completed the intensive treatment program, as compared to 5 (31.3%) of participants in the control group.

Treatment condition and self-reported motivation

Twenty-six participants (81%) completed questionnaires at the second assessment. A series of repeated measures ANOVAs were conducted on each of the self-report measures, comparing participants' scores at the second assessment to their scores at the first assessment. None of the interactions were significant at an α of 0.01; however, there were trends towards differences between the groups across time in the total score of the PCED Cons scale (F (1, 24) = 4.21, $p = .05$, partial $\eta^2 = .15$), in that scores for the MI group increased over the four-week treatment period, whereas the same scores for the control group decreased over this time period. As well, there was a trend towards participants in the MI group having decreased confidence in their ability to stop being preoccupied with weight and shape, and the control group having increased confidence across time (F (1, 24) = 4.72, $p = .04$, partial $\eta^2 = .16$). There was also a significant main effect for time: confidence in changing eating increased in both groups between filling out the first set of questionnaires and filling out the second (F (1, 23) = 12.97, $p = .002$, partial $\eta^2 = .36$).

Discussion

Eating disorders typically involve very low motivation to change and high rates of treatment drop out. The present study was a preliminary investigation of the impact of a brief MI intervention on subsequent completion rates of an intensive hospital treatment program for eating disorders. Findings indicated that patients who were randomly assigned to receive MI pre-treatment had a significantly higher rate of completion of the intensive treatment program compared to those who received treatment as usual. This was true despite the fact that the MI intervention was brief (three or four 50-minute sessions). These findings are among the first to empirical support for the utility of MI in improving later intensive treatment completion. They are consistent with the results of Treasure and colleagues [13], who found that motivational enhancement therapy was an effective first phase treatment for BN, and were in contrast to the results of Wade and colleagues [19], who did not find that a motivational interviewing pre-treatment led to improvements in subsequent treatment completion. The contrast between the intensive treatment completion rates of the two groups was impressive (i.e., 69% in the MI group vs. 31% in the control group). Odds ratio analysis revealed that participants in the MI condition were 4.8 times more likely to complete intensive treatment than were those in the control condition. Past research

Table 2 Means and SDs for all measures across time by treatment group (n = 26)

Measure and condition	Baseline			After pre-treatment		
	Mean	SD	Partial η^2	Mean	SD	Partial η^2
PCED – pros subscale						
MI group	8.96	18.19	.001	1.60	23.41	.01
Control group	10.33	23.87		7.50	26.86	
PCED – cons subscale						
MI group	36.79	9.76	.001	40.27	9.23	.10
Control group	36.05	14.99		32.18	14.61	
MTC importance of eating						
MI group	8.09	2.74	.01	8.64	2.16	.000
Control group	7.60	2.23		8.60	1.80	
MTC confidence eating[a]						
MI group	6.09	2.12	.01	7.64	1.63	.04
Control group	5.57	2.38		6.86	2.07	
MTC readiness eating						
MI group	7.73	2.15	.16	8.73	2.15	.20
Control group	5.80	2.37		6.77	1.94	
MTC importance restriction						
MI group	8.18	2.27	.21	8.27	2.49	.04
Control group	5.53	2.90		7.47	2.31	
MTC confidence restriction						
MI group	6.05	2.49	.01	6.73	2.49	.01
Control group	6.47	2.31		7.27	2.31	
MTC readiness restriction						
MI group	6.80	1.79	.10	9.60	.89	.41
Control group	5.71	1.70		6.14	2.79	
MTC importance weight/shape						
MI group	9.00	1.00	.16	9.45	1.04	.14
Control group	7.47	2.23		8.33	1.68	
MTC confidence weight/shape						
MI group	6.73	1.95	.09	5.82	1.78	.04
Control group	5.00	3.21		6.67	2.19	
MTC readiness weight/shape[b]						
MI group	6.80	1.64	.06	9.80	.45	.29
Control group	5.71	2.63		7.29	2.69	

No analyses were significant at an α of 0.01.
[a](n = 25).
[b](n = 12).

that has shown that completion of intensive hospital-based eating disorder treatment programs range from 32% to 51% [31,32]. The current study provides support for an association between an MI pre-treatment and increased likelihood of completing a subsequent intensive treatment program. Geller and colleagues recently concluded that MI may be of most benefit to improving the motivation levels of highly ambivalent patients with disordered eating [33], which may be similar to the population in this study. At the present time, we do not have any long-term follow-up data on the participants in the two groups. However, based on past research it is reasonable to assume that a large proportion of the participants who dropped out of the intensive treatment program will return for another admission of intensive treatment [34]. Thus, clinically speaking, there is a meaningful contrast between 31% of the MI group falling into this category of high risk for re-admission, as compared to 69% in the control group.

All of the participants in the current study were admitted into a well-established, intensive hospital-based treatment program for eating disorders where normalization of eating and weight are required. It would be interesting for future research to examine the impact of the type of program patients attend following MI. It may be that nature of the program and, more specifically, the degree to which there are behavioural change expectations, impacts on the apparent effectiveness of MI. Programs that require very high levels of behavioural change (including most inpatient and day hospital programs) may be those whose completion rates benefit most from MI pre-treatment.

Treatment condition and measures of motivation

Although the current analysis determined that the MI intervention was associated with a higher probability of intensive treatment completion than no intervention, the mechanisms involved in this relationship are not yet clear. There were no significant differences found between the groups in terms of the measures of motivation across time, as had been predicted. An obvious limitation of the study was that the sample size was small, and it is possible that there was not enough statistical power to detect group differences on the self-reported measures of motivation. Also, since the majority of patients in both groups had started intensive treatment at the time that their motivation was assessed, their levels of motivation may have been equivalently heightened, which could explain why no significant differences between the treatment conditions were found. It is also important to consider that, according to the MI model; an individual's level of motivation is constantly in flux. Some participants completed the measures on their own time and it is impossible to know what other factors may have been affecting them at the moment they sat down to fill out the measures. This limitation is inherent to some degree in all self-report measures, but may be particularly problematic when measuring motivation, given its potentially capricious nature. Future research examining changes in motivation through multiple assessments and in naturalistic environments (e.g., ecological momentary assessment approaches) and the triggers for these changes, would be especially useful to future research on motivation to change and eating disorders.

Another possibility is the measures of motivation in this study did not tap the important factors involved in change in an MI treatment. Amrhein and colleagues [35] investigated the relationship between client language in an MI session and outcome in treatment for drug use. They noted that, not only was there a distinction in client language between commitment ("I won't be using."), desire ("I want to quit doing drugs."), ability ("I can do it...this is doable."), need ("I need to stop."), readiness ("I'm ready to do this."), and reasons ("I'm killing myself.") to change, but that commitment language was the only one of these categories to predict behavioural change. In addition, the remaining categories were found to predict commitment language. Using these categories, it appears that the measures of motivation used in the present study assessed participants' levels of ability, need, readiness, and reasons to change, but not their actual commitment to changing. Although the results of the current study would suggest that these variables were equivalent in both groups, it is possible that the detailed exploration of these variables in MI may have led to more commitment language on the part of the MI participants, which then predicted increased probability of behavioural change (within the intensive treatment program). In other words, the effectiveness of MI may not lie in the client's utterances of desire, ability, need, readiness, and reasons to change, but rather that making these utterances to a curious, non-judgmental therapist (who reflects these statements back to the client) may allow the client to synthesize these beliefs about change and may lead to statements of commitment to actually make a change, which would then lead to increased chances of completing a subsequent treatment program.

Strengths of the current study

The present study had a number of strengths. First, it utilized a randomized controlled trial (RCT) methodology. RCTs are rare in research on ED treatment, and the present study represents an important first step in filling this deficiency in the literature. The present study was also particularly ecologically valid in that it had very few exclusion criteria: participants had to have symptoms that met criteria for a DSM-IV diagnosis of an ED (including EDNOS) and they had to have a minimum BMI of only 13. It was also important in terms of generalizability that the current study did not exclude participants who were acutely suicidal. It is interesting to note that two of the three participants in this study with known suicidal intent (including the person who was hospitalized) went on to complete the treatment program, which would suggest that individuals at risk for suicide are still amenable to treatment. Finally, treatment integrity was high; the study involved with close supervision of the MI sessions by a highly experienced clinician and the collection measures of theoretically related psychotherapeutic constructs.

Limitations of the present study

Despite the above strengths, the current study also had a number of limitations. Importantly, participants in the "treatment as usual" control group did not receive individual therapist contact time equivalent to the MI group. Thus, it is impossible to know whether the increased likelihood of intensive treatment completion was associated with the unique components of MI specifically, or can be attributed to the opportunity for clients to simply talk with a supportive person before or during intensive treatment.

Choosing and implementing an appropriate psychotherapeutic intervention that can serve as a control group against which to compare MI should be a goal for future, larger studies in this area. This was a naturalistic study and there were opportunities for concurrent treatments. There were also varying lengths of time between completion of the MI sessions and admission into intensive treatment. In fact, the majority of the completers were admitted to hospital prior to completing their MI sessions. This confound also influenced comparison scores between baseline and the second assessment of readiness. Participants in both conditions had access to other forms of treatment while they were waiting for intensive hospital treatment. Also, participants were not blind to their group assignment. As previous research has suggested that treatment expectations can affect the course and outcome of psychotherapy [36], it is possible that individuals in the treatment group had an increased likelihood of completing the intensive treatment program because they believed they received superior treatment than did those in the control group. The sample size of this pilot study was small. Despite the fact that significant group differences on treatment completion were found with the small sample, the reduced statistical power may have limited our ability to detect the psychological mechanisms through which MI treatment was related to completion of the subsequent intensive treatment program. Different measures of readiness for change might have yielded different results. And, finally, the current study was inclusive of participants who are often excluded from clinical trials, but was not able to control for all of the variables that the literature has suggested to be associated with outcome in intensive treatment for an eating disorder (e.g., low admission BMI, past treatment failures) [37].

Conclusions

Despite the myriad risks associated with eating disorders, they are characterized by low motivation to change and high rates of treatment drop-out. Treatment dropout has negative consequences from both the perspective of the well-being of the patient and from a health economics standpoint. The current study found that a brief, pre-treatment consisting of four individual sessions of MI was associated with a significantly increased likelihood of intensive treatment completion as compared to the control group. MI can be a useful intervention to engage individuals with severe eating disorders prior to participation in intensive treatment. MI as a brief prelude to hospital-based treatment for an eating disorder may help to improve completion rates in such programs. Further research is required to determine the precise therapeutic mechanisms of change in MI as well as to explore the impact of pre-treatment on intensive treatment completion more generally.

Endnote

[a]Of potential note, this individual was eventually weight restored after attending this subsequent treatment program for the first time in her treatment history.

Competing interests
The authors have no competing interests to declare.

Authors' contributions
CW conceived of the study, carried out the data collection, performed the statistical analysis, and wrote the majority of the manuscript. JM participated in the design and supervision of the study, and co-wrote the manuscript. HW participated in the design of the study, supervised some of the clinical intervention cases, and helped edit portions of the manuscript. JC participated in the design of the study, supervised some of the clinical intervention cases, and helped edit portions of the manuscript. This study was carried out as part of CW's dissertation. All authors read and approved the final manuscript.

Acknowledgements
This study was partially funded by the Social Sciences and Humanities Research Council of Canada doctoral fellowship awarded to the first author. The authors thank Erica Tucciarone for her assistance with manuscript preparation.

Author details
[1]Department of Psychiatry, St. Joseph's Healthcare, Hamilton, Ontario, Canada. [2]Department of Psychology, York University, Toronto, Ontario, Canada. [3]Department of Psychology, Memorial University of Newfoundland, St. John's, Newfoundland, Canada.

References

1. Miller WR, Rollnick S: *Motivational interviewing: helping people change.* 3rd edition. New York: Guilford Press; 2012.
2. Carter JC, Blackmore E, Sutandar-Pinnock K, Woodside DB: **Relapse in anorexia nervosa: a survival analysis.** *Psychol Med* 2004, **34**:671–679.
3. American Psychiatric Association: *Diagnostic and statistical manual of mental disorders.* 4th edition. Washington: Author; 2000. text rev.
4. Blake W, Turnbull SJ, Treasure J: **Stages and processes of change in eating disorders: Implications for therapy.** *Clin Psychol Psychot* 1997, **4**:186–191.
5. Casasnovas C, Fernandez-Aranda F, Granero R, Krug I, Jimenez-Murcia S, Bulik CM, *et al*: **Motivation to change in eating disorders: clinical and therapeutic implications.** *Eur Eat Disord Rev* 2007, **15**:449–456.
6. Ward A, Troop N, Todd G, Treasure J: **To change or not to change—"How" is the question?** *Brit J Med Psychol* 1996, **69**:139–146.
7. Jones A, Bamford B, Ford H, Schreiber-Kounine C: **How important are motivation and initial body mass index for outcome in day therapy service for eating disorders.** *Eur Eat Disord Rev* 2007, **15**:283–289.
8. Guarda AS, Pinto AM, Coughlin JW, Hussain S, Haug NA, Heinberg LJ: **Perceived coercion and change in perceived need for admission in patients hospitalized for eating disorders.** *Am J Psychiat* 2007, **164**:108–114.
9. Geller J, Drab-Hudson DL, Whisenhunt BL, Srikameswaran S: **Readiness to change dietary restriction predicts outcomes in the eating disorders.** *Eat Disord* 2004, **12**:209–224.
10. Bewell CV, Carter JC: **Readiness to change mediates the impact of eating disorder symptomatology on treatment outcome in anorexia nervosa.** *Int J Eat Disorder* 2008, **41**:368–371.
11. McHugh MD: **Readiness for change and short-term outcomes of female adolescents in residential treatment for anorexia nervosa.** *Int J Eat Disorder* 2007, **40**:602–612.
12. Franko DL: **Ready or not? Stages of change as predictors of brief group therapy outcome in bulimia nervosa.** *Group* 1997, **21**:39–45.
13. Treasure JL, Katzman M, Schmidt U, Troop N: **Engagement and outcome in the treatment of bulimia nervosa: first phase of a sequential design comparing motivation enhancement therapy and cognitive behavioral therapy.** *Behav Res Ther* 1999, **37**:405–418.

14. Halmi KA, Agras WS, Mitchell J, Wilson GT, Crow S, Bryson SW, *et al*: **Relapse predictors of patients with bulimia nervosa who achieved abstinence through cognitive behavioral therapy.** *Arch Gen Psychiat* 2002, **59:**1105–1109.
15. Richard M, Bauer S, Kordy H: **Relapse in anorexia and bulimia nervosa-a 2.5-year follow-up study.** *Eur Eat Disord Rev* 2005, **13:**180–190.
16. Cassin SE, von Ranson KM, Heng K, Brar J, Wojtowicz AE: **Adapted motivational interviewing for women with binge eating disorder: a randomized controlled trial.** *Psychol Addict Behav* 2008, **22:**417–425.
17. Dunn EC, Neighbors C, Larimer ME: **Motivational enhancement therapy and self-help treatment for binge eaters.** *Psychol Addict Behav* 2006, **20:**44–52.
18. Feld R, Woodside DB, Kaplan AS, Olmsted MP, Carter JC: **Pretreatment motivational enhancement therapy for eating disorders: a pilot study.** *Int J Eat Disorder* 2001, **29:**393–400.
19. Wade TD, Frayne A, Edwards S-A, Robertson T, Gilchrist P: **Motivational change in an inpatient anorexia nervosa population and implications for treatment.** *Aust NZ J Psychiat* 2009, **43:**235–243.
20. Dray J, Wade T: **Is the transtheoretical model and motivational interviewing approach applicable to the treatment of eating disorders? A review.** *Clin Psych Review* 2012, **32:**558–565.
21. Knowles L, Anokhina A, Serpell L: **Motivational interventions in the eating disorders: what is the evidence?** *Int J Eat Disord* 2013, **46:**97–107.
22. Gowers SG, Smyth B: **The impact of a motivational assessment interview on initial response to treatment in adolescent anorexia nervosa.** *Eur Eat Disord Rev* 2004, **12:**87–93.
23. Olmsted MP, Woodside DB, Carter JC, McFarlane TL, Staab R, Colton PA, *et al*: **Intensive therapies for eating disorders.** In *Gabbard's Treatments of psychiatric disorders.* Edited by Gabbard GO. Washington: American Psychiatric Press; 2007.
24. Forcano L, Fernández-Aranda F, Álvarez-Moya E, Bulik C, Granero R, Gratacòs M, *et al*: **Suicide attempts in bulimia nervosa: personality and psychopathological correlates.** *Eur Psychiat* 2009, **24:**91–97.
25. Gale C, Holliday J, Troop NA, Serpell L, Treasure J: **The pros and cons of change in individuals with eating disorders: a broader perspective.** *Int J Eat Disorder* 2006, **39:**394–403.
26. Walsh BT, Kaplan AS, Attia E, Olmsted M, Parides M, Carter JC, *et al*: **Fluoxetine after weight restoration in anorexia nervosa: a randomized controlled trial.** *J Amer Med Assoc* 2006, **295:**2605–2612.
27. Boudreaux ED, Sullivan A, Abar B, Bernstein SL, Ginde AA, Camargo CA Jr: **Motivation rulers for smoking cessation: a prospective observational examination of construct and predictive validity.** *Addict Sci Clin Pract* 2012, **7:**8.
28. Moyers TB, Martin T, Manuel JK, Hendrickson SML, Miller WR: **Assessing competence in the use of motivational interviewing.** *J Subst Abuse Treat* 2005, **28:**19–26.
29. Westra HA, Arkowitz H, Dozois DJA: **Adding a motivational interviewing pre-treatment to cognitive behavioral therapy for generalized anxiety disorder: a preliminary randomized controlled trial.** *J Anxiety Disord* 2009, **23:**1106–1117.
30. Hernán MA, Hernández-Diaz S: **Beyond the intention-to-treat in comparative effectiveness research.** *Clin Trials* 2012, **9:**48–55.
31. Woodside DB, Carter JC, Blackmore E: **Predictors of premature termination of inpatient treatment for anorexia nervosa.** *Amer J Psychiat* 2004, **161:**2277–2281.
32. Zeeck A, Hartmann A, Buchholz C, Herzog T: **Drop outs from in-patient treatment of anorexia nervosa.** *Acta Psychiat Scand* 2005, **111:**29–37.
33. Geller J, Brown KE, Srikameswaran S: **The efficacy of a brief motivational intervention for individuals with eating disorders: a randomized control trial.** *Int J Eat Disorder* 2011, **44:**497–505.
34. Lock J, Litt I: **What predicts maintenance of weight for adolescents medically hospitalized for anorexia nervosa?** *Eat Disord* 2003, **11:**1–7.
35. Amrhein PC, Miller WR, Yahne CE, Palmer M, Fulcher L: **Client commitment language during motivational interviewing predicts drug use outcomes.** *J Consult Clin Psych* 2003, **71:**862–878.
36. Greenberg RP, Constantino MJ, Bruce N: **Are patient expectations still relevant for psychotherapy process and outcome?** *Clin Psychol Rev* 2006, **26:**657–678.
37. Guarda AS: **Treatment of anorexia nervosa: insights and obstacles.** *Physiol Behav* 2008, **94:**113–120.

Medication and psychotherapy in eating disorders: is there a gap between research and practice?

Myra Cooper* and Hannah Kelland

Abstract

Background: Little research has investigated the use of evidence-based guidelines by eating disorder (ED) therapists, or prescribing of psychotropic medication. Moreover, people with EDs have rarely been surveyed on these topics, and their clinical and demographic features have not been presented. This study investigated perception of psychotherapy, psychotropic medication and the clinical characteristics of a community sample of people with EDs.

Method: An online survey methodology was used to recruit 253 people with eating disorders in the community. Where feasible, comparisons were made between four types of eating disorder, anorexia nervosa, bulimia nervosa, and two types of atypical or 'sub-threshold' eating disorder.

Results: Unlike medication, reported psychotherapy showed some congruence with evidence based and other guidance. Most participants were currently receiving either psychotherapy, medication or both, and most had a severe and chronic ED.

Conclusions: Findings are considered in light of use of evidence-based treatment for EDs, calls for greater dissemination of cognitive behaviour therapy (CBT); indications that much may be poor quality; and the importance of what treatments to offer those who are chronically and severely ill. Development of theory and novel treatments is considered a priority.

Keywords: Eating disorders, Psychotherapy, Medication

Background

Eating disorders (EDs) are associated with significant mortality and morbidity [1]. They can be difficult to treat, and there is room for improvement [2]. Not all community cases receive treatment [3], and not all receive "evidence-based" treatment [4]. Practice guidelines [5–8] identify cognitive behaviour therapy (CBT), and fluoxetine as the best evidence based treatments for bulimia nervosa (BN). CBT is recommended for adult anorexia nervosa (AN), "based on strong consensus but weak evidence"([6], p4). Interpersonal psychotherapy (IPT), cognitive analytic therapy (CAT) and psychodynamic therapies may be useful for AN but 'evidence for each of these is modest' ([8], p14). Guidelines recommend sub-threshold EDs be treated in line with the disorder they most resemble [5], although an evidence base is lacking. No drugs are specifically recommended for AN. Use of a range of psychotropic medication in is discussed in AN [5, 6, 8], but guidelines urge extreme caution, and highlight potentially serious hazards.

Few studies have investigated what treatment people with EDs in the community receive, and whether or not it meets practice guidelines. Most survey therapists not patients. Therapists report high use of psychotherapy, particularly CBT. One study [9] found 196 (74.5 %) of ED therapists employed CBT for AN, and 181 (83.8 %) for BN. However, among community clinicians there was a wider range of approaches. Few used evidence-based treatment [10], and less than a quarter, 27 (22.9 %), used CBT. When those with EDs in the

* Correspondence: myra.cooper@hmc.ox.ac.uk
Isis Education Centre, University of Oxford, Warneford Hospital, Oxford OX3 7JX, UK

community replied to a research notice, 220 (62.4 %) with probable BN reported receiving psychotherapy, although few (N = 23, 6.7 %) had received narrowly defined CBT [11]. Psychotherapy received by those with AN or sub-threshold EDs has not been studied from the patient's perspective. Moreover, it has not always been clear whether therapy was designed to treat the ED. This is important as EDs have been associated with high co-morbidity [3].

In relation to psychotropic medication, chart review found ED patients had often received antidepressants, N = 102 (50 %), and anxiolytics, N = 32 (16 %), in the preceding 12 months, although no details of the drugs, ED or other diagnosis being treated, was provided [12]. A study of patients with AN found 278 (53 %) reported current use of psychotropic medication (N = 254, 48.4 %, antidepressants and N = 68, 13 %, antipsychotics) [13]. Exact figures are not provided, but a wide range of drugs was being taken. In the only study to report on medication and psychotherapy, 225 (63.7 %) with probable BN had received pharmacological treatment (vs N = 220, 62.4 %, psychotherapy), and 129 (36.6 %) were judged to have had an adequate course of fluoxetine [11]. As in other studies, sub-threshold EDs were not studied, no detail was provided on the drugs taken and whether the ED, or a different problem, was the target.

Importantly, no study has reported demographic and clinical information, including data collected using standardised self-report measures. This would establish a baseline against which to compare future studies as well as aid interpretation of findings. The current study therefore investigated medication and type of psychotherapy perceived to have been received by those with an ED, including sub-threshold diagnoses. Participants were questioned about treatment specifically for their ED. Information on demographic characteristics, including height and weight, and psychiatric symptoms, using standardised measures, was collected.

Methods

Participants

A community sample (aged 18-65) was recruited through internet advertisements on websites such as Facebook and Beating Eating Disorders (a UK charity). The text noted "we are looking for women and men who are currently suffering from an eating disorder (anorexia nervosa, bulimia nervosa and eating disorder not otherwise specified). To take part you must be 18–65 years of age and speak fluent English".

Design

The study was an internet-based self-report survey.

Procedure

Approval was obtained from the University ethics board. Participants were provided with a link to the online survey. An option of completing paper copies of the questionnaires was available. All participants gave informed consent.

Measures

Participants were asked their height and weight to calculate current BMI. They were asked details of age, ethnicity, and occupation and any psychiatric diagnoses, apart from an ED. Participants completed the following self-report questionnaires.

Eating disorder diagnostic scale (EDDS; 14)

This brief scale diagnoses EDs. The items map onto the Diagnostic and Statistical Manual, fifth edition (DSM-V) criteria [15] for AN and BN, and permit diagnosis of sub-threshold AN and BN (i.e. where full criteria are not met). The EDDS possesses good test-retest reliability (r = .87) and internal consistency (alpha = .89) [14].

Hospital anxiety and depression scale (HADS;16)

This questionnaire contains seven statements related to anxiety and seven related to depression. A score of 11 or more indicates probable mood disorder. The sub-scales are independent, and have good homogeneity and reliability [17].

Eating attitudes test (EAT; 18)

This measure of eating disturbance is an abbreviated (26-item) version of the 40-item EAT [19], and the two are highly correlated (r = .98; 18). Scores above 20 indicate potential eating disturbance. It has good reliability and validity [18].

Eating disorder examination questionnaire (EDE-Q; 20)

This is a self-report version of the Eating Disorder Examination [21]. It has 4 subscales, and concerns behaviour over the past 28 days. A global score can be computed. A review indicates good reliability, and supports its use in identifying cases [22].

Medication and psychotherapy use

Medication use

Participants were asked whether or not they were currently taking medication in relation to their ED. They were asked to list all these.

Psychotherapy use

Participants were asked whether or not they had received or were currently receiving psychotherapy for their ED. They were asked to list the type of therapy/ therapies.

Results

Data analysis

Demographic data were analysed by diagnostic group using one way analysis of variance for continuous variables and chi square for categorical data. Chi square was used to examine group differences in total number receiving psychotropic medication and current and past psychotherapy. Further statistical testing was not undertaken due to small numbers in most categories.

Response

Four hundred and fifty four people started, and 260 (57 %) completed, the survey. Two hundred and fifty three (97.3 %) were diagnosed with AN, BN, or sub-threshold ED using the EDDS.

Diagnosis

Extracting data from the EDDS, and using the algorithm [13], forty-four participants had a DSM-V [15] diagnosis of AN; 30 a diagnosis of atypical (sub-threshold) AN, 126 a diagnosis of BN, and 53 a diagnosis of BN of low frequency and/or duration (sub-threshold BN).

Demographic results

Two hundred and forty six participants were female and seven were male (one AN, three BN and three sub-threshold BN). Demographic details (continuous variables) for each diagnostic group are in Table 1 and (categorical variables) in Table 2. There was no significant difference between the four groups in age (F = 1.53, df = 3, 248, $p = .21$). Most participants were in their late 20s. There was a significant difference between groups in BMI (F = 13.3, df = 3, 250, $p < .001$). Post hoc Tukey tests indicated those with AN had a lower mean BMI than all other groups (all p values < .03). The distribution of Caucasian/non Caucasian participants did not differ ($chi^2 = 1.62$ df = 3, $p = .65$), and most were Caucasian. The majority lived in the United Kingdom or USA. Socioeconomic Status (SES) was classified using the Office of National Statistics Standard Occupational Classification [23]. Extra categories were added for students, the unemployed and retired. The majority were students although a significant number were managers/professionals or unemployed. There were no significant differences in occupation in the four groups ($chi^2 = 6.62$, df = 9, $p = .67$). Over a third had been a psychiatric inpatient, particularly those with AN and sub-threshold AN ($chi^2 = 13.9$, df = 3, $p = .003$). Mean duration of ED was similar across the sample (11.3 years, SD = 9.37), (F = 1.64, df = 3, 249, $p = .18$). Twenty four (11.3 %) reported a current psychiatric diagnosis other than an ED, with no differences between the groups ($chi^2 = 3.96$, df = 3, $p = .27$).

Self-report questionnaires

Scores for the diagnostic groups on the questionnaires are in Table 1. There was a significant difference between the groups in EAT scores (F = 10.29, df = 3252, $p = <.001$). Post hoc Tukey tests found the sub-threshold BN group had a significantly lower score than the other groups (all p values < .002). There was a significant difference between groups in EDE-Q total score (F = 13.76, df = 3, 252, $p < .001$). Post hoc Tukey tests indicated a lower score in the sub-threshold BN group compared to all other groups (all p values < =.001). There was no significant difference between the four groups in HADS depression (F = 1.8, df = 3252, $p = .15$) or anxiety (F = 1.59, df = 3, 252, $p = .19$).

Medication use

Table 3 displays psychotropic medication use for the four diagnostic groups and whole sample. There was a significant difference between the groups ($chi^2 = 9.62$, df = 3, $p = .02$) in whether or not any psychotropic medication was being taken. It was most

Table 1 Demographic and clinical characteristics of the sample – continuous variables

	AN (N = 44)		AN-sub-threshold (N = 30)		BN (N = 126)		BN-sub-threshold (N = 53)		Total (N = 253)	
	Mean	SD	Mean	SD	Mean	SD	Mean	SD	Mean	SD
Age	28.0	10.3	26.3	9.4	26.1	8.5	29.4	12.3	27.1	9.8
Body Mass Index	15.8	1.2	20.2	6.1	23.1	8.1	22.8	6.8	21.4	7.3
EAT	49.4	13.3	46.8	14.7	42.6	14.0	33.5	18.4	42.4	15.8
EDE-Q	4.6	1.1	4.8	0.9	4.8	0.9	3.7	1.6	4.6	1.2
HADS-depression	11.0	4.5	10.6	4.3	10.0	4.6	8.9	4.9	10.0	4.6
HADS-anxiety	15.1	4.4	14.6	3.6	14.0	3.9	13.3	4.8	14.1	4.2
Duration of ED (years)	13.3	9.4	9.3	7.5	10.6	9.0	12.5	9.4	11.3	9.4

Key: *AN* Anorexia Nervosa, AN-sub-threshold, *BN* Bulimia Nervosa, BN-sub-threshold, *EAT* Eating Attitudes Test, *EDE-Q* Eating Disorder Examination – Questionnaire, *HADS* Hospital Anxiety and Depression Scale

Table 2 Demographic and clinical characteristic of the sample – categorical variables

	AN (N = 44)		AN-sub-threshold (N = 30)		BN (N = 126)		BN-sub-threshold (N = 53)		Total (N = 253)	
	N	%	N	%	N	%	N	%	N	%
Ethnicity										
Caucasian	41	93.2	29	96.7	114	90.5	46	86.8	230	90.9
Non Caucasian	3	6.8	1	2.3	12	9.5	3	5.7	19	7.5
Country										
United Kingdom	21	47.8	11	36.7	47	37.5	27	50.9	91	36.0
USA	12	27.3	15	50.0	44	35.0	16	30.2	78	30.8
Canada, Australia, New Zealand	8	18.2	4	13.3	18	14.3	3	5.7	31	12.3
SES										
Managers/professionals	8	18.2	4	13.3	20	15.9	6	11.3	38	15.0
Associate professionals	3	6.8	2	6.7	5	4.0	6	11.3	16	6.3
Students	14	31.8	15	50.0	44	35.0	22	41.5	95	37.5
Unemployed	6	13.6	6	20.0	23	18.3	6	11.3	41	16.2
ED/psychiatric variables										
Been a psychiatric inpatient	26	59.0	14	46.7	37	29.4	16	30.2	93	36.8
Other psychiatric diagnosis										
Depression	3	6.8	1	2.3	7	5.6	2	3.8	13	5.1
Anxiety	3	6.8	0	0	2	1.6	0	0	5	2.0
Borderline personality disorder	2	4.5	0	0	4	3.2	0	0	6	2.4
Bipolar disorder	1	2.3	1	2.3	4	3.2	0	0	6	2.4
PTSD	3	6.8	0	0	3	2.4	1	1.9	7	2.8
OCD	0	0	0	0	3	2.4	0	0	3	1.2
Self-harm	0	0	0	0	1	0.8	0	0	1	0.4
ADHD	0	0	0	0	0	0	0	0	1	0.4

Key: *AN* Anorexia Nervosa, AN-sub-threshold, *BN* Bulimia Nervosa, BN-sub-threshold *SSRIs* Selective

common in AN (N = 26, 59 %), and least common in BN (N = 41, 32.5 %). Overall, a substantial minority (N = 54, 10.2 %) were taking two or more psychotropic drugs. Antidepressants were the most common (taken by N = 107, 42.3 %), with N = 50, 19.8 % on Selective Serotonin Reuptake Inhibitors and N = 21, 8.3 %, on Selective Norepinephrine Reuptake Inhibitors. A minority were taking fluoxetine (N = 15, 5.9 %); four (3.2 %) had BN and two (3.8 %) had sub-threshold BN. A significant minority were taking anti-anxiety drugs (N = 36, 14.2 %), mood stabilisers (N = 26, 10.3 %) and antipsychotics (N = 21, 8.3 %).

Psychotherapy use

Table 4 displays current and past psychotherapy use for the whole sample and each ED diagnosis. Just under half were receiving current psychotherapy (N = 123, 48.6 %), with no group differences ($chi^2 = 4.97$, df = 3, $p = .17$). CBT was being received by N = 110, 23.3 % of the total sample, and family therapy by a small number of those with AN (N = 6, 13.6 %) and sub-threshold AN (N = 3, 10 %). Overall, few were receiving Cognitive Analytic Therapy (CAT) (N = 2, 0.8 %), Dialectical Behaviour Therapy (DBT) (N = 9, 3.6 %), Interpersonal Psychotherapy (IPT) or Counselling (N = 8, 3.2 %). A number did not know what type of psychotherapy they were receiving (N = 44, 17.4 %). Some were receiving a range of "other" forms of therapy (N – 25, 9.9 %).

81.8 % (N = 207) had received past psychotherapy, with no group differences ($chi^2 = 4.0$, $p = .26$). Just under half had received CBT (N = 110, 47 %). A number with AN (N = 14, 31.8 %), or sub-threshold AN (N = 12, 40 %) had received family therapy. A significant minority had received psychodynamic therapy (N = 43, 17 %), some had received CAT (N = 13, 5.1 %), DBT (N = 3, 1.2 %), IPT or Counselling (N = 7, 2.8 %). A number did not know what type of therapy they had received (N = 61, 24.1 %).

Combination therapies

Just under half who had received past psychological therapy were currently receiving it. Nearly one third (N = 75,

Table 3 Summary of medication taken by sample

	AN (N = 44)		AN-sub-threshold (N = 30)		BN (N = 126)		BN-sub-threshold (N = 53)		Total (N = 253)	
	N	%	N	%	N	%	N	%	N	%
No medication	17	38.6	14	46.7	77	69.1	31	58.5	139	54.9
One psychiatric drug	14	31.8	9	30	22	17.5	8	15.1	53	20.9
Two psychiatric drugs	5	11.4	3	10.0	13	10.3	5	9.4	26	10.3
Three psychiatric drugs	3	6.8	4	13.3	7	5.6	3	5.7	17	6.7
Four psychiatric drugs	4	9.1	0	0	2	1.6	2	3.8	8	3.2
Five psychiatric drugs	0	0	0	0	3	2.4	0	0	3	1.2
Total on any psychiatric medication	26	59.0	16	53.3	41	32.5	25	47.2	108	42.7
Anti-anxiety	7	15.9	5	16.7	12	9.5	6	11.3	36	14.2
Hypnotics	0	0	0	0	4	3.2	2	3.8	6	2.4
Psycho-stimulants	2	4.5	0	0	3	2.4	2	3.8	7	2.8
Tricyclic antidepressants	1	2.3	0	0	1	0.8	1	1.9	3	1.2
SSRIs	20	45.5	11	36.7	8	14.3	11	20.8	50	19.8
Fluoxetine	4	9.1	5	16.7	4	3.2	2	3.8	15	5.9
SARIs	2	4.5	0	0	3	2.4	0	0	5	2.0
SNRIs	1	2.3	2	6.7	15	11.9	3	3.8	21	8.3
NaSSRAs	1	2.3	1	3.3	4	3.2	1	1.9	7	2.8
NDRIs	1	2.3	0	0	5	4.0	0	0	6	2.4
Melatonergic agonists	0	0	0	0	1	0.8	0	0	1	0.4
Antidepressant (unspecified)	1	2.3	0	0	0	0	1	1.9	2	0.8
Total on anti-depressants	27	61.4	14	46.7	41	32.5	25	47.2	107	42.3
Mood stabilisers	3	6.8	4	13.3	16	12.7	3	3.8	26	10.3
Antipsychotics	7	15.9	2	6.7	8	6.3	4	7.5	21	8.3

Key: *AN* Anorexia Nervosa, AN-sub-threshold, *BN* Bulimia Nervosa, BN-sub-threshold, *SSRIs* Selective Serotonin Reuptake Inhibitors, *SARIs* Serotonin Antagonist and Reuptake Inhibitor, *SNRIs* Serotonin Norepinephrine Reuptake Inhibitor, *NaSSAs* Noradrenergic and Specific Serotinergic Antidepressant, *NDRIs* Norepinephrine Dopamine Reuptake Inhibitor

29.6 %) was currently receiving both psychological therapy and psychotropic medication (highest in AN, N = 19, 43.2 %). Thirty people (11.9 %) were currently taking medication only (highest in sub-threshold BN, N = 9, 17 %). Thirty-nine people (18.3 %) were receiving psychotherapy only (highest in AN, N = 27, 61.4 %). Overall, just over one quarter were not receiving current treatment (N = 72, 28.5 %), highest in BN (N = 47, 37.3 %) and sub-threshold AN (N = 10, 33.3 %), and lowest in AN (N = 8, 18.2 %), and sub-threshold BN (N = 7, 13.2 %).

Discussion

A community sample was asked about treatment for their ED. Just under half were taking psychotropic medicine, with few taking fluoxetine. Nearly half were receiving psychotherapy, often CBT. A wide range of psychotropic and psychological therapies was being received. Most had previously received psychotherapy. Just under a third was receiving both medication and psychotherapy.

The sample was demographically similar to clinical samples (including AN, BN and sub-threshold diagnoses in the community, 24), but with more severe psychopathology and longer illness duration. Indeed, our sample had severe and chronic EDs, and the findings should be interpreted in this light. Interestingly, those with sub-threshold diagnoses had symptom scores similar to those with AN or BN, and illness of similar duration, suggesting sub-threshold disorders can also be severe and chronic. To date, treatment received has usually been studied only in AN or BN, has not investigated medication and psychotherapy, nor reported ED symptom severity, thus enabling therapy data to be contextualised. Unlike most studies we asked patients (not clinicians) what treatment was received, gaining a view of what patients perceived (particularly important for type of psychotherapy). Most had previously received psychotherapy for their ED, including those with sub-threshold diagnoses. This is consistent with the finding that many who present to services have such diagnoses, and that these are relatively common ED diagnoses [25]. Nearly half were currently taking psychotropic medication, and just over half were receiving psychotherapy. Some (32.9 %) were

Table 4 Summary of psychotherapy received by sample

	AN (N = 44)		AN-sub-threshold (N = 30)		BN (N = 126)		BN-sub-threshold (N = 53)		Total (N = 253)	
	N	%	N	%	N	%	N	%	N	%
Current therapy	27	61.4	16	53.3	61	48.4	19	35.8	123	48.6
CBT	14	31.8	10	33.3	25	19.8	10	18.9	110	23.3
Schema focussed therapy	1	2.3	0	0	0	0	0		1	0.4
Family therapy	6	13.6	3	10.0	5	4.0	2	3.8	16	6.3
Psychodynamic therapy	2	4.5	2	6.7	7	5.6	2	3.8	13	5.1
CAT	1	2.3	0	0	1	0.8	0	0	2	0.8
DBT	1	2.3	2	6.7	6	4.8	0	0	9	3.6
Counselling	1	4.5	2	6.7	3	2.4	2	3.8	8	3.2
Other	7	15.9	5	16.7	10	7.9	3	5.7	25	9.9
Don't know type of therapy	5	11.4	6	20.0	21	16.7	12	22.4	44	17.4
Past therapy	41	93	25	83.3	102	81	39	73.6	207	81.8
CBT	23	52.3	19	63.3	52	41.3	25	47.2	119	47.0
Schema focussed therapy	1	2.3	2	6.7	4	3.2	1	1.9	8	3.2
Family therapy	14	31.8	12	40.0	22	17.5	12	22.4	60	23.7
Psychodynamic therapy	11	25.0	4	13.3	18	14.3	10	18.9	43	17.0
CAT	3	6.8	1	3.3	4	3.2	5	9.4	13	5.1
DBT	2	4.5	0	0	2	1.6	1	1.9	3	1.2
Counselling	2	4.5	2	6.7	2	1.6	1	1.9	7	2.8
Other	3	6.8	1	3.3	9	7.1	4	7.5	17	6.7
Don't know type of therapy	8	18.2	5	16.7	38	30.2	10	18.9	61	24.1
Current and past psychological therapy	27	61.4	13	43.3	53	42.1	17	32.1	110	43.5
Combination therapy	19	43.2	11	36.7	36	28.6	9	17.0	75	29.6
Psychotherapy only	27	61.4	5	16.7	23	18.2	10	18.9	56	39.5
Medication only	7	15.9	5	16.7	13	10.3	9	17.0	30	11.9
No therapy	8	18.2	10	33.3	47	37.4	7	13.2	72	28.5

Key: *AN* Anorexia Nervosa, AN-sub-threshold, *BN* Bulimia Nervosa, BN-sub-threshold, *CBT* Cognitive Behaviour Therapy, *CAT* Cognitive Analytic Therapy, *DBT* Dialectical Behaviour Therapy

receiving both. Receipt of psychotropic medication is similar to previous studies [12, 13]. However, the percent (7 %) receiving fluoxetine was markedly lower [11]. Indeed, it is surprisingly low, given fluoxetine is recommended by NICE for BN and sub-threshold BN. However, some guidelines are less enthusiastic about prescribing fluoxetine, highlighting lack of follow-up, and high attrition [8]. Overall, however, nearly half was taking an antidepressant, often an SSRI, but like previous studies, a wide range of other antidepressants [13]. A significant minority were taking anti-anxiety drugs, mood stabilisers, and antipsychotics. This is consistent with in-patients with AN [13] and extends these findings to other diagnoses and the community. However, it is important to note that none of these medications has an evidence base in EDs, and some may be contraindicated because of safety, particularly in AN [6–8, 13]. Just over half our sample was receiving CBT, and some with AN or sub-threshold AN, family therapy. This is consistent with the evidence base in BN, and recommendations for AN. However, several other psychological therapies were being received, most with minimal evidence base in EDs. Worryingly, many did not know what type of psychological therapy they were, or had been, receiving. Over half receiving psychotherapy had previously received psychotherapy, suggesting it had not resolved the ED, they had experienced a recurrence of symptoms or perhaps had not completed or engaged with treatment, all of which are known problems in EDs. These possibilities seem particularly likely given the chronicity and severity of the sample. For example, use of non-evidence based therapy currently may be due to previous failure of evidence-based treatment. One particular limitation here is that while we asked about previous psychotherapy we did not ask about previous medication; thus previous use of evidence-based medication could not be evaluated, and it may be that fluoxetine (for example) had not proved helpful for our patients in the past and thus more diverse drugs had been prescribed. Self-reported comorbidity was low, and the reason for this is unclear. One possibility is that it is less likely to be identified and labelled outside highly structured research, another that it is often considered a secondary problem.

Despite encouraging trends for CBT and family therapy, the fit between our data and ED (evidence-based) practice guidelines is not close. A plethora of different treatments (some evidence based, but many not) had been, and were being, received. Explanations for treatment failure in EDs vary from lack of dissemination of CBT to poor patient motivation/engagement [26]. While these may play a role, what is striking about the current sample is that all had a severe and chronic ED. An alternative to these different explanations for treatment failure may be that, in fact, we currently lack effective, powerful treatments for EDs. The question is not, why don't more people receive CBT or fluoxetine? It may not be why is better quality treatment not available? The question may be why is there not more emphasis on the development of theory to inform novel treatment approaches? For some with a chronic and severe ED the range of treatments tried (understandably given failure to recover) is truly staggering.

The study has limitations. The majority of participants had received treatment; the sample is unlikely therefore to represent all those with EDs in the community (27). Diagnosis was completed using self-report questionnaire, likely less valid than clinician obtained diagnosis. The sample was relatively ill with severe symptoms and a chronic course, thus not representative of those with less severe symptoms and recent onset. Indeed, there may have been a selection bias in that the survey appealed to those with chronic and severe EDs. Self-report of medication and psychotherapy may be less reliable and valid than chart review. Data on quality, frequency, duration or dosage of the interventions, or individual adherence, was not obtained. Finally, given clinician self-report of evidence based treatment may lack validity [4], this may also be problematic for patient self-report of these.

Conclusions

It is easy to criticise non-evidence based psychotherapy, and the apparently widespread use of psychotropic medication that lacks an evidence base for EDs. As their scores and history indicate, this sample is seriously and chronically ill. It is not easy for therapists and services to do nothing. If CBT has failed (however well delivered), it is hard to justify providing it again, and perhaps understandably, patients and therapists may seek alternative psychotherapies. It is not clear why fluoxetine is given or taken so rarely (some suggestions are given above). However, it is clear that cautious and carefully monitored use of a number of non-evidenced based psychotropic medications can, as suggested by the APA Practice Guidelines for the Treatment of Patients with EDs [6], provide some relief from troubling symptoms, even if not directly treating the ED. In the absence of any real ED specific medication this is likely to be a useful option for some, and one that it would not be appropriate to withhold from patients. The same may also be true of some non-evidence based psychotherapy. Finally, it may be mistaken to conclude that individuals in our sample have not benefitted from at least some of the interventions received. While efficacy studies focus on modifying diagnostic features, clinicians treating those who are very ill, are likely to be rather more concerned with quality of life. A wide range of therapies may be needed to achieve this, including those not specifically focussed on the ED.

Competing interests

The authors declare that they have no competing interests.

Authors' contributions

HK designed the study, undertook data collection and performed some of the data analysis. MJC helped design the study, conducted some of the data analysis, reviewed the literature and prepared the manuscript. Both authors read and approved the final manuscript.

Authors' information

The data were collected in part fulfilment of HK's doctorate in clinical psychology at the University of Oxford.

References

1. Arcelus J, Mitchell JA, Wales J, Nielsen S. Mortality rates in patients with anorexia nervosa and other eating disorders: a meta-analysis of 36 studies. Arch Gen Psych. 2011;68:724–31.
2. Jansen A. Towards effective treatment of eating disorders: nothing is as practical as a good theory. Beh Res Ther. 2001;39:1007–22.
3. Hudson JI, Hiripi E, Pope HG, Kessler RC. The prevalence and correlates of eating disorders in the National Comorbidity Survey Replication. Biol Psych. 2007;61:348–58.
4. Waller G, Stringer H, Meyer C. What cognitive behavioural techniques do therapists report using when delivering cognitive behavioural therapy for the eating disorders? J Cons Clin Psych. 2012;80:171–5.
5. National Institute for Clinical Excellence. Eating disorders. London: British Psychological Society and the Royal College of Psychiatrists; 2004.
6. American Psychiatric Association. Guideline watch (August). Practice guideline for the treatment of patients with eating disorders. 3rd ed. New York: American Psychiatric Association; 2012.
7. American Psychiatric Association. Practice guideline for the treatment of patients with eating disorders. 3rd ed. New York: American Psychiatric Association; 2006.
8. Hay P, Chinn D, Forbes D, Madden S, Newton R, Surgenor L, et al. Australian and New Zealand College of Psychiatrists clinical practice guidelines for the treatment of eating disorders. Aust NZ J Psych. 2014;48:1–62.
9. Wallace LM, von Ranson KM. Perceptions and use of empirically-supported psychotherapies among eating disorder professionals. Beh Res Ther. 2012;50:215–22.
10. Von Ranson KM, Wallace LM, Stevenson A. Psychotherapies provided for eating disorders by community clinicians: infrequent use of evidence-based treatment. Eat Dis. 2013;23:333–43.

11. Crow S, Mussell MP, Peterson CM, Knopke A, Mitchell J. Prior treatment received by patients with bulimia nervosa. Int J of Eat Dis. 1999;25:39–44.
12. Striegel-Moore RH, DeBar L, Wilson GT, Dickerson J, Rosselli F, Perrin N, et al. Health services use in eating disorders. Psychol Med. 2008;38:1465–74.
13. Fazeli PK, Caldeer GL, Miller KK, Misra M, Lawson EA, Meenaghn E, et al. Psychotropic medication use in anorexia nervosa between 1997 and 2009. Int J Eat Dis. 2012;45:970–6.
14. Stice E, Telch CF, Rizvi SL. Development and validation of the Eating Disorder Diagnostic Scale: a brief self-report measure of anorexia, bulimia, and binge-eating disorder. Psychol Ass. 2000;12:123–31.
15. American Psychiatric Association. Diagnostic and statistical manual of mental disorders. 5th ed. New York: American Psychiatric Association; 2013.
16. Zigmond AS, Snaith RP. The hospital anxiety and depression scale. Acta Psych Scand. 1983;67:361–70.
17. Spinhoven PH, Ormel J, Sloekers PPA, Kempen GIJM, Speckens AEM, Van Hemert AM. A validation study of the Hospital Anxiety and Depression Scale (HADS) in different groups of Dutch subjects. Psychol Med. 1997;27:363–70.
18. Garner D, Olmsted M, Bohr Y, Garfinkel P. The eating attitudes test: psychometric features and clinical correlates. Psychol Med. 1982;12:871–8.
19. Garner D, Garfinkel P. The eating attitudes test: an index of the symptoms of anorexia nervosa. Psychol Med. 1979;9:273–9.
20. Fairburn CG, Beglin SJ. Assessment of eating disorder psychopathology: interview or self-report questionnaire? Int J Eat Dis. 1994;16:363–70.
21. Fairburn CG, Cooper Z. The Eating Disorder Examination. In: Fairburn CG, Wilson GT, editors. Eating disorders and obesity. New York: Guilford Press; 1993. p. 1993.
22. Berg KC, Peterson CB, Frazier P, Crow SJ. Psychometric evaluation of the eating disorder examination and eating disorder examination-questionnaire: a systematic review of the literature. Int J Eat Dis. 2012;45:428–38.
23. Office of National Statistics. The national statistics socio-economic classification. London: Office of National Statistics; 2010.
24. Fairburn CG, Cooper Z, Doll HA, O'Connor ME, Bohn K, Hawker DM, et al. Trans-diagnostic cognitive-behavioural therapy for patients with eating disorders: a two-site trial with 60-week follow-up. Am J Psych. 2009;166:311–9.
25. Turner H, Bryant-Waugh R. Eating disorder not otherwise specified (EDNOS): profiles of clients presenting at a community eating disorder service. Eur Eat Dis Rev. 2004;12:18–26.
26. Shafran R, Clark DM, Fairburn CG, Arntz A, Barlow DH, Ehlers A, et al. Mind the gap: Improving the dissemination of CBT. Beh Res Ther. 2009;47:902–9.
27. Haas HL, Clopton JR. Comparing clinical and research treatments for eating disorders. Int J Eat Dis. 2003;33:412–20.

Dimensions of control and their relation to disordered eating behaviours and obsessive-compulsive symptoms

Franzisca V. Froreich[1*], Lenny R. Vartanian[1], Jessica R. Grisham[1] and Stephen W. Touyz[2]

Abstract

Background: Issues of personal control have been proposed to play a central role in the aetiology and maintenance of eating disorders. Empirical evidence supporting this relationship is inconsistent, partly due to the multiplicity of constructs used to define "control". This study compares six commonly used measures of control with the aim of determining which operationalisation of control is most centrally relevant to eating pathology. Given the high level of comorbidity between eating disorders and obsessive-compulsive disorder and the potentially common risk/maintenance factors for the two disorders, we also examine the relationship between control and obsessive-compulsive symptomatology.

Methods: Female community participants ($N = 175$) completed self-report measures of control, eating disorder pathology and obsessive-compulsive symptoms.

Results: Multivariate analyses of variance indicated significant differences between individuals with high vs. low levels of psychopathology on most of the measures of control. Using regression analyses, we found that a sense of ineffectiveness and fear of losing self-control were the only significant independent predictors of eating pathology, and fear of losing self-control was the most significant predictor of obsessive-compulsive symptoms.

Conclusions: This study highlights the importance of issues of control, particularly feelings of ineffectiveness and fear of losing self-control, in eating disorder symptoms. Furthermore, our findings suggest that there may be a similar underlying fear of losing self-control among individuals who engage in disordered eating and obsessive-compulsive behaviours. Thus, ineffectiveness and fear of losing self-control are two dimensions that are important to consider in maintenance and treatment models of disordered eating behaviours.

Keywords: Assessment of control, Disordered eating, Fear of losing self-control, Ineffectiveness, Obsessive-compulsive symptoms

Background

Issues of personal control have been proposed to play a central role in the aetiology and maintenance of eating disorders (ED), in particular Anorexia Nervosa (AN). For example, Bruch defined AN as a "struggle for control, for a sense of identity, competence, and effectiveness" ([1] p. 251). In her view, AN symptomatology can be understood as a desperate attempt to compensate for an underlying sense of ineffectiveness and lack of control experienced in the rest of the individual's life. Similarly, Slade hypothesised that control in weight loss enables individuals with AN to avoid negative affect associated with general life dissatisfaction and interpersonal problems. Control over eating becomes the primary focus because it is perceived as "successful behaviour in the context of perceived failure in all other areas of functioning" ([2] p. 173). Several other authors have proposed models of AN maintenance that emphasise the role of control within the disorder, noting that individuals use control over weight and shape as an index of overall self-control and self-worth [3], that they control their environment, especially close family members through their illness [4], and that the condition is reinforced through the individual's intense fear of loss of

* Correspondence: franzisca.froreich@gmail.com
[1]School of Psychology, UNSW Australia, Sydney, New South Wales 2052, Australia
Full list of author information is available at the end of the article

control [5]. Although the representation of control within these accounts do vary to some extent, they share the underlying premise that obsessive restriction over food and weight represent strategies to cope with generalised feelings of perceived lack of control. In the absence of adaptive personal control strategies, the individual may be driven to enact ritualistic body control as an auxiliary control mechanism.

Although most research on psychological control has been conducted with AN patients, those studies that have included individuals with Bulimia Nervosa (BN) have generally found no significant difference between AN and BN on the basis of control variables [6–8]. Slade [2] highlighted that a subset of individuals who develop BN have transitioned from AN. He argued that, at least for these patients, bulimic behaviour is an attempted alternative method of weight control that does not involve self-starvation and therefore bypasses direct confrontation with other people. Indeed, longitudinal research finds that 20–50 % of individuals with AN will develop BN over time [9–11], which speaks to the instability of ED diagnoses and why it may be difficult to find risk factors that differentiate between ED syndromes. Thus, control issues may be relevant not only for AN but across the ED spectrum.

Studies using qualitative methods provide support for the notion that perceived lack of control is a major contributing factor to the development of ED (see [12] for an example). Many patients recall starting dieting at a time when they perceived life to be chaotic and out of control. In this context, controlling one's food intake is seen as the "solution". As one patient described: "When I started changing my eating habits it was... because I didn't feel in control of my life or of myself. Controlling what I ate was one way of controlling at least part of my life... I felt that if I could control what went in and out and how much exercise I did then I could control other things in my life" ([13] p. 16).

Despite the strong theoretical and qualitative link between issues of control and ED, evidence from quantitative studies is limited and inconsistent. One difficulty in this area of research is that there is considerable heterogeneity in how the construct "control" is defined (see [14] for a review). A cursory review of research in the area reveals a large number of terms that have been used to conceptualise control, including *sense of control, locus of control, fear of losing control, desire for control, mastery,* and *ineffectiveness.* Although these terms may be interrelated and partially overlapping, they have been found to produce different results in relation to ED, thus complicating our understanding of the link between ED and control. For example, a sense of *ineffectiveness,* which reflects feelings of deficient control and worthlessness, and a low *sense of control* have consistently been found to influence risk and maintenance of ED [15–17]. In fact, Ineffectiveness is one of the subscales of the Eating Disorders Inventory [18], a measure of ED attitudes and behaviours that is widely used in research settings and clinical practice. Furthermore, in one study that compared multiple measures of control, *fear of losing self-control* was the most significant predictor of ED symptomatology [7] but this finding still awaits replication.

In contrast to the constructs described above that have shown consistent results across studies, other constructs have received inconsistent support. Studies assessing *locus of control,* which refers to an individual's belief about the source of control over reinforcement [19], have found that women who report engaging in disordered eating behaviours show greater externality [20], greater internality [21], and even no difference compared to healthy controls [22]. Similarly, studies exploring *desire for control* have found that ED patients have lower [7] or similar levels [16] of motivation to control the events in their lives compared to healthy controls.

In short, control appears to be a concept of importance in relation to ED but some of its dimensions are more consistently related to ED symptoms than are others. Determining which operationalisation of control is most centrally relevant to ED is important, not only because it will aid with the accumulation of research findings, but also because it could help clinicians understand which specific aspects of control (if any) need to be assessed and perhaps addressed in treatment. Past research in this domain has predominantly examined a single aspect of control in relation to ED symptomatology [20, 23], with only a few studies comparing up to three dimensions of control [7, 21]. Thus, the primary aim of the current study was to build on previous research by examining a broader range of constructs in order to determine which form (or forms) of control are most strongly associated with eating pathology. Specifically, this study compares six constructs commonly used in the eating-disorder literature to assess issues of control: locus of control, sense of control, fear of losing self-control, desire for control, sense of mastery, and ineffectiveness. We predicted that women who score high on a measure of disordered eating would show a weaker sense of personal control than would women who score low on the measure of disordered eating. We also assessed which specific measure(s) would emerge as the strongest predictor(s) of ED symptomatology but, given the inconsistencies in previous research, no firm predictions were made in this case.

A secondary aim of this study was to explore the relationship between control and obsessive-compulsive symptomatology. Obsessive-compulsive disorder (OCD) and ED are highly comorbid [24] and a number of authors have suggested that there may be common risk factors and/or shared mechanisms for maintenance of the two disorders [25, 26]. Similar to ED, phenomenological descriptions of OCD have often highlighted the role of control within the disorder. For example, individuals exhibiting OCD symptoms have been noted to "dislike spontaneity and prefer safety and predictability in order to appease their strong need for control over the environment" ([27] p. 756). Furthermore, OCD symptoms have been associated with a lower sense of control over the self and the environment, and this discrepancy between desire for control and perceived control is thought to motivate compulsive symptoms [28]. In these ways, it appears that both conditions, OCD and ED, may have functionally similar clinical presentations; that is, both represent attempts to reassert control, albeit through different means. In light of these apparent similarities between ED and OCD, we examined whether the constructs of control that are relevant to ED are also related to OCD symptoms. Because of the lack of research in this domain, no firm predictions were made.

Methods

Participants

Data were collected through Amazon Mechanical Turk (MTurk), a crowdsourcing website. Female MTurk registered users residing in the United States between the ages of 18 and 40 were eligible to participate. Participants were excluded if they provided incomplete data or if they failed any of the validity checks that were included in the survey. Valid and usable data were available for 175 female participants, aged 19–40 years ($M = 30.25$, $SD = 5.7$). Their mean body mass index (BMI [kg/m^2], based on self-reported height and weight) was 22.95 ($SD = 6.81$). Participants identified primarily as White/Caucasian ($n = 138$; 78.9 %), followed by African-American ($n = 15$; 8.6 %), Hispanic ($n = 9$; 5.1 %), Asian ($n = 6$; 3.4 %), and "other" ($n = 7$; 4.0 %).

Materials and procedure

Participants signed up for an online study that was described as an investigation of peoples' experiences of control in their lives. After reading an introductory information page and indicating their consent, participants completed the questionnaires described below. Control-related questionnaires were presented first, in randomised order, followed by measures assessing ED and OCD symptoms. Participants were also asked to report their age, height, weight, and ethnicity. After completing all of the measures, participants read a debriefing page providing further information about the study, and received credit on their Amazon account as compensation for their participation. This study was approved by the University's ethics committee.

Locus of control

Locus of control was assessed using Levenson's Internal, Powerful Others and Chance Scale (IPC) [29]. The IPC incorporates three subscales that measure the extent to which individuals believe that outcomes are due to their own actions (I: Internal Control), to powerful others (P: Powerful Others), or to chance or fate (C: Chance). Each subscale includes eight items that are rated on a 7-point Likert scale (−3 = *Strongly disagree*, +3 = *Strongly agree*), and items were summed and a constant of 24 added to each scale to eliminate negative sums. This measure has demonstrated moderate internal consistency and good construct validity [30]. For the current study, Cronbach's alpha for each subscale was .70, .79 and .82, respectively.

Sense of control

The Shapiro Control Inventory (SCI) [31] measures domain-general and domain-specific perceived control, positive and negative control mechanism, and motivation for control. For this study, we focused on participants' domain-general psychological sense of control by administering the 11-item positive sense of control scale (which measures perceived self-efficacy and self-control) and the 5-item negative sense of control scale (which captures loss of control, feelings of passivity and helplessness). A sample item from the positive sense of control scale (PSC) is, "If I decide to, I have the ability to make changes in order to gain more control over my life". A sample item from the negative sense of control scale (NSC) is, "I lack control of my environment (other people, situations)". For both subscales, each item is rated on a 6-point scale (1 = *Never*, 6 = *Very Often*). However, due to an administrative error, some of the items had 5 response options instead of 6, so scores were standardised and averaged. Both scales have yielded evidence of internal consistency and construct validity among clinical and normative populations [15, 31]. In the current study, Cronbach's alpha was .90 for PSC and .76 for NSC.

Fear of losing self-control

Fear of losing self-control was measured using an adapted version of the Self-Control subscale of Reid and Ware's Internal-External questionnaire [32]. Tiggemann and Raven [7] adapted the original 8-item scale to express fear of losing self-control by adding "I fear", "I am afraid" or "I worry" to the beginning of each item. A sample item of the original scale is, "Sometimes I impulsively do things, which at other times I definitely would not let myself do", and this item was changed to, "I worry that I sometimes will impulsively do things, which at other times I definitely would not let myself do." Each item was rated on a 7-point scale that ranged from 1 (*Doesn't apply to me at all*) to 7 (*Always applies to me*), with higher scores indicating greater doubts about being able to control one's own impulses, desires, and emotional behaviour. This scale has been shown to be related to other measures of control and also to greater eating psychopathology [7]. Consistent with prior work [7], internal consistency was excellent in the current sample (Cronbach's $\alpha = .94$).

Desire for control

Burger and Cooper's Desirability of Control Scale (DCS) [33] was administered to assess individual differences in general desire or need for control over life events. This measure contains 20 items with response options ranging from 1 (*This statement doesn't apply to me at all*) to 7 (*This statement always applies to me*), and with higher scores indicating greater desire for control. A sample item is, "I try to avoid situations where someone else tells me what to do". In previous studies, this measure has demonstrated evidence of internal consistency, test-retest reliability, and criterion validity [33]. For the current study, Cronbach's alpha was .83.

Sense of mastery

Mastery was assessed using the Personal Mastery Scale developed by Pearlin and Schooler (PMS) [34]. This scale consists of seven items that are rated on a 5-point scale ranging from 1 (*Strongly disagree*) to 5 (*Strongly agree*). A sample item is, "I can do about anything I really set my mind to". The total of the seven items was used as a measure of overall mastery, with higher scores reflecting greater personal mastery. For the current study, Cronbach's alpha was .83.

Ineffectiveness

Participants completed the 10-item Ineffectiveness subscale of the Eating Disorder Inventory-2 (EDI-2-I) [35]. This subscale assesses feelings of general inadequacy, insecurity, worthlessness and lack of control over one's life. Participants rate each item on a 6-point scale from 1(*Never*) to 5 (*Always*), with higher scores indicating a greater sense of ineffectiveness. High internal reliability estimates for the Ineffectiveness subscale have been demonstrated in both clinical and non-clinical samples [36, 37]. Consistent with previous research, Cronbach's alpha in this study was high ($\alpha = .94$).

Eating pathology

The Eating Disorder Diagnostic Scale (EDDS) [38] was used to assess ED psychopathology. This measure consists of 19 questions capturing ED symptoms, as described in 4th edition of the *Diagnostic and Statistical Manual for Mental Disorders* (DSM–IV) [39]. The EDDS provides diagnoses for full threshold AN, full threshold BN, and full threshold Binge Eating Disorder (BED), as well as subthreshold AN, subthreshold BN, and subthreshold BED. Items can also be standardised and summed (excluding items asking about weight, height, and birth control pill use) to create a continuous ED symptom composite score (SCS). The current study utilised the EDDS diagnoses to delineate individuals who are free from ED symptoms versus those who are symptomatic, and the SCS to index participants' overall level of eating pathology. Previous studies have yielded evidence of criterion validity, convergent validity, and internal consistency of the EDDS diagnoses and symptom composite [38, 40]. Cronbach's alpha for the SCS in this study was .90.

Obsessive-compulsive symptoms

Participants completed the Obsessive–Compulsive Inventory - Revised (OCI-R) [41], an 18-item self-report measure of OCD and its various symptom presentations. The OCI-R has excellent reliability and validity and is widely used in clinical research [42]. Higher scores indicate a greater degree of obsessive-compulsive symptoms. Cronbach's alpha in this study was .90.

Statistical analyses

Prior to conducting the primary analyses, univariate and multivariate outliers were identified following the procedure described by Tabachnick and Fidell [43] and were excluded from all further analyses ($n = 22$). Univariate outliers were defined as those with Z scores > 3.00. Mahalanobis distance for the complete set of predictors was used to detect multivariate outliers; cases exceeding the critical chi-square value were omitted. The final sample consisted of 175 participants, and all analyses reported below are based on this final sample. The sample size was based on Tabachnick and Fidell's [43] recommendation that a sample of $N \geq 104 + m$ is needed for adequate power in linear regression. With nine predictors included in the regression model, the sample size was more than adequate. All variables satisfied the assumptions of normality, linearity, homoscedasticity, and multicollinearity. Re-analysis of the data including outliers produced an identical pattern of results.

The first step in our analyses was to conduct bivariate correlations among all the variables included in the study. Next, in order to compare individuals high vs. low in psychopathology on the measures of control, we divided the sample into groups based on their scores on the EDDS and on the OCI-R. For the EDDS, we used the code developed by the scale's authors to differentiate individuals meeting an ED diagnosis (full and subthreshold; ED group) from those who were symptom free (no-ED group). The ED group ($n = 55$; full diagnosis $n = 34$ and subthreshold diagnoses $n = 21$) consisted of 16 individuals with AN, 25 with BN, and

14 with BED. The remaining 120 participants did not fulfil one of the three main (or subthreshold) diagnoses. For the OCI-R, we utilised the cut-off score of 21 [41] to divide participants into those who scored high (OCD group; $n = 39$) and those who scored low on obsessive-compulsive symptoms (no-OCD group; $n = 136$). The high prevalence of psychopathology found in this study is consistent with recent work showing that MTurk participants endorse clinical symptoms to a substantially greater degree than do traditional nonclinical samples (e.g., undergraduate subject pools) [44]. Multivariate analyses of variance (MANOVA) was then used to examine significant differences between these groups on the dependent measures, with a Bonferroni correction applied to the follow-up univariate analyses. Although BMI was correlated with EDDS scores, the pattern of results did not change when controlling for participants' BMI, and therefore BMI was not included in the analysis. Finally, we used multiple regression analyses to determine which measures of control were the strongest predictors of ED symptoms and OCD symptoms, separately. Because our predictors were all significantly correlated with one another (range = |.32| to |.74|), in addition to providing standardised regression weights, we also provided other indices of predictor importance that allow for more accurate variance partitioning among correlated predictors, including incremental R^2, general dominance weights, and relative importance weights [45, 46].

Results

Correlation analyses

The bivariate correlations among all of the variables in this study are shown in Table 1, as are the means, standard deviations, and range for those variables. ED and OCD symptom severity were positively associated with external locus of control, negative sense of control, feelings of ineffectiveness, and fear of losing self-control, and were negatively associated with sense of mastery. Both eating pathology and obsessive-compulsive pathology were also negatively associated with internal locus of control, but the correlation with EDDS scores was not significant. Desire for control had a negligible zero-order correlation with both EDDS scores and OCI-R scores. It should also be noted that EDDS scores and OCI-R scores were positively correlated.

Multivariate analyses of variance

A MANOVA indicated a significant overall difference between the ED group and the no-ED group, $F(9, 165) = 4.09$, $p < .001$, $\eta_p^2 = .18$. Follow-up univariate analyses yielded significant group differences on five of the nine subscales (see Table 2). Participants in the ED group scored significantly higher than did those in the no-ED group on external LOC-powerful others, negative sense of control, ineffectiveness, and fear of losing self-control. They also reported significantly lower positive sense of control.

Table 1 Bivariate correlations, means, and standard deviations for all variables included in the analyses

	1	2	3	4	5	6	7	8	9	10	11	12
1. BMI	–											
2. LOC-I	−.07	–										
3. LOC-P	.05	−.46***	-									
4. LOC-C	.09	−.53***	.68***	–								
5. PSC	−.16*	.58***	−.48***	−.43***	–							
6. NSC	.20**	−.42***	.50***	.43***	−.67***	–						
7. FLC	.22**	−.39***	.51***	.45***	−.52***	.67***	–					
8. DCS	−.09	.37***	−.34***	−.32***	.53***	−.48***	−.36***	–				
9. PMS	−.13	.62***	−.53***	−.54***	.69***	−.66***	−.51***	.51***	–			
10. EDI-I	.24**	−.49***	.47***	.40***	−.73***	.71***	.58***	−.50***	−.74***	–		
11. SCS	.35***	−.13	.29***	.23**	−.26**	.32***	.50***	−.13	−.25**	.46***	–	
12. OCI-R	.14	−.26***	.24**	.18*	−.31***	.33***	.44***	−.06	−.30***	.36***	.37***	–
M	22.95	35.62	19.67	18.66	0	0	23.44	98.30	26.53	24.04	−.09	12.33
SD	6.81	5.97	8.58	8.78	0.70	0.72	10.43	14.09	4.46	9.76	0.55	10.30
Min	13.64	19	0	0	−2.02	−1.23	8	63	15	10	−.80	0
Max	45.77	48	42	43	1.35	2.14	52	137	35	51	1.16	41

BMI body mass index, *I-LOC* Locus of Control- Internal, *P-LOC* Powerful Others Locus of Control, *C-LOC* Chance Locus of Control, *PSC* Positive Sense of Control, *NSC* Negative Sense of Control, *FLC* Fear of Losing Self-Control, *DCS* Desirability of Control Scale, *PMS* Personal Mastery Scale, *EDI-I* Eating Disorder Inventory-Ineffectiveness, *SCS* Symptom Composite Score, *OCI-R* Obsessive-Compulsive Inventory-Revised

*$p < .05$. **$p < .01$. ***$p < .001$

Table 2 Means (SD) and pairwise comparisons of each measure of control for EDDS and OCI-R groups

	EDDS				OCI-R			
	No-ED group	ED group	*p*-value[a]	η_p^2	No-OCD group	OCD group	*p*-value[a]	η_p^2
LOC-I	35.73 (6.26)	35.40 (5.33)	.74	.001	36.34 (5.76)	33.13 (6.07)	.003	.05
LOC-P	18.61 (8.47)	21.98 (8.43)	.02	.03	19.07 (8.85)	21.74 (7.29)	.09	.02
LOC-C	18.12 (8.97)	19.86 (8.30)	.23	.01	17.84 (8.93)	21.54 (7.66)	.02	.03
PSC	0.07 (0.70)	−0.16 (0.67)	.05	.02	0.08 (0.66)	−.29 (0.76)	.004	.05
NSC	−0.10 (0.69)	0.22 (0.74)	.01	.04	−.08 (0.68)	.27 (0.77)	.01	.04
FLC	20.90 (9.20)	28.98 (10.89)	< .001	.13	21.93 (9.84)	28.69 (10.86)	< .001	.07
DCS	98.25 (14.17)	98.40 (14.04)	.95	< .001	98.79 (14.24)	96.59 (13.58)	.39	.004
PMS	26.82 (4.33)	25.91 (4.74)	.21	.01	27.02 (4.27)	24.82 (4.75)	.01	.04
EDI-I	22.57 (8.76)	27.24 (11.09)	.003	.05	22.97 (9.46)	27.77 (10.03)	.01	.04

I-LOC Locus of Control- Internal, *P-LOC* Powerful Others Locus of Control, *C-LOC* Chance Locus of Control, *PSC* Positive Sense of Control, *NSC* Negative Sense of Control, *FLC* Fear of Losing Self-Control, *DCS* Desirability of Control Scale, *PMS* Personal Mastery Scale, *EDI-I* Eating Disorder Inventory-Ineffectiveness, *EDDS* Eating Disorder Diagnostic Scale, *OCI-R* Obsessive-Compulsive Inventory-Revised

[a]Adjusted by Bonferroni criteria for multiple comparisons

For the OCD groups, the MANOVA was also statistically significant, F (9, 165) = 2.12, $p = .03$, $\eta_p^2 = .10$, with seven of the nine measures of control yielding significant univariate differences between groups (Table 2). Notably, the pattern of results among the variables was quite similar between EDDS and OCI-R groups, with the OCD group scoring significantly lower than the no-OCD group on internal LOC, positive sense of control, and mastery, and scoring significantly higher on LOC-chance, negative sense of control, ineffectiveness, and fear of losing self-control.

Regression analyses

Linear regressions analyses were conducted separately for EDDS SCS and OCI-R. For eating pathology, the overall model was significant, F (9, 165) = 10.36, $p < .001$, explaining 36 % of the variance in EDDS scores. Ineffectiveness and fear of losing self-control were the only significant independent predictors of EDDS scores (Table 3). To gain a broader and fuller perspective on the contributions that the control variables made to each regression equation, we also report incremental R^2, general dominance weights, and relative importance weights. Consistent with the beta coefficients, ineffectiveness and fear of losing self-control were the strongest predictors of ED pathology across all three indices. They obtained the largest incremental R^2, both on their own and when taking all other predictors into account. Dominance analysis results demonstrated complete dominance of ineffectiveness and fear of losing self-control over all other variables, as they contributed more unique variance in the regression effect across all possible model subsets in which they were included. Similarly, relative importance weights also favoured ineffectiveness and fear of losing self-control. Notably, the submodel containing only ineffectiveness and

Table 3 Summary of statistics determining independent variable contributions to regression effect

	EDDS					OCI-R				
	ß weights	Incremental R^2	Incremental R_F^2	DW	RIW	*ß* weights	Incremental R^2	Incremental R_F^2	DW	RIW
LOC-I	.11	.02	.007	.008	.007	−.10	.07	.005	.018	.019
LOC-P	.05	.08	.001	.021	.022	.02	.06	< .001	.012	.012
LOC-C	.06	.05	.002	.012	.014	−.09	.03	.004	.007	.006
PSC	.10	.07	.004	.016	.019	−.06	.10	.001	.023	.022
NSC	−.15	.10	.007	.028	.029	−.01	.11	< .001	.028	.026
FLC	.44***	.25	.094	.144	.134	.37***	.19	.066	.101	.095
DCS	.09	.02	.005	.007	.007	.21*	.004	.031	.021	.014
PMS	.17	.06	.009	.018	.019	−.03	.09	< .001	.020	.019
EDI-I	.56***	.21	.099	.127	.109	.16	.13	.009	.041	.037

Entries are standardised coefficients. R_F^2 Incremental R^2 in full model, *DW* Dominance Weights, *RIW* Relative Importance Weights, *I-LOC* Locus of Control- Internal, *P-LOC* Powerful Others Locus of Control, *C-LOC* Chance Locus of Control, *PSC* Positive Sense of Control, *NSC* Negative Sense of Control, *FLC* Fear of Losing Self-Control, *DCS* Desirability of Control Scale, *PMS* Personal Mastery Scale, *EDI-I* Eating Disorder Inventory-Ineffectiveness

*$p < .05$

***$p < .001$

fear of loss of self-control accounted for 29 % of the variance. Therefore, by eliminating all variables except for ineffectiveness and fear of losing self-control, we are able to gain a more parsimonious model with very little loss in predictive efficiency (a loss of 7 %).

For OC symptoms, the overall model was also significant, F (9, 165) = 6.09, $p < .001$, explaining 25 % of the variance in OCI-R scores. Fear of losing self-control and desire for control emerged as the only significant independent predictors of OCI-R scores (Table 3). In this case, all three indices of predictor importance identified fear of losing self-control as the strongest contributor. By itself, fear of losing self-control explained 19.4 % of the variance of OCI-scores. Although desire for control had a statistically significant beta weight in the full regression model, it was not found to directly contribute variance to the dependent variable using other predictor importance measures.

Discussion

The primary purpose of the present study was to elucidate how different control constructs relate to disordered eating behaviours. In particular, we examined the associations among sense of control, locus of control, fear of losing self-control, desire for control, mastery, ineffectiveness, and ED symptomatology. The results of this investigation provide further support for the role of control in disordered eating behaviours. When comparing women with high versus low levels of disordered eating behaviours, those with high scores on the EDDS were significantly more external in their locus of control, reported greater negative sense of control, feelings of ineffectiveness, and greater fear of losing self-control, as well as less positive sense of control. Analyses of relative predictor importance showed ineffectiveness and fear of losing self-control to be the variables that contributed the most to eating psychopathology. In fact, eliminating all other variables allowed for the most model parsimony without a substantial loss in variance explained.

The current findings suggest that, although a number of control dimensions are related to disordered eating behaviours, ineffectiveness and fear of losing self-control are the two strongest predictors of eating pathology. Ineffectiveness has received considerable research support in the ED literature [17, 47], and the present study adds to this growing body of evidence by suggesting that ineffectiveness may be critical to the development of disordered eating behaviours [48]. The second important dimension of control identified in this study, fear of losing self-control, has yet to be fully explored as a potential risk factor. Tiggemann and Raven [7] were first to report the importance of fear of losing self-control as a contributor to ED pathology when it emerged as the most potent predictor of ED symptomatology in their study. Surprisingly, this prominent result has not been further investigated and the measure of losing self-control developed by Tiggemann and Raven [7] is yet to be subjected to rigorous psychometric evaluation. The present study thus adds to the literature on the assessment of fear of losing self-control by providing additional evidence for the reliability and validity of the measure.

It is important to note that none of the items in any of the control scales administered in this study directly refer to eating, weight or shape. This suggests that the underlying control beliefs are not disorder-specific but are more general in nature, further supporting the "functional analysis" of ED [2]. The direction of causality between control and ED cannot be determined by the present result. We can speculate, however, that the need to control eating is a product of these individuals' internalised sense of ineffectiveness and a fear of losing self-control. In response to feeling ill-prepared to function effectively in their lives, individuals with ED resort to auxiliary control mechanisms to ward off the fear of having no control at all [49]. In this respect, the illness can be understood as a functional response (albeit a maladaptive one) that derives from the failure of more appropriate mechanisms and sources of control [50].

The secondary aim of this research was to explore whether the constructs of control that are relevant to ED are also related to OCD symptoms. The results revealed a similar pattern to that observed with eating pathology. In comparison to the group with low OCI-R scores, women with high scores displayed significantly more externality, negative sense of control, feelings of ineffectiveness, fear of losing self-control, and less sense of mastery, positive sense of control, and internal LOC. Relative importance analysis identified fear of losing self-control to be the most important predictor of OCI-R scores. It is interesting to note that desire for control was not related to OCD symptoms in the bivariate correlations, but was a significant predictor in the regression model. This pattern of results has been reported previously [28] and suggested a possible suppression effect. Overall, the results support the contention that both disorders may have similar underlying issues of control. On the one hand, the findings suggest that both disorders are characterised by a fear of losing self-control. This is consistent with other studies that found marked fear of losing control over mental activities, impulses, and emotions in patients with OCD [51]. On the other hand, feelings of inadequacy, worthlessness and lack of control, as measured by the EDI-Ineffectiveness scale, seem to be aspects that are especially characteristic of ED [52].

The results of the present study should be interpreted in the context of their limitations. First, we conducted the study with a female, non-clinical sample and so the results await replication in males and clinical samples.

However, research on non-clinical populations in this domain is important given the prevalence of disordered eating in today's society [53] and the potential for such research to contribute to prevention and intervention efforts. Furthermore, research suggests that obsessive-compulsive symptoms in non-clinical community samples are qualitatively indistinguishable from those in clinically diagnosed samples of OCD patients [54], thus supporting the assumption that obsessive-compulsive symptoms and dysfunctional beliefs are dimensional rather than categorical in nature. It therefore seems likely that the associations found in the current study between issues of control and ED/OCD symptoms would be similar, if not stronger, among individuals with symptoms severe enough to meet the criteria for a diagnosis. Second, another limitation of the present study was the exclusive reliance on self-reports for assessment. Future research is needed to verify the results of this study using more diverse and reliable methods. In particular, the use of interview methods to arrive at a clear-cut diagnosis of ED is advocated. Third, the present study did not explore whether different control measures differentially relate to different ED diagnoses or symptoms. Future research should explore this possibility either by including measures that capture diagnosis-specific symptoms or by conducting this study with a clinical sample that provides sufficiently large diagnostic groups to ensure adequate statistical power. Finally, the present study sought to distinguish among existing measures of control. It is possible that some measures of control include multiple dimensions of control within the same measure, or that there are higher order constructs that would be apparent across measures. A step forward for researchers would be to collect data on a much larger sample, submit all items simultaneously to a joint exploratory factor analysis, and reanalyse the relationships between the newly created factors and ED/OCD symptoms.

Conclusions

The findings provide some evidence that ineffectiveness and fear of losing self-control are two dimensions that are important to consider in maintenance and treatment models of disordered eating behaviours. Treatment approaches that solely focus on stringent behavioural goals (i.e., reduce control over eating, weight, and shape) may fail to address the deeper problem underlying and often maintaining these symptoms [55]. Helping the individual re-established adaptive mechanisms of personal control and effectiveness may reduce their need to rely on weight/shape control. Similarly, individuals vulnerable to OCD may benefit from psychotherapeutic interventions that challenge worries of losing control over one's impulses, desires and emotional behaviours (i.e., self-control). Future work should examine how these cognitions can be targeted in prevention and intervention efforts.

Ethics

All procedures performed in studies involving human participants were in accordance with the ethical standards of a medical ethics committee and with the 1964 Helsinki declaration and its later amendments or comparable ethical standards. This project (HREAP 143–132) has been approved by the Human Research Ethics Advisory Panel for the School of Psychology, UNSW.

Informed consent

Informed consent was obtained from all individual participants included in the study.

Competing interests
The authors declare that they have no competing interests.

Authors' contributions
FVF, LRV, JRG, and SWT were involved in the design of the study; FVF collected the data; FVF and LRV analysed the data; and FVF, LRV, JRG, and SWT drafted and approved the final manuscript.

Author details
[1]School of Psychology, UNSW Australia, Sydney, New South Wales 2052, Australia. [2]School of Psychology, University of Sydney, Sydney 2006, New South Wales, Australia.

References

1. Bruch H. The golden cage. The enigma of anorexia nervosa. Cambridge: Harvard University Press; 1978.
2. Slade P. Towards a functional analysis of anorexia nervosa and bulimia nervosa. Br J Clin Psychol. 1982;21:167–79.
3. Fairburn CG, Shafran R, Cooper Z. A cognitive behavioural theory of anorexia nervosa. Behav Res Ther. 1999;37:1–13.
4. Schmidt U, Treasure J. Anorexia nervosa: Valued and visible. A cognitive-interpersonal maintenance model and its implications for research and practice. Br J Clin Psychol. 2006;45:343–66.
5. Crisp AH. Anorexia nervosa: Let me be. Hove, UK: Psychology Press; 1995.
6. Jacobi C, Paul T, de Zwaan M, Nutzinger DO, Dahme B. Specificity of self-concept disturbances in eating disorders. Int J Eat Disord. 2004;35:204–10.
7. Tiggemann M, Raven M. Dimensions of control in bulimia and anorexia nervosa: Internal control, desire for control, or fear of losing self-control? Eat Disord. 1998;6:65–71.
8. Williams CJ, Power KG, Millar HR, Freeman CP, Yellowlees A, Dowds T, Jackson MA. Comparison of eating disorders and other dietary/weight groups on measures of perceived control, assertiveness, self-esteem, and self-directed hostility. Int J of Eat Disord. 1993;14:27–32.
9. Eddy KT, Dorer DJ, Franko DL, Tahilani K, Thompson-Brenner H, Herzog DB. Diagnostic crossover in anorexia nervosa and bulimia nervosa: implications for DSM-V. Am J Psychiatry. 2008;165:245–50.
10. Eckert ED, Halmi KA, Marchi P, Grove W, Crosby R. Ten-year follow-up of anorexia nervosa: clinical course and outcome. Psychol Med. 1995;25:143–56.
11. Strober M, Freeman R, Morrell W. The long-term course of severe anorexia nervosa in adolescents: survival analysis of recovery, relapse, and outcome predictors over 10–15 years in a prospective study. Int J Eat Disord. 1997;22:339–60.
12. Espindola CR, Blay SL. Anorexia nervosa's meaning to patients: a qualitative synthesis. Psychopathology. 2009;42:69–80.
13. Patching J, Lawler J. Understanding women's experiences of developing an eating disorder and recovering: a life-history approach. Nurs Inq. 2009;16:10–21.
14. Skinner EA. A guide to constructs of control. J Pers Soc Psychol. 1996;71:549–70.
15. Lee S, Chan YY, Kwok K, Hsu LK. Relationship between control and the intermediate term outcome of anorexia nervosa in Hong Kong. Aust N Z J Psychiatry. 2005;39:141–5.

16. Shapiro JR, Blinder BJ, Hagman J, Pituck S. A psychological "sense-of-control" profile of patients with anorexia nervosa and bulimia nervosa. Psychol Rep. 1993;73:531–41.
17. Wade TD, Wilksch SM, Paxton SJ, Byrne SM, Austin SB. How perfectionism and ineffectiveness influence growth of eating disorder risk in young adolescent girls. Behav Res Ther. 2015;66:56–63.
18. Garner DM, Olmstead MP, Polivy J. Development and validation of a multidimensional eating disorder inventory for anorexia nervosa and bulimia. Int J Eat Disord. 1983;2:15–34.
19. Rotter JB. Generalized expectancies for internal versus external control of reinforcement. Psychol Monogr-Gen A. 1966;80:1–28.
20. Fouts G, Vaughan K. Locus of control, television viewing, and eating disorder symptomatology in young females. J Adolesc. 2002;25:307–11.
21. Donovan CL, Penny R. In control of weight: The relationship between facets of control and weight restriction. Eat Behav. 2014;15:144–50.
22. Cachelin FM, Striegel-Moore R, Paget WB. Comparison of women with various levels of dietary restraint on body image, personality, and family environment. Eat Disord. 1997;5:205–15.
23. Waller G. Perceived control in eating disorders: Relationship with reported sexual abuse. Int J Eat Disord. 1998;23:213–6.
24. Kaye WH, Bulik CM, Thornton L, Barbarich N, Masters K, Price Foundation Collaborative Group. Comorbidity of anxiety disorders with anorexia and bulimia nervosa. Am J Psychiatry. 2004;161:2215–21.
25. Altman SE, Shankman SA. What is the association between obsessive–compulsive disorder and eating disorders? Clin Psych Rev. 2009;29:638–46.
26. Vartanian LR, Grisham JR. Obsessive–compulsive symptoms and body checking in women and men. Cognit Ther Res. 2012;36:367–74.
27. Gibbs NA. Nonclinical populations in research on obsessive-compulsive disorder: a critical review. Clin Psychol Rev. 1996;16:729–73.
28. Moulding R, Kyrios M. Desire for control, sense of control and obsessive-compulsive symptoms. Cognit Ther Res. 2007;31:759–72.
29. Levenson H. Differentiating among internality, powerful others, and chance. In: Lefcourt HM, editor. Research with the locus of control construct. New York: Academic; 1981. p. 15–63.
30. Levenson H. Reliability and Validity of the I, P, and C Scales-A Multidimensional View of Locus of Control. Montreal: Paper presented at American Psychological Association Convention; 1973. Available from: http://files.eric.ed.gov/fulltext/ED087791.pdf.
31. Shapiro DH. Manual of the Shapiro Control Inventory (SCI). Palo Alto: Behaviordata, Inc; 1994.
32. Reid DW, Ware EE. Multidimensionality of internal versus external control: addition of a third dimension and non-distinction of self versus others. Can J Behav Sci. 1974;6:131–42.
33. Burger JM, Cooper HM. The desirability of control. Motiv Emot. 1979;3:381–93.
34. Pearlin LI, Schooler C. The structure of coping. J Health Soc Behav. 1978; 19:2–21.
35. Garner DM. Eating Disorder Inventory-2. Odessa: Psychological Assessment Resources, Inc; 1991.
36. Eberenz KP, Gleaves DH. An examination of the internal consistency and factor structure of the eating disorder inventory-2 in a clinical sample. Int J Eat Disord. 1994;16:371–9.
37. Schaefer WK, Maclennan RN, Yaholnitsky-Smith SA, Stover ED. Psychometric evaluation of the Eating Disorder Inventory (EDI) in a clinical group. Psychol Health. 1998;13:873–81.
38. Stice E, Telch CF, Rizvi SL. Development and validation of the Eating Disorder Diagnostic Scale: A brief self-report measure of anorexia, bulimia, and binge-eating disorder. Psychol Assess. 2000;12:123–31.
39. American Psychiatric Association (APA). Diagnostic and Statistical Manual of Mental Disorders 4th ed.; DSM-4. 4th ed. Washington, DC: APA; 1994.
40. Stice E, Fisher M, Martinez E. Eating disorder diagnostic scale: additional evidence of reliability and validity. Psychol Assess. 2004;16:60–71.
41. Foa EB, Huppert JD, Leiberg S, Langner R, Kichic R, Hajcak G, Salkovskis PM. The Obsessive-Compulsive Inventory: development and validation of a short version. Psychol Assess. 2002;14:485–96.
42. Abramowitz JS, Deacon BJ. Psychometric properties and construct validity of the Obsessive–Compulsive Inventory—Revised: Replication and extension with a clinical sample. J Anxiety Disord. 2006;20:1016–35.
43. Tabachnick BG, Fidell LS. Using multivariate statistics. 5th ed. Boston: Allyn and Bacon; 2007.
44. Arditte KA, Çek D, Shaw AM, Timpano KR. The Importance of Assessing Clinical Phenomena in Mechanical Turk Research. Psychol Assess. 2015; doi: 10.1037/pas0000217.
45. Braun MT, Oswald FL. Exploratory regression analysis: a tool for selecting models and determining predictor importance. Behav Res Methods. 2011; 43:331–9.
46. Nathans LL, Oswald FL, Nimon K. Interpreting multiple linear regression: a guidebook of variable importance. Pract Assess Res Eval. 2012;17:1–19.
47. Jacobi C, Hayward C, de Zwaan M, Kraemer HC, Agras WS. Coming to terms with risk factors for eating disorders: application of risk terminology and suggestions for a general taxonomy. Psychol Bull. 2004;130:19–65.
48. Bruch H. Eating disorders: obesity, anorexia nervosa, and the person within. New York: Basic Books; 1973.
49. Bruch H. Anorexia Nervosa: therapy and theory. Am J Psychiatry. 1982;139: 1531–8.
50. Surgenor LJ, Horn J, Plmridge EW, Hudson SM. Anorexia nervosa and psychological control: a reexamination of selected theoretical accounts. Eur Eat Disord Rev. 2002;10:85–101.
51. Denys D, de Geus F, van Megen HJ, Westenberg HG. Symptom dimensions in obsessive-compulsive disorder: factor analysis on a clinician-rated scale and a self-report measure. Psychopathology. 2004;37:181–9.
52. Jimenez-Murcia S, Fernandez-Aranda F, Raich RM, Alonso P, Krug I, Jaurrieta N, et al. Obsessive-compulsive and eating disorders: Comparison of clinical and personality features. Psychiatry Clin Neurosci. 2007;61:385–91.
53. National Eating Disorder Collaboration. Eating Disorder Prevention, treatment, and management: An evidence review. Canberra: Prepared for the Commonwealth Department of Health and Ageing; 2010. http://www.nedc.com.au/files/pdfs/NEDC_Evidence%20Review_Final.pdf. Accessed 25 January 2016.
54. Abramowitz JS, Fabricant LE, Taylor S, Deacon BJ, McKay D, Storch EA. The relevance of analogue studies for understanding obsessions and compulsions. Clin Psychol Rev. 2014;34:206–17.
55. Bruch H. Perils of behavior modification in treatment of anorexia nervosa. J Am Med Assoc. 1974;230:1419–22.

A clinical profile of compulsive exercise in adolescent inpatients with anorexia nervosa

Melissa Noetel[1*], Jane Miskovic-Wheatley[2,3], Ross D. Crosby[4,5], Phillipa Hay[6], Sloane Madden[2,7] and Stephen Touyz[1]

Abstract

Background: The aim of the current study was to contribute to the development of a clinical profile of compulsive exercise in adolescents with Anorexia Nervosa (AN), by examining associations between compulsive exercise and eating and general psychopathology.

Method: A sample of 60 female adolescent inpatients with AN completed a self-report measure of compulsive exercise and a series of standardized self-report questionnaires assessing eating and general psychopathology.

Results: Higher levels of compulsive exercise were associated with increased levels of eating disorder psychopathology and anxiety. Specifically, the avoidance aspect (negatively reinforced) of compulsive exercise was associated with elevated scores on measures of eating disorder, anxiety, depression, and obsessive compulsiveness psychopathology, as well as lower self-esteem scores. The mood improvement value (positively reinforced) of compulsive exercise, however, did not reflect such trends.

Conclusions: Compulsive exercise driven by avoidance of negative affect is associated with more severe psychological features in adolescent inpatients with AN. The current findings emphasize the need for research and clinical efforts in the development of treatments addressing avoidance of negative affect and compulsive exercise in adolescents with AN.

Keywords: Adolescent, Eating disorders, Anorexia, Exercise, Psychopathology

Background

Adolescence is a risk period for the onset of Anorexia Nervosa (AN) [1], and as a group, adolescents present with the challenge of a unique clinical profile compared to adults with AN [2]. One particular clinical feature that seems to be indiscriminate with regard to age and presents challenges to all individuals with eating disorders is compulsive exercise. There has been an accumulating body of research focusing on the role of compulsive exercise in the pathogenesis and maintenance of eating disorders in adults. Despite the period of adolescence being a crucial time in the development of exercise- and eating-related attitudes [3, 4], research is yet to clearly define the specific psychological and clinical challenges associated with compulsive exercise in adolescents with an eating disorder [5].

There is ambiguity in the literature regarding the qualitative and quantitative dimensions that most accurately reflect the pathological nature of exercise in individuals with eating disorders [6], which is further compounded by the use of various terms to describe this behaviour such as excessive exercise, obligatory exercise, and driven exercise. Research to date, however, suggests that compulsive exercise seems to be the most theoretically and clinically sound construct of exercise observed in this population [6, 7]. Compulsive exercise is characterized by rigidity and a highly driven urge to exercise, with a perceived inability to stop exercising despite the individual being aware of its possible negative consequences

* Correspondence: mfie2396@uni.sydney.edu.au
[1]School of Psychology, The University of Sydney, Sydney, Australia
Full list of author information is available at the end of the article

in their emaciated state [8]. Research has identified compulsive exercise as playing an important role in the aetiology, development and maintenance of eating disorders [9, 10]. A recent systematic review [5] identified prevalence estimates for exclusively adolescent eating disorder samples that ranged from 16.7 % [11] to 85.3 % [12]. Compulsive exercise is transdiagnostic, however, it is most commonly reported in individuals with AN [13, 14], with prevalence estimates ranging from 44.6 to 80 % [5].

A cognitive behavioural model of compulsive exercise in the context of eating disorders highlighted four key constructs that underpin and maintain the compulsive dimension of exercise: eating psychopathology, obsessive-compulsiveness, affect-regulation and perfectionism [15]. Exercise in this population functions to compensate for caloric intake, as well as to regulate mood [16, 17]. This notion is supported by frequent patient reports that exercise is often equally being maintained for the control of negative affect as it is to account for caloric intake [18, 19]. Consistent with the addiction model of compulsive exercise [20], it is proposed that the reliance on exercise is maintained through both positive and negative reinforcement schedules. Specifically, the behaviour itself is one that serves to produce pleasure, as well as to avoid or neutralize internal distress [21]. Recent neurobiological research has evidenced the positive motivational valence of exercise for individuals with AN, which may also contribute to the development and maintenance of the disorder. Specifically, visual stimuli associated with exercise was found to be processed as rewarding by individuals with AN [22]. In summary, research to date has identified a number of key constructs that operate in the development and maintenance of compulsive exercise in eating disorders.

A number of adverse clinical outcomes have been associated with compulsive exercise in individuals with AN. Medical complications linked with compulsive exercise include an increased risk of overuse injuries, stress fractures [23], as well as functional and structural cardiac problems [24]. Furthermore, research and clinical attention has recently been given to the pathogenic aspects of compulsive exercise, as well as its association with poor treatment outcomes and increased psychological distress. Treatment outcomes in adults with AN include increased risk for relapse [25], higher energy requirements for re-feeding for equivalent levels of weight gain [26], and longer hospitalizations for adults with AN, Bulimia Nervosa, and Eating Disorder Not Otherwise Specified [27]. Within the adolescent-specific literature, research has identified that the presence of driven exercise at the commencement of treatment predicted significantly worse eating disorder symptomology, preoccupations, and rituals at the end of treatment for individuals with AN [28].

These poor treatment outcomes may be explained in part by the increased psychological distress and more severe eating disorder psychopathology that are typically found in individuals with compulsive exercise compared to those without compulsive exercise. Within an adult population, the positive relationship between compulsive exercise and eating disorder psychopathology has been well established. Specifically, increased levels of compulsive exercise have been associated with increased dietary restraint, weight and shape concerns [29, 30], drive for thinness, body dissatisfaction [27, 31], and perfectionism [30]. Compulsive exercise has also been associated with elevated levels of general psychopathology in adults with an eating disorder, including depression [17, 32], chronic negative affect [17, 33], anxiety [17, 30–32], and obsessive-compulsiveness [30, 34].

In contrast to the evidence that compulsive exercise is related to adverse physical and psychosocial outcomes in adults with an eating disorder, there is limited similar research in adolescents with an eating disorder. A recent systematic review (search date: May 2013) identified only four studies that examined this relationship in an exclusively adolescent sample, two of which included only individuals with AN [5]. Consistent with the adult literature, compulsive exercise in adolescents with an eating disorder was found to be associated with increased eating disorder pathology [35–37], and anxiety [35, 36]. The review identified inconsistent findings for other measures of psychopathology, including depressive symptoms and obsessive-compulsiveness [5]. Taken together, insufficient data exists to establish a reliable risk profile of compulsive exercise for adolescents with an eating disorder [5].

The aim of the current study was to examine the psychopathological correlates of compulsive exercise in adolescents with AN, and thus, contribute to the clinical profile of compulsive exercise. It was hypothesized that higher levels of compulsive exercise would be associated with increased eating and general psychopathology, namely anxiety, depression, obsessive compulsiveness and self-esteem.

Method

Participants

Participants were 60 adolescent females, who were recruited from the Eating Disorders Inpatient Service at the Children's Hospital at Westmead between September 2013 and January 2015. Treatment aims of this service were to achieve medical stabilization and safe eating practices under the care of a specialist, multidisciplinary eating disorders team (see [38] for additional treatment program details). The treatment program also managed co-morbid psychiatric conditions using evidence-based practice, including the prescription of psychotropic medications such as selective serotonin reuptake inhibitors (SSRIs) and atypical antipsychotics. Participants were eligible if they were aged between 12 and 17 years and met DSM-5 [39] diagnostic criteria for AN, as assessed by a specialist child and adolescent psychiatrist. Exclusion criteria were acute suicidality, evidence of psychosis or related thought disorder, non-proficiency in English, and male. Males were excluded from the current study due to the low numbers evident within this clinical population and to avoid confounds of sex on study variables. From the 118 consecutive admissions, 19 individuals met the exclusion criteria, 25 were re-admitted to the service after completing the study, eight did not consent to participate, and six individuals had incomplete data, leaving a total of 60 participants. This study gained ethical clearance from the Hunter New England Human Research Ethics Committee. Participants and their parents/legal guardian provided written informed consent.

Procedure

A specialist child and adolescent psychiatrist and paediatrician, both highly experienced in the treatment of eating disorders, conducted routine assessments at admission, including medical examinations, as well as diagnostic evaluations for eating disorder psychopathology and co-morbid conditions. All participants were then approached and completed standardized self-report questionnaires assessing eating and general psychopathology, as well as compulsive exercise features and exercise characteristics. A medical file review was conducted for each participant upon discharge to obtain necessary background and demographic information. Percentage of expected body weight (EBW) according to gender, age and height was calculated using the Centers for Disease Control and Prevention growth charts [40], and weight and height measurements were taken at admission and discharge.

Measures

Compulsive Exercise Test (CET)

The CET [8] is a 24-item self-report questionnaire that assesses the key cognitive, behavioural, and emotional features of compulsive exercise. Responses are scored on a six-point Likert scale (0 = *never true* to 5 = *always true*). The CET is comprised of five subscales, including avoidance and rule-driven behaviour (e.g., 'I feel extremely guilty if I miss an exercise session'; Cronbach's α in the current sample = .94), weight control exercise (e.g., 'I exercise to burn calories and lose weight'; Cronbach's α = .90), mood improvement (e.g., 'I feel less depressed or low after I exercise'; Cronbach's α = .75), lack of exercise enjoyment (e.g., 'I find exercise a chore'; Cronbach's α = .80), and exercise rigidity (e.g., 'My weekly pattern of exercise is repetitive'; Cronbach's α = .81). A total CET score (Cronbach's α = .93) is calculated from the sum of the mean item score for each of the five subscales, with higher scores reflecting a higher degree of pathology. The CET has demonstrated sound psychometric properties with a community sample of young adult exercisers [8], and has been validated for the use with adolescents [41].

Exercise frequency

An estimate of each participant's quantity of exercise was obtained through retrospective ratings of the number of weeks of participation, average number of sessions per week, the average duration of each session, and the self-reported intensity ('low', 'moderate', 'high') of a given exercise activity. This was rated for all of their exercise activities and assessed according to the previous 4 weeks and previous year. An overall measure of 'exercise frequency' was then estimated by multiplying each of the above four criteria and summing this measure for all of their reported exercise activities [42]. This method of assessing exercise frequency has been reliably used on inpatients with an eating disorder [42].

Athleticism

Participants were asked a series of qualitative questions regarding whether they identified themselves as a current or former athlete, as well as the highest level of competition for their given sport they had participated in.

Youth Eating Disorder Examination-Questionnaire (YEDE-Q)

The YEDE-Q [43] was adapted from the widely used measure of eating disorder symptomology, the Eating Disorder Examination-Questionnaire (EDE-Q) [44]. The 39-item self-report questionnaire assesses behavioral and attitudinal disordered eating features over the previous 28 days. The Y-EDEQ has sound psychometrics and has been validated for use with adolescents [43]. In the current study, Cronbach's α scores for each of the subscales and global score were as follows: Global Score .97, Restraint .89, Eating Concern .79, Shape Concern .96, and Weight Concern .93.

Revised Child Anxiety and Depression Scale (RCADS)

The RCADS [45] was developed to assess DSM-IV specific symptoms of anxiety disorders and depression in youth aged between 7 and 18-years-old. The self-report measure consists of 47 items, which generate five subscales: generalized anxiety disorder (GAD), separation anxiety disorder (SAD), social phobia, panic disorder, obsessive compulsive disorder (OCD), and major depressive disorder (MDD). The RCADS has sound psychometric properties, with good internal consistency, discriminant and convergent validity [46]. In the current study, Cronbach's α scores were as follows: Total Anxiety Scale .96, Total Internalizing Scale .97, GAD .89, SAD .84, Social Phobia .92, Panic Disorder .92, OCD .88, and MDD .91.

Children's Obsessional Compulsive Inventory-Revised (ChOCI-R)

OCD symptom severity and impairment was measured using the self-report version of the ChOCI-R [47], which is applicable for use with youth aged 7 to 17-year-olds. The ChOCI-R is comprised of two sections that assess compulsions and obsessions respectively. Each section includes 10 items measuring the presence of OCD symptoms and 6 items probing the severity and impairment associated with the OCD symptoms. The ChOCI-R has sound internal consistency and criterion validity [48]. Cronbach's α values within the current sample were .92 for both total scores.

Rosenberg Self Esteem Scale (RSES)

The RSES [49] is a commonly used 10-item self-report questionnaire that evaluates global trait self-esteem. Its reliability and validity are well established [50]. In the current study, the Cronbach's α for the RSES was .92.

Sample size and power

A priori power analysis estimated that a total of 60 participants would provide 80 % power to detect a medium effect size ($r = .30$; $\alpha = .05$, two-tailed). A medium effect size was derived from a risk profile analysis testing similar hypotheses within an eating disorder population ($r = .30$) [37]. Due to a number of differences when compared to the proposed study (e.g., categorical vs. continuous data), however, a marginally increased effect size ($r = .35$) was predicted for this study.

Statistical analysis

Pearson's correlations were used to test associations between compulsive exercise and clinical and physical activity characteristics. A multiple regression analysis was conducted to assess the associations between compulsive exercise and key psychopathology features (YEDE-Q Global Score, RCADS Depression and Total Anxiety subscales, CHOCI-R Total Symptom subscale). The subsequent multiple regression analysis was deemed satisfactory as inspections of all residuals demonstrated normal distributions and all assumptions were met [51]. Initial correlation analyses (Pearson's r) indicated that none of the descriptive variables were correlated with CET Total Score, and therefore, controlling for such variables was not required in the regression analysis. A significance level was set at $p < .05$ (two-tailed), and all analyses were conducted using SPSS, Version 22.0.

Results

Participant characteristics

The demographic and clinical characteristics for the final participant sample of 60 are summarised in Table 1. A majority of the sample met the diagnostic criteria for AN (90 %; $n = 54$) and retrospective classification indicated that the remaining participants met DSM-5 criteria for Atypical AN (10 %; $n = 6$). For the purpose of the final analyses, the two eating disorder diagnostic groups were pooled together. The only significant differences between the eating disorder diagnostic groups were the minimum reported weight (AN: $M = 41.54$, $SD = 5.89$; Atypical AN: $M = 59.83$, $SD = 13.42$; $t(52) = -5.75$, $p < .001$); the mean percentage EBW at admission (AN: $M = 83.89$, $SD = 9.02$; Atypical AN: $M - 111.27$, $SD = 11.85$; $t(58) = -6.84$, $p < .001$); the mean percentage EBW at discharge (AN: $M = 90.78$, $SD = 9.00$; Atypical AN: $M = 112.32$, $SD = 12.46$; $t(58) = -5.35$, $p < .001$); and the YEDE-Q Global Score (AN: $M = 3.65$, $SD = 1.69$; Atypical

Table 1 Demographics and clinical characteristics

	M (SD)	*n* (%)	Range
Demographics			
Age (years)	15.02 (1.22)		12 to 17
Ethnicity			
Caucasian		56 (93.3)	
Asian		2 (3.4)	
Other		2 (3.4)	
Clinical characteristics			
Diagnosis			
AN		54 (90.0)	
Atypical AN		6 (10.0)	
Duration of illness at admission (months)	13.4 (11.79)		1 to 66
% EBW at admission	86.6 (12.39)		
% EBW at discharge	92.9 (11.33)		
Duration of admission (days)	38 (50.17)		7 to 379
Previous hospitalizations	1 (1.29)		0 to 6
Medications prescribed throughout admission			
SSRIs		9 (15.0)	
Atypical antipsychotics		8 (13.3)	
Both SSRIs and atypical antipsychotics		16 (26.7)	
None		27 (45.0)	

AN anorexia nervosa, *%EBW* percentage expected body weight, *SSRIs* selective serotonin reuptake inhibitors, *M* mean, *SD* standard deviation

AN: $M = 5.20$, $SD = .43$; $t(58) = -2.22$, $p = .030$). There were no differences on other demographic or screening variables. Additionally, sensitivity analyses that were conducted based on eating disorder diagnostic groups revealed no differences in the interpretation of findings, and thus, all eating disorder diagnoses were analyzed simultaneously.

Relationships between compulsive exercise and participant characteristics

Pearson's correlations revealed that CET Total Score was not significantly related (all p's >.05) to any of the demographic (e.g., age) or clinical characteristic variables (e.g., duration of illness, minimum reported weight, percentage EBW at admission).

Relationships between compulsive exercise and physical activity variables

In terms of physical activity variables, CET Total Score was significantly related to the estimated frequency of physical activity over the previous month ($r = .29$, $p = .034$). CET Total Score, however, was not significantly associated with the estimated frequency of physical activity over the previous year ($r = .26$, $p = .055$) and the number of sports regularly engaged in ($r = -.13$, $p = .342$). Of the overall sample, assessment of the highest level of competition each participant had performed at identified that 13.3 % of the sample had represented their chosen sport at a national level, 25 % at a state level, and 35 % at a district or regional level. A one-way ANOVA identified that CET Total Score was unrelated to the level of sporting achievement, $F(3, 53) = 1.21$, $p = .314$, $\eta^2 = .07$. Of the current sample, 55 % identified themselves as current or former athletes in their chosen sport. An independent samples t-test revealed that CET Total Score was not associated with self-identification as a current or former athlete, $t(56) = .05$, $p = .965$, $d = .01$. Additionally, the general psychopathology profile of self-identified current or former athletes did not significantly differ from non-athletes: Y-EDEQ Global Score, $t(56) = .56$, $p = .579$, $d = .15$; RCADS Total Anxiety, $t(56) = -.12$, $p = .843$, $d = -.05$; RCADS Depression, $t(56) = .02$, $p = .983$, $d = .01$; and CHOCI-R Total Symptom, $t(56) = .29$, $p = .774$, $d = .08$.

Relationships between compulsive exercise and treatment variables

CET Total Score was not significantly associated with length of admission ($r = .20$, $p = .122$), percentage EBW at discharge ($r = .10$, $p = .438$), or readmission rate ($r = .09$, $p = .500$). A one-way ANOVA demonstrated statistically significant differences between the rates of medication prescription during admission to the treatment program according to the participant's CET Total Score, $F(3, 56) = 3.26$, $p = .028$, $\eta^2 = .17$. Planned contrasts suggested that participants who were prescribed no medication reported significantly lower levels of compulsive exercise than those prescribed any medication, $t(56) = 2.84$, $p = .006$, $g = 0.10$, with no significant differences between medication types (i.e., SSRIs, atypical antipsychotics, or both).

Associations between compulsive exercise and eating disorder symptomology and general psychopathology

As shown on Table 2, the CET Total Score was significantly associated with all measures of psychopathology and a measure of self-esteem in the expected directions. Of particular note were the significant relationships between the CET Avoidance subscale and all measures of the psychopathology and self-esteem. In contrast, the CET Mood Improvement subscale was not significantly correlated with any of these measures.

A multiple regression analysis was conducted, using CET Total Score as the outcome variable, to account for the possible shared variance between the key psychopathology measures that were selected as the predictor variables within the model. Multicollinearity was not diagnosed as a problem according to guidelines for variance inflation factors [52]. As shown on Table 3, the overall model was significant and accounted for 55 % of the CET Total Score's variance. Examination of the unique significant predictors identified that YEDE-Q Global Score and RCADS Total Anxiety were both significantly positively associated with CET Total Score once shared variance between the predictor variables was accounted for. Such results revealed that higher levels of compulsive exercise within an eating disorder inpatient sample are generally associated with increased levels of eating disorder psychopathology and anxiety. No significant associations were found between the CET Total Score and the predictor variables of RCADS Depression or CHOCI-R Total Symptom.

Discussion and conclusions

This study examined the psychopathological correlates of compulsive exercise in adolescent inpatients with AN. In support of initial hypotheses, the results demonstrated a general trend of higher levels of compulsive exercise reflecting increased psychopathology. Correlational analyses revealed increased eating disorder, depression, anxiety disorder, and obsessive compulsiveness symptomology, as well as decreased self-esteem associated with compulsive exercise.

These variables were then incorporated into a single regression model in order to assess the contribution of each variable while accounting for the shared variance. Consistent with the findings of a recent systematic review examining the psychopathological correlates of compulsive exercise in adolescents with an eating disorder [5], eating disorder symptomology and anxiety

Table 2 Pearson's correlations between measures of compulsive exercise and psychopathology measures

Measure		1	2	3	4	5	6	7	8	9	10	11	12	13	14	15	16	17	18	19
1	CET Total Score	-																		
2	CET avoidance	.93***	-																	
3	CET weight control exercise	.90***	.85***	-																
4	CET mood improvement	.31*	.27*	.08	-															
5	CET lack of exercise enjoyment	.37**	.24	.43**	-.43**	-														
6	CET exercise rigidity	.79***	.69***	.59***	.29*	-.01	-													
7	YEDE-Q restraint	.69***	**.63*** **	.78***	**.01**	.39**	.44***	-												
8	YEDE-Q eating concern	.65***	**.53*** **	.74***	**.04**	.45***	.38**	.82***	-											
9	YEDE-Q shape concern	.64***	**.60*** **	.72***	**-.01**	.36**	.40**	.81***	.79***	-										
10	YEDE-Q weight concern	.68***	**.64*** **	.74***	**.07**	.33*	.44***	.85***	.80***	.93***	-									
11	CHOCI-R total symptom	.49***	**.48*** **	.48***	**.06**	.25	.34**	.51***	.67***	.49***	.53***	-								
12	CHOCI-R total impairment	.51***	**.57*** **	.46***	**-.01**	.10	.49***	.41**	.35**	.44***	.46***	.51***	-							
13	RCADS SAD	.50***	**.52*** **	.57***	**.00**	.26**	.27**	.59***	.58***	.50***	.55***	.55***	.46***	-						
14	RCADS GAD	.61***	**.61*** **	.63***	**-.06**	.31**	.46***	.64***	.66***	.64***	.64***	.70***	.54***	.70***	-					
15	RCADS panic disorder	.65***	**.66*** **	.64***	**.03**	.27**	.49***	.67***	.67***	.69***	.70***	.73***	.59***	.60***	.80***	-				
16	RCADS social phobia	.68***	**.69*** **	.64***	**.11**	.28**	.50***	.67***	.70***	.76***	.77***	.66***	.49***	.57***	.65***	.71***	-			
17	RCADS obsessions compulsions	.50***	**.54*** **	.44***	**.08**	.19	.39**	.42**	.51***	.47***	.49***	.81***	.57***	.55***	.78***	.78***	.57***	-		
18	RCADS depression	.62***	**.60*** **	.73***	**-.12**	.42**	.37**	.74***	.67***	.77***	.79***	.55***	.57***	.65***	.74***	.80***	.65***	.62***	-	
19	RSES	-.63***	**-.66*** **	-.68***	**-.04**	-.28*	-.40**	-.71***	-.72***	-.81***	-.83***	-.60***	-.54***	-.59***	-.76***	-.74***	-.76***	-.61***	-.83***	-

CET compulsive exercise test, *YEDE-Q* youth eating disorder examination-questionnaire, *CHOCI-R* children's obsessional compulsive inventory-revised, *RCADS* revised child anxiety and depression scale, *GAD* generalized anxiety disorder, *SAD* separation anxiety disorder, *RSES* Rosenberg self esteem scale

Significance of the text in boldface (columns 2 and 4) is discussed in text

*p<.05, **p <.01, ***p <.001

Table 3 Multiple regression analysis of the relationship between compulsive exercise (outcome variable) and eating disorder and general psychopathology (predictor variables) in the current sample

Model	*F* (*df*)	R^2	Adj. R^2	β	*t*	*p* (2-sided)
1.	17.11 (4, 55)	.55	.52			<.001
YEDE-Q global score				.42	2.59	.012
RCADS total anxiety scale				.55	2.37	.021
RCADS MDD scale				-.08	-.43	.667
CHOCI-R total symptoms scale				-.15	-.93	.356

df degrees of freedom, *Adj.* adjusted, *YEDE-Q* youth eating disorder examination-questionnaire, *RCADS* revised child anxiety and depression scale, *MDD* major depressive disorder, *CHOCI-R* children's obsessional compulsive inventory-revised

were identified as significant unique predictors of compulsive exercise. Increased levels of compulsive exercise accompanying an increased severity of eating disorder symptomology is aligned with previous studies assessing this relationship in adolescents with AN who were inpatients [35], and adolescents with an eating disorder [36] or treatment seeking [37] at the time of assessment. This compounding effect compulsive exercise seems to pose to the overall eating disorder presentation is established in both the adolescent and adult literature [29–31]. Also concordant with past adolescent [35, 36] and adult [17, 30–32] research, participants who reported higher levels of compulsive exercise exhibited higher scores on a measure of anxiety symptomology. Taken together, the reliability and clinical significance of these associations emphasizes the need for compulsive exercise to be carefully assessed and considered in treatment decisions.

Of the assessed predictor variables, depression and obsessive compulsiveness symptomology were not significantly associated with compulsive exercise. Although higher depression scores have been linked to compulsive exercise in the adult literature [17, 32], this finding is yet to be reliably established in the adolescent research. To date inconsistent findings exist, with Stiles-Shields and colleagues [37] identifying a positive relationship and Holtkamp and colleagues' study [35] reporting no significant relationship. Both the current study and Holtkamp and colleagues [35] demonstrated no relationship between compulsive exercise and depression using similar analyses in which the shared variance was considered, whereas Stiles-Shields and colleagues' [37] conducted analyses that did not account for shared variance between the predictor variables. Moreover, the participants assessed in Holtkamp and colleagues' study [35] and the current study were comparable, while Stiles-Shields and colleagues [37] examined the relationship in a sample of adolescents that contained the three primary eating disorder diagnostic categories. Similar to the aforementioned literature on depression and compulsive exercise, the results in the current study pertaining to obsessive compulsiveness symptomology did not reflect the adolescent [10] and adult [30, 34] literature reporting a significant positive relationship with compulsive exercise. Once again, however, there is evidence to suggest that when the shared variance between psychopathological variables is accounted for, obsessive compulsiveness does not hold as a significant predictor of compulsive exercise in adolescent [35] or adult [32] eating disorder samples.

Going beyond the psychopathological risk profile of compulsive exercise in adolescent inpatients with eating disorders, the findings of the current study failed to reveal any effect of compulsive exercise on clinical characteristics (e.g., duration of illness, minimum reported weight, percentage EBW at admission) or treatment outcomes (e.g., length of admission, percentage EBW at discharge). These findings are inconsistent with past research that has found many poor treatment outcomes to be associated with compulsive exercise features in adults with AN [25, 26]. To the author's knowledge, only one study to date has specifically examined the influence of compulsive exercise on treatment outcomes for adolescents diagnosed with an eating disorder [28]. It therefore seems premature to derive any conclusions regarding the risks compulsive exercise may pose to treatment outcomes. Nevertheless, there remains a need for research to examine this relationship in order to assist with clarifying the diagnostic and prognostic profile of compulsive exercise in this young clinical population, and to further inform treatment efforts.

Of particular interest to treatment decisions, was the novel finding that participants who were prescribed no form of psychotropic medication throughout their inpatient admission reported significantly lower levels of compulsive exercise. Although the direction and underlying mechanism of this relationship is unable to be derived from the present data, this finding seems to support the increased severity of anxiety and eating disorder symptomology that is exhibited by participants reporting more severe compulsive exercise features. Particularly, the higher levels of agitation and arousal that may accompany the increased psychopathology may reflect the treatment team's decision to incorporate medication into the individual's treatment plan.

Consistent with previous research suggesting compulsive exercise is utilized to regulate and manage the individual's affective state [15–17], the current study found that the avoidance subscale of the compulsive exercise measure, which reflects the negative reinforcement value of exercise, was significantly associated with all of the psychopathology measures. In contrast, the mood improvement subscale that corresponds with the positive reinforcement value of exercise was not significantly associated with the psychopathology measures. This trend is consistent with results from a study that utilized the same measure of compulsive exercise within a nonclinical sample of young women [53], as well as evidence that negative affect regulation is the primary reinforcing factor and motivator for compulsive exercise [54, 55]. Although it has been suggested that compulsive exercise is maintained through both positive and negative reinforcement schedules [20, 21], such findings suggest that the role of avoiding or neutralizing internal distress through compulsive exercise is largely responsible for the pathological aspects of the behaviour. This finding reveals a possible treatment target in the management of compulsive exercise. Specifically, alternative and more functional methods for managing negative affective states could provide the individual with both short- and long-term benefits in terms of emotional regulation.

There were several strengths to this study, namely the use of an empirically derived and clinically sound measure of compulsive exercise thus avoiding the shortcomings of categorizing compulsive exercise according to arbitrary and inconsistent definitions. Additionally, key psychopathology variables were included within a single regression model to ascertain which measures were independent predictors of compulsive exercise while accounting for the shared variance. Replication of this model is required in order to determine its integrity in other samples.

A limitation of this study was that the exclusively female sample was comprised largely of individuals who met diagnostic criteria for AN and were inpatients actively engaged in treatment at the time of assessment. This compromises the generalizability of the findings, both in terms of extending the findings to males, other eating disorder diagnostic groups, as well as community samples of individuals with an eating disorder. The current study relied on retrospective data, particularly when assessing frequency of exercise engaged in over the previous 4 weeks and 1 year. This method of data collection is prone to recall bias [42], and individuals with AN have specifically been found to underreport the physical activity they have engaged in [53]. Results pertaining to retrospective assessment measures should therefore be interpreted with caution. The use of objective measures of physical activity, such as accelerometers, may have addressed these previously mentioned limitations. Such methods, however, are prone to compliance problems and may have adversely impacted upon recruitment, particularly in an adolescent population. Future studies may consider the use of objective measures; nevertheless, the compliance, recruitment, and attrition issues surrounding the use of such methods [56] warrant attention. Another limitation is the cross-sectional nature of the results, which precludes conclusions about causality and the temporal order of the identified relationships. Future research is indicated to replicate these findings utilizing a prospective design.

To conclude, the current findings suggest that adolescents with AN who endorse compulsive exercise traits have increased psychopathology, particularly eating disorder symptoms and anxiety. Such risks and the added strain of the physical activity itself can lead to or compound the physical and psychological consequences of the eating disorder. Clinical attention is therefore needed in the early detection of compulsive exercise, alongside further research to assist with the development of clinical practice guidelines and prevention programs.

Abbreviations

AN: anorexia nervosa; CET: compulsive exercise test; ChOCI-R: children's obsessional compulsive inventory-revised; DSM-5: diagnostic and statistical manual of mental disorders, fifth edition; EBW: expected body weight; EDE-Q: eating disorder examination-questionnaire; GAD: generalized anxiety disorder; MDD: major depressive disorder; OCD: obsessive compulsive disorder; RCADS: revised child anxiety and depression scale; RSES: Rosenberg self esteem scale; SAD: separation anxiety disorder; SSRIs: selective serotonin reuptake inhibitors; YEDE-Q: youth eating disorder examination-questionnaire.

Competing interests

ST and PH receive royalties from Hogrefe, and Huber and McGraw-Hill publishers for contributions on eating disorders. ST receives an honorarium from Shire Pharmaceuticals. PH received royalties form Oxford University Press and receives sessional fees and lecture fees from the Australian Medical Council, Therapeutic Guidelines publication, and New South Wales Institute of Psychiatry.

Authors' contributions

MN participated in the conceptualization of the study, conducted the majority of the data collection, the data analysis, as well as the writing of the manuscript. JM and SM participated in the conceptualization of the study, the data collection, and the editing of the manuscript. PH and ST participated in the conceptualization of the study and the editing of the manuscript. RC participated in the data analysis and the editing of the manuscript. All authors read and approved the final manuscript.

Acknowledgements

The authors thank the staff of the Eating Disorder Service, the Hospital School, and the Physiotherapy Department at The Children's Hospital at Westmead for providing support surrounding recruitment and data collection.

Author details

[1]School of Psychology, The University of Sydney, Sydney, Australia. [2]Eating Disorder Service at The Sydney Children's Hospitals Network, Westmead, Australia. [3]Westmead Clinical School, The University of Sydney, Sydney, Australia. [4]Department of Psychiatry and Behavioral Science, University of North Dakota School of Medicine and Health Sciences, Fargo, USA. [5]Neuropsychiatric Research Institute, Fargo, USA. [6]Centre for Health Research, School of Medicine, Western Sydney University, Penrith, Australia. [7]Discipline of Pediatrics, Faculty of Medicine, The University of Sydney, Sydney, Australia.

References

1. Hudson JI, Hiripi E, Pope HG, Kessler RC. The prevalence and correlates of eating disorders in the national comorbidity survey replication. Soc Biol Psychiatry. 2007;61:348–58.
2. Scott L, Van Blyderveen S. Physical activity recommendations for adolescents with anorexia nervosa: an existing protocol based on physical activity risk. Ment Health Phys Act. 2014;7:163–70.
3. Striegel-Moore RH, Bulik CM. Risk factors for eating disorders. Am Psychol. 2007;62:181–98.
4. Tremblay L, Lariviere M. The influence of puberty onset, body mass index, and pressure to be thin on disordered eating behaviours in children and adolescents. Eat Behav. 2009;10:75–83.
5. Fietz M, Touyz S, Hay P. A risk profile of compulsive exercise in adolescents with an eating disorder: a systematic review. Adv Eat Disord. 2014;2:241–63.
6. Meyer C, Taranis L. Exercise in the eating disorders. Terms and definitions. Eur Eat Disord Rev. 2011;19:169–73.
7. Holland LA, Brown TA, Keel PK. Defining features of unhealthy exercise associated with disordered eating and eating disorder diagnoses. Psychol Sport Exerc. 2014;15:116–23.
8. Taranis L, Touyz S, Meyer C. Disordered eating and exercise: development and preliminary validation of the Compulsive Exercise Test (CET). Eur Eat Disord Rev. 2011;19:256–68.
9. Davis C, Katzman DK, Kaptein S, Kirsh C, Brewer H, Kalmbach K, et al. The prevalence of high-level exercise in the eating disorders: etiological implications. Compr Psychiatry. 1997;38:321–26.
10. Davis C, Katzman DK, Kirsh C. Compulsive physical activity in adolescents with anorexia nervosa: a psychobehavioral spiral of pathology. J Nerv Ment Dis. 1999;187:336–42.
11. Machado PPP, Machado BC, Gonçalves S, Hoek HW. The prevalence of eating disorders not otherwise specified. Int J Eat Disord. 2007;40:212–17.
12. Stiles-Shields EC, Labuschagne Z, Goldschmidt AB, Doyle AC, Le Grange D. The use of multiple methods of compensatory behaviors as an indicator of eating disorder severity in treatment-seeking youth. Int J Eat Disord. 2012; 45:704–10.
13. Beumont PJV, Arthur B, Russel JD, Touyz SW. Excessive physical activity in dieting disorder patients: proposals for supervised exercise program. Int J Eat Disord. 1994;15:21–36.
14. Thien V, Thomas A, Markin D, Birmingham CL. Pilot study of a graded exercise program for the treatment of anorexia nervosa. Int J Eat Disord. 2000;28:101–6.
15. Meyer C, Taranis L, Goodwin H, Haycraft E. Compulsive exercise and eating disorders. Eur Eat Disord Rev. 2011;19:174–89.
16. Fairburn CG. Cognitive behavior therapy and eating disorders. New York: NY Guilford Press; 2008.
17. Penas-Lledo E, Vaz Leal FJ, Waller G. Excessive exercise in anorexia nervosa and bulimia nervosa: relation to eating characteristics and general psychopathology. Int J Eat Disord. 2002;31:370–5.
18. Davis C, Woodside DB. Sensitivity to the rewarding effects of food and exercise in the eating disorders. Compr Psychiatry. 2002;43:189–94.
19. Long CG, Smith J, Midgley M, Cassidy T. Over-exercising in anorexic and normal samples: behaviour and attitudes. J Ment Health. 1993;2:321–27.
20. Davis C. Exercise abuse. Int J Sport Psychol. 2000;31:278–89.
21. Goodman A. Addiction: definition and implications. Br J Addict. 1990;85:1402–8.
22. Giel KE, Kullmann S, Preißl H, Bischoff SC, Thiel A, Schmidt U, et al. Understanding the reward system functioning in anorexia nervosa: crucial role of physical activity. Biol Psychol. 2013;94:575–81.
23. Haddad FS, Bann S, Hill RA, Jones DH. Displaced stress fracture of the femoral neck in an active amenorrhoeic adolescent. Br J Sports Med. 1997;31:70–2.
24. Olivares JL, Vazquez M, Fleta J, Moreno LA, Perez-Gonzalez JM, Bueno M. Cardiac findings in adolescents with anorexia nervosa at diagnosis and after weight restoration. Eur J Pediatr. 2005;164:383–6.
25. Carter JC, Blackmore E, Sutandar-Pinnock K, Woodside DB. Relapse in anorexia nervosa: a survival analysis. Psychol Med. 2004;34:671–9.
26. Kaye WH, Gwirtsman HE, Obarzanek E, George DT. Relative importance of calorie intake needed to gain weight and level of physical activity in anorexia nervosa. Am J Clin Nutr. 1998;47:989–94.
27. Solenberger SE. Exercise and eating disorders: a 3-year inpatient hospital records analysis. Eat Behav. 2001;2:151–68.
28. Stiles-Shields C, Bamford B, Lock J, Le Grange D. The effect of driven exercise on treatment outcomes for adolescents with anorexia and bulimia nervosa. Int J Eat Disord. 2015;48:392–6.
29. Dalle Grave R, Calugi S, Marchesini G. Compulsive exercise to control shape or weight in eating disorders: prevalence, associated features and treatment outcome. Compr Psychiatry. 2008;49:346–52.
30. Shroff H, Reba L, Thornton LM, Tozzi F, Klump KL, Berretini WH, et al. Features associated with excessive exercise in women with eating disorders. Int J Eat Disord. 2006;39:454–61.
31. Brewerton TD, Stellefson EJ, Hibbs N, Hodges EL, Cochrane CE. Comparison of eating disorder patients with and without compulsive exercising. Int J Eat Disord. 1995;17:413–6.
32. Bewell-Weiss CV, Carter JC. Predictors of excessive exercise in anorexia nervosa. Compr Psychiatry. 2010;51:566–71.
33. Vansteelandt K, Rijmen F, Pieters G, Probst M, Vanderlinden J. Drive for thinness, affect regulation and physical activity in eating disorders: a daily life study. Behav Res Ther. 2007;45:1717–34.
34. Davis C, Kaptein S, Kaplan AS, Olmsted MP, Woodside DB. Obsessionality in anorexia nervosa: the moderating influence of exercise. Psychosom Med. 1998;60:192–7.
35. Holtkamp K, Hebebrand J, Herpertz-Dahlmann B. The contribution of anxiety and food restriction on physical activity levels in acute anorexia nervosa. Int J Eat Disord. 2004;36:163–71.
36. Madison JK, Ruma SL. Exercise and athletic involvement as moderators of severity in adolescents with eating disorders. J Appl Sport Psychol. 2003;15:213–22.
37. Stiles-Shields EC, Goldschmidt AB, Boepple L, Glunz C, Le Grange D. Driven exercise among treatment-seeking youth with eating disorders. Eat Behav. 2011;12:328–31.
38. Madden S, Miskovic-Whealtey J, Wallis A, Kohn M, Lock J, Le Grange D, et al. A randomized controlled trial of in-patient treatment for anorexia nervosa in medically unstable adolescents. Psychol Med. 2015;45:415–27.
39. American Psychiatric Association. Diagnostic and statistical manual of mental disorders. 5th ed. Washington: American Psychiatric Association; 2013.
40. Kuczmarski RJ, Ogden CL, Grummer-Strawn LM, Flegal KM, Guo SS, Wei R, et al. CDC growth charts: United States. Adv Data. 2000;8:1–27.
41. Goodwin H, Haycraft E, Taranis L, Meyer C. Psychometric evaluation of the Compulsive Exercise Test (CET) in an adolescent population: links with eating psychopathology. Eur Eat Disord Rev. 2011;19:269–79.
42. Davis C, Kennedy SH, Ralevski E, Dionne M. The role of physical activity in the development and maintenance of eating disorders. Psychol Med. 1994; 24:957–67.
43. Goldschmidt AB, Doyle AC, Wilfley DE. Assessment of binge eating in overweight youth using a questionnaire version of the child eating disorder examination with instructions. Int J Eat Disord. 2007;40:460–67.
44. Fairburn CG, Beglin SJ. Assessment of eating disorders: interview or self-report questionnaire? Int J Eat Disord. 1994;16:363–70.
45. Chorpita BF, Yim L, Moffitt C, Umemoto LA, Francis SE. Assessment of symptoms of DSM-IV anxiety and depression in children: a revised child and depression scale. Behav Res Ther. 2000;38:835–55.
46. Chorpita BF, Moffitt C, Gray J. Psychometric properties of the revised child anxiety and depression scale in a clinical sample. Behav Res Ther. 2005;43:309–22.
47. Shafran R, Frampton I, Heyman I, Reynolds M, Teachman B, et al. The preliminary development of a new self-report measure for OCD in young people. J Adolesc. 2003;26:137–42.
48. Uher R, Heyman I, Turner C, Shafran R. Self-, parent-report and interview measures of obsessive-compulsive disorder in children and adolescents. J Anxiety Disord. 2007;22:979–90.
49. Rosenberg M. Conceiving the self. New York: Basic Books; 1979.
50. Fleming JS, Courtney BE. The dimensionality of self-esteem: II. Hierarchical facet model for revised measurements scales. J Pers Soc Psychol. 1984;46:404–21.
51. Field A. Discovering statistics using SPSS. 3rd ed. London: Sage; 2009.
52. Hair JF, Anderson RE, Tatham RL, Black WC. Multivariate data analysis. 3rd ed. New York: Macmillan; 1995.
53. Taranis L, Meyer C. Associations between specific components of compulsive exercise and eating disordered cognitions and behaviors among women. Int J Eat Disord. 2011;44:452–8.

54. BratlandSanda S, SundgotBorgen J, Rø Ø, Rosenvinge JH, Hoffart A, Martinesen EW. Physical activity and exercise dependence during inpatient treatment of longstanding eating disorders: an exploratory study of excessive and nonexcessive exercisers. Int J Eat Disord. 2010;43:266–73.
55. Geller J, Cockell SJ, Goldner EM. Inhibited expression of negative emotions and interpersonal orientation in anorexia nervosa. Int J Eat Disord. 2000;28:8–19.
56. Gümmer R, Giel KE, Schag K, Resmark G, Junne FP, Becker S, et al. High levels of physical activity in anorexia nervosa: a systematic review. Eur Eat Disord Rev. 2015;23:333–44.

Socio-cultural context of eating disorders in Poland

Maciej Wojciech Pilecki[1*], Kinga Sałapa[2†] and Barbara Józefik[3†]

Abstract

Background: The goal of this study was to assess the relationship between sociocultural factors and clinical eating disorders during the intensive process of Westernisation in Poland that occurred after 1989. The study population included girls diagnosed with an eating disorder according to DSM-IV criteria ($n = 47$ anorexia nervosa restrictive type [ANR], $n = 16$ anorexia binge/purge type [ANBP], $n = 34$ bulimia nervosa [BN], $n = 19$ eating disorder not otherwise specified [EDNOS]) who received consultation for the first time between 2002 and 2004 in the Department of Clinical Child and Adolescent Psychiatry, University Hospital, Kraków, Poland. The study included an age-matched normal control group [NOR] of 85 schoolgirls from Kraków.

Methods: Relationships between two given qualitative features were investigated using the chi-square test or Fisher's exact test. Correspondence analysis was applied to graphically explore the relationship. The Kruskal-Wallis test with the Bonferroni was performed to compare quantitative results across groups.

Results: Objective sociodemographic variables and responses to the 62-item Questionnaire of Socio-cultural Context were measured. The mothers of ANBP and BN patients were less professionally active than mothers of ANR patients and NOR subjects. Subjective socio-cultural factors were more relevant for the BN group than the ANR group. Questionnaire responses in the ANBP group were more similar to those in the BN group than to those in the ANR group. The most unambiguous and specific characteristic of the ANR group was a sense of belonging to the middle class. Variables that differentiated the BN group from the NOR group included the importance attached to thinness treated as an expression of power and control over one's self, as well as a multifaceted negative evaluation of one's own family, including a negative assessment of the position of women and parental lack of concern for appearance and principles of nutrition. All patients, regardless of diagnosis, identified with other people with similar problems and considered anorexia and bulimia to be a major issue of their generation and social environment.

Conclusions: The results of this first in Poland exploratory study of socio-cultural context of eating disorders indicate the importance of both objective and subjective socio-cultural factors in eating disorders in the group studied.

Keywords: Anorexia nervosa, Bulimia nervosa, Westernisation, Culture

Background

Socio-cultural context is acknowledged as an important risk factor for the development and specificity of clinical eating disorders [EDs] [1, 2].

Although EDs are not exclusive to contemporary Western culture, process of Westernisation in Japan after the Second World War and in countries of the former Eastern Bloc after the lifting of the Iron Curtain is accompanied by the increase of EDs prevalence in this countries [3, 4]. The same applies for the process of acculturation and over-identification to the occurrence of EDs after immigration to countries of Western culture [5] or changes in race identity within the sphere of Western countries [6, 7]. In this context, EDs are sometimes referred to as culture-bound syndromes [8].

Over the years, the dominant view has been that the highest risk of EDs occurs among girls that attend private schools in large cities and that come from families who place a high value on achievement and adaptability [9, 10]. Currently, however, it is difficult to discern a

* Correspondence: maciej.pilecki@uj.edu.pl
†Equal contributors
[1]Department of Child and Adolescent Psychiatry, Jagiellonian University Medical College, ul. Kopernika 21a, 31-501 Kraków, Poland
Full list of author information is available at the end of the article

clear relationship between the occurrence of EDs and the social class of patients, and studies of different populations (e.g. clinical, community) contradict each other [11]. This may be due to recent expansion of the disease across different social strata [12], or to erroneous conclusions in the initial stages of research that relied on the analysis of data collected from private clinics, which would have been attended by only rich patients [4, 13]. Social class may be significant not only as a risk factor, but also as a factor in the course of EDs [14].

More conclusive evidence of the importance of cultural context in EDs is provided by research that has looked for mechanisms linking general characteristics of Western culture with the risk of EDs occurring in specific individuals. Socio-cultural pressure to be thin is a relevant risk factor for EDs that acts on an individual level [15]. Experimental findings have confirmed that the perceived pressure to be thin and the internalisation of the thin ideal is a causal risk factor for body dissatisfaction, dieting, negative affect and eating pathology [16, 17]. Body preoccupation and the fear of weight gain correspond with the above phenomena and are also a significant risk factor for eating problems [17, 18].

Although the importance of thin ideal can be observed in different cultures, it is notably associated with Western culture values [19]. It may be responsible for dieting, even in the absence of body dissatisfaction, as the result of a desire to adapt to applicable standards [15]. Researchers suggest that the construction of an ideal body has become mandatory for modern women and cause a deep sense of imperfections of one's own body and a sense of guilt and shame [20–22]. From this perspective, thinness may be regarded as a body modification specific to Western culture [23, 24].

Mass media, family communication and the peer group all have an important impact on the construction of the sociocultural pressure to be thin [25–29]. Many studies have shown that mass media is an important element influencing body dissatisfaction [30], or at least awareness and attention to one's body [31, 32]. However, assigning a significant role to media exposure may provide too narrow a view of the problem. Mass media can exert influence through complementary stimuli, for example, the confrontation of one's own body with the bodies of models seen in advertisements, participation in the lives of celebrities through social media and celebrity gossip portals, coveting things advertised by models.

EDs have become a separate aspect of mass culture. They have gained independent, culture-forming significance as Internet phenomena such as *Thinspiration*, *Pro-ana* and *Mia* [33–35]. One may wonder about the importance of cultural factors as risk factors, or at the very least maintenance factors, in the development of AN and BN.

Some research confirms the importance parental attitudes towards body standards and weight loss on the development of an eating pathology [27, 36], especially the critical comments of loved ones on body shape, weight and food [37]. However, there is an absence of convincing evidence that this dependency, which has been confirmed in the general population, is significant as a risk factor for EDs [25, 29]. On the other hand, EDs in mothers do constitute an important factor for development of eating pathology in daughter [38].

Persons who constitute a peer group frequently have similar problems associated with their relationship to their bodies and their dietary behaviour [39] Peer group can have a significant impact on body image, dieting attitudes and eating pathology, especially among individuals with BN [29], and that the influence of peers is one of the strongest cultural factors correlated with body dissatisfaction [28].

Despite some doubts about the importance of culture in EDs, some of its aspects appear to be an important risk factor [40]. However, it should be noted that the majority of convincing empirical studies address socio-cultural risk factors for binge eating and symptoms of bulimia or general symptoms of eating pathology, rather than symptoms of anorexia [15]. The importance of cultural factors in the development of EDs has been confirmed in prospective studies [41], and indirect confirmation has been provided by the development of effective prevention programs [42]. However, it is not clear why, despite much evidence supporting the significance of socio-cultural pressure on women to be thin in the aetiology of EDs, relatively few women living in contemporary Western cultures are affected by EDs [43].

Countries in the former Eastern Bloc, such as Poland, pose an interesting problem for the role of sociocultural context in development of EDs. Clinical cases of eating disorders prior to political change of 1989 were rare. Prevalence of eating disorders in general population was not studied, or methodology of this studies is unknown or unreliable [4, 44]. After 1989 EDs have become one of the most common mental disorders faced by young girls in Poland [45]. In Rathner's opinion, countries of the former Eastern Bloc undergoing Westernisation are challenged with "first, the transition to capitalism with all the imponderables of early capitalist accumulation within a few years, and second, the immediate confrontation with globalisation and modernisation with their attendant disruptions" ([4], p. 94). One may assume that the socio-cultural connotations of these disorders in Poland may differ from those observed in Western countries, where they have been observed and studied much longer [46]. Significant differences may include the low percentage of patients diagnosed with EDs in earlier generations, the ethnic coherence of the contemporary Polish population, very low immigration, the high percentage of persons of the Catholic faith, the dynamic process of political transformation and major class-related changes after 1989, as well as other meanings attributed to body weight and shape in the generations raised in communist Poland [46–48]. The dynamic development of the media from 1989 up to the beginning of the 21st century may also be an important factor. During this time, Poland recorded a three-fold increase in the number of press titles to more than 6000 and an increase from two to 80 television stations, and witnessed the dynamic growth of the Internet [49, 50], including the emergence of phenomena related to the *Pro-ana* and *Mia* movements [51].

The aims of this research were to investigate socio-cultural risk factors for ED previously identified in Western societies, now within a Polish context. The study focused on objective measures of the socio-demographic situation of patients and the self-rated importance of socio-cultural context.

Methods

The presented research was a part of a larger research project entitled "Socio-cultural, familial, and individual factors in anorexia and bulimia nervosa", which was financed by a scientific grant from the State Committee for Scientific Research (Grant Number: 6 POSE 09021).

Participants

The study was conducted between 2002 and 2004 on a group of teenage female patients who presented with an ED for the first time to the Child and Adolescent Psychiatry Clinic of the University Hospital in Krakow. The parents of the enrolled patients also participated. Patients and their parents were asked to fill in questionnaires used in the study. EDs diagnoses, based on clinical interview, were made according to DSM-IV criteria [52]. No one refused to participate in the study. Patients with uncertain diagnosis (20 persons), mentally handicapped (4 persons) and being in foster care (10 persons) were not included in the study.

The study included 47 female patients with restrictive anorexia nervosa [ANR], 16 patients with binge/purge anorexia [ANBP], 34 patients with bulimia nervosa (BN) and 19 patients with an eating disorder not otherwise specified [EDNOS]. The study also included an age-matched control group (NOR) of 85 girls (and theirs parents) from Krakow schools. Schools were selected based on a stratified sampling of all the Krakow schools. All chosen schools were public. Voluntary participation in the study was proposed during parent-teachers nights.

Assessment

The objective socio-demographic situation was quantified using family structure, age, education and employment status of parents. The cultural factors were evaluated using the statements' form Questionnaire of Socio-Cultural Context (QSCC) designed by M. Pilecki and B. Józefik [53, 54]. The QSCC consists of 62 statements related to the respondent's views and beliefs on issues that are considered significant cultural risk factors in the development and course of ED, and included statements of Polish specificity (Table **1**). The statements are presented in a random order and responses are made using a six-point Likert scale ranging from 1 (the statement does not apply to me at all) to 6 (the statement describes me very well).

Statistical analysis

Categorical results are presented as number and percentage. Relationships between two given categorical features were investigated using the chi-square test or Fisher's exact test in case of insufficient theoretical size. The decomposition of chi-squre test was applied in case of significant results to give a better understanding of the relationship between the two variables. A contingency table which gives rise to a chi-square with p degrees of freedom were decomposed into as many as p smaller tables. Quantitative results, such as the girls' age and questionnaire responses are presented as mean ± standard deviation, median (lower, Q_1, and upper, Q_3, quartile) and minimum and maximum value. Those data were compared across groups (NOR, ANR, ANBP, BN, EDNOS) using the Kruskal-Wallis test due to the lack of normality in case of the age and the overall QSCC scores or due to the ordinal scale of responses of each item. The Shapiro-Wilk test was used to assess normality. In this case the Bonferroni correction was applied to resolve the problem of multiple testing and of finding at least one significant result just due to chance. The significance level was adjusted by the number of tests corresponding with the number of analysed items and the cut-off point was set to be less than .0001.

In any other case p value < .05 was considered statistically significant. The analyses were performed using SPSS Statistics v.21 (IBM, New York, USA).

Ethics

The study was approved by the Bioethics Commission UJ CM No: KBET/26/B/2001.

Results

The percentage of patients with complete and incomplete families was significantly different across groups (p = .013, Fisher's exact test, Table **2**). The proportion of girls with complete families was higher in the control group than in the other groups. Significant differences were observed between median of patients' age (p = .022, Kruskal-Wallis test, Table **2**). The post-hoc test showed that the ANR group (16.34 (15.0–18.0)

Table 1 Items in the Questionnaire of Socio-Cultural Context

1. A person should control his various weaknesses.
2. It is important to the members of my family that we be "up-to-date".
3. **I know many people who have problems with food.**
4. Sex is decidedly a much more enjoyable experience for men than for women.
5. **The principles governing my family could be a model for others.**
6. **In my social circles, appearance is crucial to a successful social life.**
7. **Anorexia and bulimia nervosa are an important issue nowadays.**
8. Currently, fashion sets the rules of conduct in many areas.
9. **It can happen that I carry on an internal struggle with myself.**
10. **Women in my family do not have an easy life.**
11. We live in times when people are guided more by their own interests than, for example, loyalty and friendship.
12. **When I see a thin model, I feel fat and unattractive.**
13. **A slim figure may sometimes help more in life than high intelligence.**
14. **If someone is not able to control how much and what they eat, they are not able to control anything at all.**
15. Lately, everything is changing so fast, it is difficult to keep up.
16. **To be more attractive, I should be skinnier.**
17. **My mother has a more difficult life than my father does.**
18. **I am jealous of a model's slim appearance.**
19. Boys can be themselves to a greater degree than girls can.
20. **My father pays attention to his figure.**
21. Often, an attractive appearance can only be achieved through hard work on your body.
22. I am sometimes guided in my decisions by advertisements.
23. In life, you should be striving for perfection.
24. **Anorexia and bulimia are a problem of my generation.**
25. My father attaches great importance to his external appearance.
26. In today's times, it is difficult to be yourself in relations with boys.
27. I am religious person.
28. **Sometimes, I do not know what is appropriate and what not in relations with others.**
29. **I try to eat "healthy food".**
30. **My greatest desire is to know how to control my life.**
31. **My mother pays attention to her figure.**
32. I believe that my family is materially better off than other families.
33. **Currently, fashionable clothing is tailored so that only thin girls can fit into it.**
34. People who devote themselves to others are fools.
35. **If I could get my weight lower or higher by a few kilograms, my female classmates would immediately notice.**
36. **A woman should strive to have a profession that allows her to be independent.**
37. **Sometimes I succumb to the temptations of my body.**
38. In my social circle, friendliness is what decides your social success.
39. **What my family considers delicious food is unhealthy in my opinion.**
40. I believe that observing fasts for religious reasons has deep meaning.
41. **True excellence is the ability to have full control over all your feelings.**
42. **When I hear about people who have problems with eating, such as anorexia and bulimia, I understand them very well.**
43. Religion is very important in the life of my family.
44. In the world of film and fashion, there are people I would like to resemble.
45. Sometimes it seems to me that there is a large gap between how my parents think and how my grandparents think.
46. It has happened that I have allowed my decisions to be guided by the tastes of well-known models and actresses.
47. Intuition directs us better than logic and planning.
48. Adjusting to today's times requires a great deal of effort on the part of my family.
49. Healthy competition can be fun.50. It happens that others are jealous of my good grades.
51. I know at least a few people that are trying to lose weight.
52. Faith does not have great significance for me.
53. **The opinion of others is very important to members of my family.**
54. Sons have it easier in Polish families than daughters.
55. **I feel that my peers pay attention to how much I eat.**
56. If I am not successful in life, my parents will be disappointed.
57. My mother attaches great importance to her external appearance.
58. Food advertisements are the most difficult to resist.
59. I learn more about how to live from my father than my mother.
60. We will be punished for our sins.
61. **My family belongs to the "middle-class".**
62. **If pregnancy were to make my body less attractive, then I would give some thought to whether I want to have any children at all.**

Items statistically differed between groups are presented in bold

years) differed significantly from the BN group (17.53 (17.0–18.0) years) ($p = .013$).

Maternal and paternal age did not differ significantly between the groups ($p = .570$ and $p = .154$, respectively, Fisher's exact test, Table **2**). Likewise, maternal and paternal level of education did not differ significantly between groups ($p = .740$ and $p = .317$, respectively, Fisher's exact test; Table **2**).

The percentage of patients living in villages, small towns and large cities was significantly different across groups

Table 2 Socio-demographic characteristics of patient and control groups

		NOR	ANR	ANBP	BN	EDNOS	*p*-value
Number		85	47	16	34	19	
Age (years)	mean ± SD	17.00 ± 1.59	16.34 ± 1.58	16.75 ± 1.29	17.53 ± .96	17.0 ± 1.37	.022
	Q1-Q3	17 (16–18)	16 (15–18)	17 (15.25–18)	17.5 (17–18)	17 (16-18)	
	min-max	13–19	13–19	15–18	15–20	15–19	
	n	85	47	16	34	19	
No. of families with both biological parents		70 (89.7 %)	34 (72.3 %)	12 (75.0 %)	21 (63.3 %)	15 (83.3 %)	.013
n		78	47	16	33	18	
Mother's age	<35 years	2 (2.4 %)	1 (2.1 %)	1 (6.3 %)	1 (2.9 %)	0 (0 %)	.570
	36–45 years	48 (57.8 %)	29 (61.7 %)	9 (56.3 %)	25 (73.5 %)	14 (73.7 %)	
	46–55 years	31 (37.3 %)	13 (27.7 %)	6 (37.5 %)	8 (23.5 %)	5 (26.3 %)	
	>56 years	2 (2.4 %)	4 (8.5 %)	0 (0 %)	0 (0 %)	0 (0 %)	
	n	83	47	16	34	19	
Father's age	<35 years	0 (0 %)	0 (0 %)	1 (7.7 %)	1 (4.0 %)	0 (0 %)	.154
	36–45 years	28 (35.0 %)	17 (43.6 %)	3 (23.1 %)	14 (56.0 %)	9 (50.0 %)	
	46–55 years	45 (56.3 %)	20 (51.3 %)	9 (69.2 %)	8 (32.0 %)	9 (50.0 %)	
	>56 years	7 (8.8 %)	2 (5.1 %)	0 (0 %)	2 (8.0 %)	0 (0 %)	
	n	80	39	13	25	18	
Mother's education level	Primary	14 (16.9 %)	7 (25.9 %)	3 (18.8 %)	8 (25.0 %)	2 (11.1 %)	.740
	Secondary	41 (49.4 %)	16 (36.4 %)	8 (50.0 %)	12 (37.5 %)	10 (55.6 %)	
	Higher	28 (33.7 %)	21 (29.6 %)	5 (31.3 %)	12 (37.5 %)	6 (33.3 %)	
	n	83	44	16	32	18	
Father's education level	Primary	20 (27.8 %)	10 (27.8 %)	7 (53.8 %)	12 (50.0 %)	6 (35.3 %)	.317
	Secondary	26 (36.1 %)	14 (38.9 %)	2 (15.4 %)	7 (29.2 %)	8 (47.1 %)	
	Higher	26 (36.1 %)	12 (33.3 %)	4 (30.8 %)	5 (20.8 %)	3 (17.6 %)	
	n	72	36	13	24	17	
Place of residence	Village	13 (16.5 %)	13 (31.0 %)	3 (18.8 %)	10 (32.3 %)	4 (26.7 %)	<.001
	Small town	5 (6.3 %)	14 (33.3 %)	9 (56.3 %)	9 (29.0 %)	5 (33.3 %)	
	Large city	61 (77.2 %)	15 (35.7 %)	4 (25.0 %)	12 (38.7 %)	6 (40.0 %)	
	n	79	42	16	31	15	
Mother's professional circumstance	Employed	69 (84.1 %)	36 (81.8 %)	8 (50.0 %)	21 (65.6 %)	16 (88.9 %)	.031
	Pension	3 (3.7 %)	2 (4.5 %)	3 (18.8 %)	6 (18.8 %)	0 (0 %)	
	Retired	0 (0 %)	2 (4.5 %)	0 (0 %)	0 (0 %)	0 (0 %)	
	Unemployed	7 (8.5 %)	2 (4.5 %)	4 (25.0 %)	4 (12.5 %)	2 (11.1 %)	
	Other	3 (3.7 %)	2 (4.5 %)	1 (6.3 %)	1 (3.1 %)	0 (0 %)	
	n	82	44	16	32	18	
Father's professional circumstance	Employed	58 (81.7 %)	29 (87.9 %)	8 (72.7 %)	19 (86.4 %)	17 (94.4 %)	.435
	Pension	3 (4.2 %)	2 (6.1 %)	0 (0 %)	1 (4.5 %)	0 (0 %)	
	Retired	2 (2.8 %)	0 (0 %)	0 (0 %)	2 (9.1 %)	0 (0 %)	
	Unemployed	7 (9.9 %)	1 (3.0 %)	3 (27.3 %)	0 (0 %)	1 (5.6 %)	
	Other	1 (1.4 %)	1 (3.0 %)	0 (0 %)	0 (0 %)	0 (0 %)	
	n	71	33	11	22	18	

Quantitative data are presented as mean ± SD, median (interquartile range) and min–max value. Qualitative data as N (%)
Abbreviations: *NOR* controls, *ANR* anorexia nervosa restrictive type, *ANBP* anorexia binge/purge type, *BN* bulimia nervosa, *EDNOS* eating disorder not otherwise specified

($p < .001$, chi-square test, Table **2**). Most patients in the BN and ANR groups lived in a rural village (ca. 30 %), the most patients in the ANBP groups lived in a small town (ca. 56 %), and the most controls lived in Krakow, a large city (ca. 77 %). The proportion of mothers who were living on a pension, retired or unemployed was significantly different across groups ($p = .031$, Fisher's exact test; Table **2**). In all groups, the vast majority of mothers worked (81–89 % in the NOR, ANR and EDNOS groups, 66 % in the BN group and 50 % in the ANBP group). The proportion of fathers who were living on a pension, retired or unemployed was not significantly different across groups ($p = .435$, Fisher's exact test; Table **2**).

29 of the 62 items on the QSCC were able to statistically distinguish between groups. Those items are shown in bold in Table **1**, whereas descriptive statistics of the items with results of post-hoc tests are presented in Table 3.

Discussion

The aim of this study was to assess the relationship between the clinical characteristics of EDs and socio-cultural factors in Poland. We considered factors that objectively describe the socio-economic status of patients as well as the importance that patients attached to various culture aspects described as important risk factors for the development and course of EDs. This is the first exploratory study of socio-cultural aspects of Eds in Poland and one of the firsts in Eastern Europe.

Objective descriptors of social affiliation did not distinguish girls with EDs from the control group. An important source of potential bias is the recruitment of the control group from female high school students in Krakow. The girls in the EDs groups more frequently came from villages and small towns. This may mean that living in smaller populated areas, for some reason, may be connected with the significant cultural risk of developing eating disorders in Poland. Other possibility is that girls from larger cities, especially Krakow, have access to private healthcare. Althought interpreting this result is not simple. It does not necessarily define a different membership to social groups of people living in various areas. After the year 1989, living in the countryside or in a smaller town may be a social advancement and moving to a detached house build outside large urban agglomerations may be interpreted as such. There was a significant difference in the professional activity of mothers across different diagnoses. The proportion of mothers that worked was lower in the BN and ANBP groups than in the NOR and ANR groups. The most common reason for the lack of professional activity was a pension. The comparatively higher percentage of single parent families, especially in the patients with BN, may indicate a significant level of socio-economic crisis in this families. An objective analysis of the family situation does not allow clear conclusions regarding social class and the occurrence of EDs. However, our patients tended to come from a particular group. According to Central Statistical Office of Poland in 2002, 9.3 % of men and 10.4 % of women in Poland had higher education, 30.1 % of men and 16.9 % of women had basic vocational training, and 28 % of men and 31.4 % of women had primary education [55]. Compared to these sociological data, the education level of the parents of our patients was higher than average, with an over-representation of parents having a high level of education and an under-representation of those with vocational and primary education. This confirms data from research from other countries [11].

Only a subset of the QSCC variables significantly distinguished patients with EDs from the control group. The NOR group was distinguishable from the BN group by the greatest number of items (23), whereas the ANR group was distinguishable from NOR by 7 items, and ANBP and EDNOS by 9.

A negative assessment of the dietary rules prevailing in the family house in comparison with control group (item 39 on the QSCC) was common to all the girls with EDs diagnosis. For the BN and ANR groups, this was associated with the belief that the father cared very little about his figure (item 20). In the EDNOS group, a similar relationship was observed with respect to mothers (item 31). One possible interpretation is that the patients came from homes where diet and appearance were not important. Given Poland's history, it does not mean that the patients came from families of a lower social class. The parents of the patients grew up in communist Poland. The early 1980s was a time of deep economic crisis in Poland, with rationing of food and a chronic shortage of supplies. Therefore, the relationship that people of this generation have with food has been subject to the same processes as any society emerging from poverty and shortage, where obesity, once a signifier of high economic status, becomes a symbol of poverty and backwardness. This change is slower in men than in women [56].

A focus on eating and appearance may also be the result of patient attitudes that are not shared by their parents. In the BN group, in particular, the meaning ascribed to thinness may be an expression of an attempt to distinguish oneself from one's parents and not follow them. In addition, the response of the patients may not be an objective perception of parental attitudes, but rather an expression of strict standards and rules these girls apply to their diets and their personal hygiene. No interviews were conducted during the study to determine the real attitudes of parents. However, the studied mothers achieved very low scores in the EAT26 test, indicating an absence of problems with eating and their relationship to their own bodies, although this did include a lack of interest in

Table 3 Descriptive characteristics of items that differ significantly between groups

Item	NOR	ANR	ANBP	BUL	EDNOS	*p* value*
3	2.96 ± 1.45	3.07 ± 1.60	3.36 ± 1.45	4.03 ± 1.66	3.33 ± 1.68	NOR–BN p = .030
	3 (2–4)	3 (2–4)	3 (2–5)	4 (2.5–6)	3.5 (2–5)	
	1–6	1–6	1–6	1–6	1–6	
5	3.78 ± 1.41	3.17 ± 1.27	2.53 ± 1.25	2.71 ± 1.53	2.72 ± 1.45	NOR–BN p = .005 NOR–ANBP p = .033
	4 (3–5)	3 (2–4)	3 (1–4)	3 (1–4)	3 (1–4)	
	1–6	1–6	1–4	1–6	1–6	
6	3.14 ± 1.42	2.74 ± 1.35	3.67 ± 1.29	3.61 ± 1.45	3.94 ± 1.52	NOR–BN p = .005 NOR–ANBP p = .033
	3 (2–4)	2.5 (2–4)	4 (3–5)	3 (2–5)	4 (3–5)	
	1–6	1–6	1–6	1–6	1–6	
7	4.49 ± 1.52	5.30 ± 1.04	5.0 ± 1.25	5.45 ± 0.77	5.28 ± 0.75	NOR–ANR p = .010 NOR–BN p = .011
	5 (3–6)	6 (5–6)	5 (5–6)	6 (5–6)	5 (5–6)	
	1–6	2–6	1–6	3–6	4–6	
9	4.07 ± 1.52	4.72 ± 1.22	5.33 ± 1.05	5.45 ± 1.09	4.94 ± 1.47	NOR–ANBP p = .010 NOR–BN p < .001
	4 (3–5)	5 (4–6)	6 (5–6)	6 (5–6)	5.5 (4–6)	
	1–6	2–6	3–6	1–6	1–6	
10	2.58 ± 1.53	3.17 ± 1.56	3.53 ± 1.46	4.26 ± 1.69	3.67 ± 1.24	NOR–BN p < .001
	2 (1–4)	3 (2–4)	4 (3–5)	5 (3–6)	3.5 (3–4.25)	
	1–6	1–6	1–6	1–6	2–6	
12	3.38 ± 1.64	3.19 ± 1.76	5.07 ± 1.39	4.84 ± 1.44	4.67 ± 1.50	ANR–BN p = .001 ANR–ANBP p = .002 ANR-EDNOS p = .026 NOR–BN p = .001 NOR–ANBP p = .004 NOR-EDNOS p = .043
	3 (2–5)	3 (1–5)	6 (5–6)	5 (4–6)	5 (4–6)	
	1–6	1–6	2–6	1–6	1–6	
13	3.77 ± 1.40	3.28 ± 1.52	5.07 ± 1.39	4.03 ± 1.56	4.44 ± 1.58	ANR-EDNOS p = .048
	4 (3–5)	3 (2–4)	6 (5–6)	4 (3–5)	5 (3.75–6)	
	1–6	1–6	2–6	1–6	1–6	
14	2.78 ± 1.19	2.58 ± 1.22	3.73 ± 1.67	4.0 ± 1.59	4.28 ± 1.41	ANR–BN p = .001 ANR–EDNOS p = .001 NOR–BN p = .002 NOR–EDNOS p = .002
	3 (2–4)	3 (2–3)	3 (2–5)	4 (3–5)	4 (3–6)	
	1–6	1–5	1–6	1–6	1–6	
16	3.46 ± 1.75	2.50 ± 1.49	4.07 ± 1.79	4.74 ± 1.46	4.50 ± 1.79	ANR–NOR p = .049 ANR–ANBP p = .037 ANR–EDNOS p = .001 ANR–BN p < .001 NOR–BN p = .010
	3 (2–5)	2 (1–4)	4 (2–6)	5 (4–6)	5 (3.5–6)	
	1–6	1–6	1–6	1–6	1–6	
17	2.91 ± 1.69	3.10 ± 1.99	4.13 ± 1.41	4.29 ± 1.72	3.82 ± 1.85	NOR–BN p = .005

Table 3 Descriptive characteristics of items that differ significantly between groups *(Continued)*

	3 (1–4)	3 (1–5)	4 (3–6)	4 (3–6)	4 (2–5.5)	
	1–6	1–6	2–6	1–6	1–6	
18	3.42 ± 1.72	3.09 ± 1.57	4.73 ± 1.53	4.77 ± 1.67	4.72 ± 1.74	ANR–ANBP p = .017 ANR–BN p < .001 ANR-EDNOS p = .008 NOR–BN p = .002 NOR-EDNOS p = .043
	3 (2–5)	3 (1–4)	5 (4–6)	6 (4–6)	5.5 (3–6)	
	1–6	1–6	1–6	1–6	1–6	
20	2.78 ± 1.45	2.14 ± 1.52	2.0 ± 1.0	1.77 ± 1.04	1.94 ± 1.09	NOR–BN p = .006 NOR–ANR p = .044
	3 (2–4)	1 (1–3)	2 (1–3)	1 (1–2.25)	2 (1–3)	
	1–6	1–6	1–4	1–4	1–4	
24	3.961.45	4.60 ± 1.50	4.80 ± 1.37	5.13 ± 1.31	4.83 ± 1.54	NOR–BN p = .001
	4 (3–5)	5 (3–6)	5 (4–6)	6 (5–6)	5.5 (4–6)	
	1–6	1–6	1–6	1–6	1–6	
28	3.13 ± 1.39	4.09 ± 1.56	3.47 ± 1.13	3.65 ± 1.52	3.44 ± 1.50	NOR–ANR p = .009
	3 (2–4)	4 (3–6)	4 (2–4)	4 (2–5)	3.5 (2–4.25)	
	1–6	1–6	2–5	1–6	1–6	
29	3.62 ± 1.23	5.0 ± 1.16	5.13 ± 0.99	4.39 ± 1.26	4.89 ± 1.41	NOR–EDNOS p = .002 NOR–ANR p < .001 NOR–ANBP p = .001
	4 (3–4.5)	5 (4–6)	5 (4–6)	4 (3–6)	5.5 (4–6)	
	1–6	1–6	3–6	2–6	1–6	
30	3.90 ± 1.31	4.12 ± 1.55	5.33 ± 0.90	5.32 ± 0.95	4.67 ± 1.41	NOR–BN p < .001 NOR–ANBP p = .002 ANR–BN p = .003 ANR–ANBP p = .039
	4 (3–5)	4 (3–6)	6 (5–6)	6 (5–6)	5 (4–6)	
	1–6	1–6	3–6	3–6	1–6	
31	3.59 ± 1.35	2.98 ± 1.42	2.93 ± 1.34	3.16 ± 1.53	2.39 ± 1.46	NOR–EDNOS p = .014
	4 (2.5–5)	3 (2–4)	3 (2–3)	3 (2–4)	2 (1–4)	
	1–6	1–6	1–6	1–6	1–5	
33	3.67 ± 1.56	3.33 ± 1.60	4.33 ± 1.80	4.39 ± 1.61	4.61 ± 1.46	ANR-EDNOS p = .048
	3 (3–5)	3 (2–5)	5 (3–6)	5 (3–6)	5 (4–6)	
	1–6	1–6	1–6	1–6	1–5	
35	3.49 ± 1.67	4.16 ± 1.60	4.73 ± 1.39	4.57 ± 1.52	4.33 ± 1.78	NOR–BN p = .030
	3 (2–5)	4 (3–6)	5 (4–6)	5 (3–6)	5 (2.75–6)	
	1–6	1–6	2–6	1–6	1–6	
36	4.51 ± 1.19	4.86 ± 1.22	5.33 ± 0.90	5.33 ± 0.96	5.11 ± 1.13	NOR–BN p = .005
	5 (4–5)	5 (4–6)	6 (5–6)	6 (5–6)	5.5 (4.75–6)	
	1–6	1–6	3–6	2–6	3–6	
37	3.19 ± 1.46	3.40 ± 1.28	3.93 ± 1.39	4.17 ± 1.20	3.78 ± 1.48	NOR–BN p = .026

Table 3 Descriptive characteristics of items that differ significantly between groups *(Continued)*

	3 (2–4)	4 (2–4)	4 (3–5)	4 (3–5)	4 (2.75–5)	
	1–6	1–6	1–6	2–6	1–6	
39	2.73 ± 1.26	3.86 ± 1.34	4.80 ± 1.27	3.87 ± 1.57	4.50 ± 1.25	NOR–BN p = .006
	3 (2–3)	4 (3–5)	5 (4–6)	4 (2–5)	4.5 (3.75–6)	NOR–ANR p = .001 NOR–EDNOS p < .001
	1–6	1–6	2–6	1–6	2–6	NOR–ANBP p < .001
41	3.78 ± 1.26	4.02 ± 1.35	4.27 ± 1.62	4.73 ± 1.39	4.50 ± 1.43	NOR–BN p = .009
	4 (3–5)	4 (3–5)	5 (3–6)	5 (3–6)	5 (3.75–5.25)	
	1–6	1–6	1–6	1–6	1–6	
42	2.88 ± 1.33	5.02 ± 1.24	5.47 ± 1.[illegible]3	5.47 ± 1.04	5.06 ± 1.39	NOR–EDNOS p < .001
	3 (2–4)	6 (4–6)	6 (5–6)	6 (5–6)	6 (4.75–6)	NOR–ANR p < .001 NOR–ANBP p < .001
	1–6	2–6	2–6	2–6	2–6	NOR–BN p < .001
53	3.11 ± 1.26	3.33 ± 1.24	3.80 ± 1.08	4.17 ± 1.28	3.67 ± 1.46	NOR–BN p = .004
	3 (2–4)	3 (2–4)	4 (3–5)	4 (3–5)	4 (2–5)	
	1–6	1–6	2–6	2–6	1–6	
55	2.38 ± 1.52	4.05 ± 1.55	4.53 ± 1.46	4.13 ± 1.66	4.06 ± 1.70	NOR–EDNOS p = .003
	2 (1–3.5)	4 (3–5)	5 (4–6)	5 (3–5.25)	3.5 (3–6)	NOR–ANR p < .001 NOR–BN p < .001
	1–6	1–6	2–6	1–6	1–6	NOR–ANBP p < .001
61	3.99 ± 1.48	4.78 ± 1.28	4.0 ± 1.62	4.77 ± 1.04	4.94 ± 0.94	NOR–ANR p =,027
	4 (3–5)	5 (4–6)	4 (3–5.25)	5 (4–6)	5 (4.75–6)	
	1–6	1–6	1–6	3–6	3–6	
62	1.78 ± 1.22	2.21 ± 1.47	2.47 ± 1.51	3.13 ± 1.85	2.56 ± 1.62	NOR–BN p = .002
	1 (1–2)	2 (1–3)	2 (1–4)	3 (1–5)	2 (1–4)	
	1–6	1–6	1–6	1–6	1–4	

Quantitative data are presented as mean ± SD, median (interquartile range) and min–max value

Abbreviations: *NOR* controls, *ANR* anorexia nervosa, *ANBP* anorexia binge/purge type, *BN* bulimia nervosa, *EDNOS* eating disorder not otherwise specified

*p-value obtained from the post-hoc tests. The numbers presented in the table indicate the amount of answers received. Information regarding the lack of data was omitted

dietary standards and principles [47]. In particular, in the BN group, a negative evaluation of dietary standards in the family was associated with an equally negative assessment of family relations and behaviour, including the position of women and mothers in the family (items 53, 39, 10, and 17). In the ANR group, there was an association with the belief in the family's membership that they are in the middle class (item 61). Two additional items characteristic of all patient groups concerned peer groups and included understanding other people suffering from similar problems (item 42) and a belief that peers pay attention to how much the patients eat (item 55). In the BN group, patients knew other people who have problems with food (item 3) and felt that their peers would notice even small changes in their weight (item 35). This confirms previous observations of the importance of peer relationships to problems associated with the relationship to one's own body and with eating, including in their pathological forms [28, 29, 39]. The response to item 55 (I feel that my peers pay attention to how much I eat) may be an expression of a real interest in ways of losing weight (ANR and ANBP groups) or concern for a gorging-and-vomiting classmate (BN and ANBP groups). The perception of EDs as a major problem of modern teenagers (item 24 for the BN group and item 7 for the ANR and BN groups) was also able to distinguish patients with ED from controls. On several items, the ANBP group behaved in a manner similar to the BN group, supporting the intermediate character of this group [57]. The variation in the responses of the EDNOS group points to internal inconsistencies associated with the inclusion of patients diagnosed with different subclinical states [58].

There were no statistically significant differences between groups for any item related to the importance of advertising or religious context. In the case of advertising, this result is different from majority of results within the Western cultural sphere [30], and this difference may be due to the fact that, at the time of the study, the media market in Poland was less developed than in Western countries.

Would the results suggest that cultural context is relevant for BN but not for ANR? For Hilde Bruch [59], a distorted body image is central to the symptomology of ED, and the more body image is distorted, the more pronounced are the symptoms. What may be significant here are the relationships identified by items 12, 16 and 18, which indicate the irrelevance of thin pressure in the ANR group. It is possible that thin pressure was relevant before the manifestation of ED, but then lost its relevance following significant weight loss. This is not however observed in ANBP group. This indicates an interpretive trap, which similar studies may fall, not taking into account the type of eating disorders or anorexia nervosa.

These results may simply show that girls with restrictive type anorexia came from families without relationship problems [60, 61] and did not deviate significantly from the standard self-image [57]. However, EDs patients' images of family relationships are not generally as optimistic when one asks their parents [61]. Symptom denial is an important aspect of ED, and may affect not only the patient's somatic state, but also other relevant aspects of the patient's self-image and perception of relation to the world [62, 63]. This brings the credibility of any self-assessment test performed by girls suffering from ANR into question, including self-assessment tests of cultural issues.

Our study has some important limitations. Data were collected only from one university hospital. The sociocultural factors in samples from other clinical centres, community mental centres or private practises located in different areas of Poland could have been different. The recruitment of the control group based on parents volunteering and limited to girls from public schools within Krakow only can influence the results too.

It should be noticed that QSCC is a quite new tool and needs further exploration. The previous study [54] presents the results of the factor analysis of QSCC based on 614 schoolgirls from Krakow, aged 15–19 (mean: 16,83 years; SD: 1,04 years). The results of Cronbach's alphas (≥.7) and loadings (≥.35) of created 7 subscales were satisfactory and reflect 50.4 % of the total variability, but there were a lot of doubts about applying these subscales among girls with eating disorders. According to this the current paper presents the results based only on each item separately.

Conclusions

The results of this study indicate the importance of both objective social data and subjective cultural factors in EDs in the group studied. However, whether the cultural context is a true risk factor, proxy risk factor, mediating factor, potentiating factor, causal factor, maintenance factor or — in some dimensions — a protective factor cannot be determined from this type of analysis. A more clear-cut understanding of the meaning of the examined factors requires a longitudinal study that allows the emergence of EDs to be associated with an earlier interaction of variables (e.g., attitude towards one's body and eating habits) in persons without an initially occurring pathology.

Competing interests

The authors declare that they have no competing interests.

Authors' contributions

MP and BJ equally participated in: funds collection, study design, data collection, statistical analysis, data interpretation, literature search and manuscript preparation. KS participated in: statistical analysis, data interpretation, manuscript preparation. All authors read and approved the final manuscript.

Author details
[1]Department of Child and Adolescent Psychiatry, Jagiellonian University Medical College, ul. Kopernika 21a, 31-501 Kraków, Poland. [2]Department of Bioinformatics and Telemedicine, Jagiellonian University Medical College, ul. Św. Łazarza 16, 31-530 Kraków, Poland. [3]Department of Child and Adolescent Psychiatry, Laboratory of Psychology and Systemic Psychotherapy, Jagiellonian University Medical College, ul. Kopernika 21a, 31-501 Kraków, Poland.

References

1. Prince R. The concept of culture-bound syndromes: Anorexia nervosa and brain-fag. Soc Sci Med. 1985;21:197–203.
2. Swartz L. Anorexia nervosa as a culture-bound syndrome. Soc Sci Med. 1985;20:725–30.
3. Gordon RA. Eating disorders East and West: A culture bound syndrome unbound. In: Nasser M, Katzman MA, Gordon RA, editors. Eating disorders and cultures in transition. New York: Brunner-Routledge; 2001. p. 1–22.
4. Rathner G. Post-communism and the marketing of the thin ideal. In: Nasser M, Katzman MA, Gordon RA, editors. Eating disorders and cultures in transition. New York: Brunner-Routledge; 2001. p. 93–110.
5. Bulik CM. Eating disorders in immigrants: Two case reports. Int J Eat Disorder. 1987;6:133–41.
6. Dolan B. Cross cultural aspects of anorexia and bulimia: a review. Int J Eat Disorder. 1991;10:67–8.
7. Aruguete MS, Nickleberry LD, Yates A. Acculturation, body image and eating attitudes among black and white students. North Am J Psychol. 2004;6(3): 393–404.
8. DiNicola VF. Anorexia multiforme: self-starvation in historical and cultural context. Part II: Anorexia nervosa as a culture-reactive syndrome. Transcult Psychiatr. 1990;27:245–86.
9. Weiss MG. Eating disorders and disordered eating in different cultures. Psychiatr Clinics North Am. 1995;18(3):537–53.
10. Szmukler GI, Paton G. Sociocultural models of eating disorders. In: Szmukler GI, Dare C, Treasure J, editors. Handbook of eating disorders. Theory, treatment and research. New York: Wiley; 1995. p. 177–92.
11. Mitchison D, Hay PJ. The epidemiology of eating disorders: genetic, environmental, and societal factors. Clinical Epidemiology. 2014;6:89–97.
12. McClelland L, Crisp A. Anorexia nervosa and social class. Int J Eat Disord. 2001;29:150–6.
13. Gard MC, Freeman CP. The dismantling of a myth: a review of eating disorders and socioeconomic status. Int Eat Disorder. 1996;20:1–12.
14. Ahrén JC, Chiesa F, Af Klinteberg B, Koupil I. Psychosocial determinants and family background in anorexia nervosa – results from the Stockholm birth cohort study. Int Eat Disorder. 2012;45:362–9.
15. Stice E. Risk and maintenance factors for eating pathology, a meta-analytic review. Psychol Bull. 2002;128:825–48.
16. Stice E, Maxfield J, Wells T. Adverse effects of social pressure to be thin on young women: An experimental investigation of the effects of "fat talk". 21 May 2003 DOI: 10.1002/eat.10171.
17. Uher R, Rutter M. Classification of feeding and eating disorders: review of evidence and proposals for ICD-11. World Psychiatr. 2012;11:80–92.
18. McKnight I. Risk factors for the onset of eating disorders in adolescent girls: results of the McKnight longitudinal risk factor study. Am J Psychiatr. 2003; 160:248–54.
19. McCabe MP, Fuller-Tyszkiewicz M, Mellor D, Ricciardelli L, Skouteris H, Mussap A. Body satisfaction among adolescents in eight different countries. J Health Psychol. 2012;17(5):693–701.
20. Fallon P, Katzman MA, Wooley SC. Feminist perspective on eating disorders. New York-London: The Guilford Press; 1994.
21. Malson H. The thin woman. Feminism, post-structuralism and the social psychology of anorexia nervosa. London: Routledge; 1998.
22. Orbach S. Bodies. New York: Picador; 2009.
23. Bemporad JR. Cultural and historical aspects of eating disorders. Theor Med. 1997;18:401–20.
24. Schildkrout E. Body art as visual language. Anthro Notes. 2001;22:1–8.
25. Rodgers R, Chabrol H. Parental attitudes, body image disturbance and disordered eating amongst adolescents and young adults: a review. Eur Eat Disorders Rev. 2009;17:137–51.
26. Tiggemann M, Ruutel E. A cross-cultural comparison of body dissatisfaction in Estonian and Australian young adults and its relationship with media exposure. J Cross-Cult Psychol. 2001;32:736–42.
27. Woodside DB, Bulik CM, Halmi KA, Fichter MM, Kaplan A, Berrettini WH, et al. Personality, perfectionism, and attitudes toward eating in parents of children with eating disorders. Int J Eat Disorder. 2002;31:290–9.
28. Ferguson CJ, Winegard B, Winegard BM. Who is the fairest one of all? How evolution guides peer and media influences on female body dissatisfaction. Rev Gen Psychol. 2011;15:11–28.
29. Linville D, Stice E, Gau J, O'Neil M. Predictive effects of mother and peer influences on increases in adolescent eating disorder risk factors and symptoms: a 3–year longitudinal study. Int Eat Disord. 2011;44:745–51.
30. Grabe S, Ward L, Hyde J. The role of the media in body image concerns among women: a meta-analysis of experimental and correlational studies. Psych Bull. 2008;134:460–76.
31. Smolak L, Levine MP, Thompson JK. The use of the Sociocultural Attitudes Towards Appearance Questionnaire with middle school boys and girls. Int J Eat Disord. 2001;29:216–23.
32. Groesz LM, Levine MP, Murnen SK. The effect of experimental presentation of thin media images on body satisfaction: A meta-analytic review. Int J Eat Disord. 2002;31:1–16.
33. Fox N, Ward K, O'Rourke A. Pro-anorexia, weight-loss drugs and the internet: an 'anti-recovery' explanatory model of anorexia. Sociol Health Illness. 2005; 27:944–71.
34. Lipczynska S. Discovering the cult of Ana and Mia: A review of pro-anorexia websites. J Ment Health. 2007;16:545–8.
35. Dias K. The Ana sanctuary: Women's pro-anorexic narratives in cyberspace. In: Moore LJ, Kosut M, editors. The body reader: Essential social and cultural readings. New York: New York University Press; 2010. p. 399–412.
36. Benninghoven D, Tetsch N, Kunzendorf S, Jantschek G. Body image in patients with eating disorders and their mothers, and the role of family functioning. Compr Psychiatry. 2007;48:118–23.
37. Le Grange D, Lock J, Loeb K, Nicholls D. Academy for eating disorders position paper: The role of the family in eating disorders. Int J Eat Disord. 2010;43:1–5.
38. Park JP, Senior R, Stein A. The offspring of mothers with eating disorders. Eur Child Adolesc Psychiatry. 2003;12:110–9.
39. Paxton SJ, Schultz HK, Wertheim EH, Muir SL. Friendship clique and peer influences on body image concerns, dietary restraint, extreme weight loss behaviours, and binge eating in adolescent girls. J Abnorm Psychol. 1999; 108:255–66.
40. Fairburn CG, Harrison PJ. Eating disorders. Lancet. 2003;361:407–16.
41. Stice E, Marti N, Durant S. Risk factors for onset of eating disorders: Evidence of multiple risk pathways from an 8-year prospective study. Behav Res Ther. 2011;49:622–7.
42. Stice E, Ng J, Shaw H. Risk factors and prodromal eating pathology. J Child Psychol Psychiatry. 2010;51(4):518–25.
43. Polivy J, Herman CP. Sociocultural idealization of thin female body shapes: an introduction to the special issue on body image and eating disorders. J Soc Clin Psychol. 2004;23:1–6.
44. Włodarczyk-Bisaga K, Dolan B, McCluskey S, Lacey H. Disordered eating behaviour and attitudes towards weight and shape in Polish women. Eur Eat Disorders Rev. 1995;3(4):205–16.
45. Pilecki MW, Nowak A, Pilecka-Zdenkowska M. Change in the frequency of consultations concerning eating disorders in the Department of Child and Adolescent Psychiatry in Kraków (Poland) in the years 1988–2004. Arch Psychiatr Psychother. 2009;2:35–40.
46. Pilecki MW, Józefik B, Sałapa K. Disordered eating among mothers of Polish patients with eating disorders. Med Sci Monit. 2012;18:758–64.
47. Pilecki MW, Kowal M, Woronkowicz A, Kryst Ł, Sobiecki J. The socioeconomic status and family context of eating attitudes and dietary behaviours of children in Polish primary schools. Arch Psychiatr Psychother. 2014;1:5–13.
48. Pilecki MW, Józefik B, Sałapa K. : Kontekst kulturowy zaburzeń odżywiania się – badania własne. The cultural context of eating disorders – the authors'own research. Psychiatr Pol. 2012;46:189–200.
49. Filas R: Dziesięć lat przemian mediów masowych w Polsce (1989–1999). Propozycja periodyzacji. [Ten years of mass media changes in Poland (1989–1999). The periodisation proposal]. Zeszyty Prasoznawcze 1999, 157–158:31–158.
50. Filas R. Dwadzieścia lat przemian polskich mediów (1989–2009) w ujęciu periodycznym. [Twenty years of Polish media changes (1989–2009 in periodical frames]. Zeszyty Prasoznawcze 2009, 203–204.

51. Stochel M, Janas-Kozik M. Friends of virtual Ana — the phenomenon of pro-anorexia in the Internet. Psychiatr Pol. 2010;44:693–702.
52. American Psychiatric Association. Diagnostic and statistical manual of mental disorders (4th ed.). Washington, DC: American Psychiatric Association; 1994.
53. Pilecki MW, Józefik B, Sałapa K. Kontekst kulturowy zaburzeń odżywiania się — badania własne. Cultural context of eating disorders – summary of research program. Psychiatr Pol. 2012;46:189–200.
54. Pilecki M, Sałapa K, Józefik B, Kozłowska-Jasnos M. Kwestionariusz kontekstu socjo-kulturowego w zaburzeniach odżywiania autorstwa Macieja Pileckiego i Barbary Józefik – podsumowanie obecnego etapu prac nad narzędziem. [The questionnaire on sociocultural context in eating disorders developed by Maciej Pilecki and Barbara Józefik – a summary of the current stage of work on the research instrument]. Psychiatr Psychoter. 2014;10(2):3–17.
55. Mały rocznik statystyczny 2005. [Little statistical yearbook]. Główny Urząd Statystyczny. Warszawa 2005.
56. Brown PJ, Konner M. An anthropological perspective on obesity. Ann New York Acad Sci. 1987;499(1):29–46.
57. Pilęcki M, Józefik B. Self-image of girls with different subtypes of eating disorders. Arch Psychiat Psychother. 2008;10(3):17–22.
58. Pilecki MW, Sałapa K, Józefik B. Factors affecting self-image in patients with a diagnosis of eating disorders on the basis of a cluster analysis. Int J Stat Med Res. 2013;2:263–74.
59. Bruch H. Anorexia nervosa: therapy and theory. Am J Psychiatr. 1982;139:1531–8.
60. Józefik B, Pilecki M: Raport z programu badawczego z 2004. A report of the research program 2004. KBN 6PO5E09021. Kraków, Poland: Jagiellonian University Medical College, Department of Scientific Research and Structural Funds of Medical College, Jagiellonian University; 2004.
61. Józefik B. Relacje rodzinne w anoreksji i bulimii psychicznej. [Family relations in anorexia and bulimia nervosa.]. Kraków: Wydawnictwo Uniwersytetu Jagiellońskiego; 2006.
62. Vandereycken W. Denial of illness in anorexia nervosa – a conceptual review: part 1. Diagnostic significance and assessment. Eur Eat Disord Rev. 2006;14:341–51.
63. Konstantakopoulos G, Tchanturia K, Surguladze SA, David AS. Insight in eating disorders: clinical and cognitive correlates. Psychol Med. 2011;41:1951–61.

Pro-eating disorder search patterns: the possible influence of celebrity eating disorder stories in the media

Stephen P. Lewis*, Laura Klauninger and Ivana Marcincinova

Abstract

Pro eating disorder websites often contain celebrity-focused content (e.g., images) used as *thinspiration* to engage in unhealthy eating disorder behaviours. The current study was conducted to examine whether news media stories covering eating disorder disclosures of celebrities corresponded with increases in Internet searches for pro eating disorder material. Results indicated that search volumes for pro eating disorder terms spiked in the month immediately following such news coverage but only for particularly high-profile celebrities. Hence, there may be utility in providing recovery-oriented resources within the search results for pro-eating disorder Internet searches and within news stories of this nature.

Keywords: Pro-eating disorder, Thinspiration, Celebrity, Website, Internet, Online

Pro-eating disorder (pro-ED) websites are prevalent and typically involve individuals sharing strategies and messages that promote or encourage eating disorder (ED) behaviours; this includes sharing images of emaciated celebrities, which serve as "thinspiration" for extreme weight loss [1–3]. Researchers have documented that youth and emerging adults are the primary users of these websites and that exposure to pro-ED websites is associated with ED pathology [1–3].

One solution to mitigate the potential impact of pro-ED websites is to provide pro-recovery resources in the search results corresponding to pro-ED Internet searches [2, 4]. In this way, access to (and the potential impact of) pro-ED websites may be circumvented - or at least delayed. Similar strategies are currently in place for suicide web-searches on Google [5]. To do this effectively, however, it may be important to not just consider *what* pro-ED terms may be sought out on popular search engines but to also consider *fluctuations* in pro-ED web-searches [2, 4]; in particular, there may be merit in considering what might account for such changes [2]. To date, no study has examined what factors may influence pro-ED search patterns online.

* Correspondence: stephen.lewis@uoguelph.ca
University of Guelph, Guelph, ON N1G 2W1, Canada

As celebrities are used as sources of *thinspiration* [1–3], and a number of celebrities have publicly disclosed ED histories via news media [6], it is possible that public ED disclosures by celebrities represent one factor influencing pro-ED search patterns online. Findings from research examining media coverage of suicide add support for this possibility. Specifically, pursuant to media coverage of several suicides, and within the geographic region of the stories, increases in Google search patterns for the suicide methods reported in the stories have been documented [7].

Should stories covering celebrity ED disclosures impact pro-ED search patterns, it may be necessary to provide resources promoting ED prevention and recovery within people's search results, before potentially harmful content is accessed. Accordingly, we conducted the present study to determine whether Internet searches for pro-ED keywords changed pursuant to dissemination of a celebrity ED disclosures covered by news media. To do this, we examined pro-ED search trends on Google, the most used search engine worldwide [8]. We anticipated that the timing of at least some news stories would correspond with increases in pro-ED searches soon after the story was published; furthermore, we expected that this would be especially the case for high-profile celebrities, who ostensibly have a larger following and thus a possible greater influence on others.

Methods

We first identified high-profile media stories in which celebrities disclosed past ED experiences using Google News [6]. To index individual celebrity popularity, we consulted popular social networks. Specifically, we examined the number of *likes* these celebrities' official pages received on Facebook and the number of followers they accumulated on Twitter. From these efforts, one celebrity was shown to have a significant following, namely Lady Gaga. Her likes on Facebook were approximately 25 million more, and she had over 15 million more Twitter followers, than the next celebrity on our list. Although we focused most of our attention on her story in our analysis, we also compared changes in pro-ED search patterns associated with her story with those of other celebrity stories involving public ED disclosures.

To determine whether there were changes in search patterns for pro-ED terms around the timing of news stories reporting Lady Gaga's public ED disclosure, Google Trends was used [9]. After initially entering relevant keywords, this program allows users to generate frequency data for individual Google search terms by narrowing the results to particular time periods and locations. Past research has used this program to identify pro-ED search terms (e.g., *pro ana, pro thinspiration*) associated with particularly harmful pro-ED content [2]. We therefore used these search terms in the current study to determine whether the search volumes associated with each one changed when comparing the month before, the month of, and the month after news stories reported Lady Gaga's ED history. We attenuated focus to searches in the United States for two reasons. First, Lady Gaga is from the United States, as were other celebrities we identified. Second, celebrities may be used as sources of *thinspiration* [1–3] and Google Search terms related to *thinspiration* may be especially sought out in the United States [2].

Results

Analyses

Data from Google Trends pertaining to various search terms are normalized and scaled out of 100; they do not represent raw search volumes. For instance, if one term (e.g., Term X) received a value of 100 and another term (e.g., Term Y) had a value of 50, the latter (Term Y) would have received one half of the searches as the former (Term X) over a designated period of time. Upon obtaining search data for the above mentioned terms and following approaches used in other research using Google Trends to examine search term fluctuation following news stories [8], we compared search volumes for the terms noted above by examining the change (if any) between: a) the month prior to the news story, b) the month of the story and c) the month after the story was published. To do this, a series of paired t-tests[1] were computed to determine if there were significant changes in pro-ED search patterns between the above months of interest. [7]. Changes in pro-ED search term volumes from January to March of 2012 are depicted in Fig. 1.

Main findings

As an initial step in our analyses, we compared pro-ED terms search volumes for the month prior to and at the month of news coverage involving Lady Gaga's public ED disclosure. Findings indicated that there was a modest but non-significant increase in pro-ED terms search volumes from January 2012 ($M = 38.50$; $SD = 14.98$) to February 2012 ($M = 45.83$; $SD = 22.21$), $p >$. 05.

Next, we compared pro-ED search volumes for the month prior to and after publication of these news stories. Here, there was a statistically significant increase in pro-ED search volumes from January 2012 ($M = 38.50$; SD = 14.98) to March 2012 ($M = 76.17$; $SD = 15.34$), $t(5) = 9.14$; $p < .05$. Cohen's d was 3.74, indicating a large effect size. On average, the search volumes increased by 37 % with term *pro ana websites* exhibiting the largest increase (52 %).

Finally, we compared pro-ED search volumes for the month at the time of and after publication of these news stories. Here, there was a significant increase in pro-ED search term volumes from February 2012 ($M = 45.83$; $SD = 22.21$) to March 2012 ($M = 76.17$; $SD = 15.34$), $t(5) = 4.51$; $p <$. 05. Cohen's d was 2.03, indicating a large effect size. On average, the search volumes increased by 30 % per term with *pro ana websites* again exhibiting the largest increase (52 %).

To determine if the above findings were an artefact of the time of year, we examined the same search terms over the same time frame one year later. As shown in Fig. 2, there was no substantive change in pro-ED search patterns at this time. Paired t-tests comparing mean pro-ED search volumes between any months of interest (January, February, March) confirmed that changes were non-significant ($p > .05$). Finally, to examine if there were changes in pro-ED search patterns following stories involving ED disclosures of lower-profile celebrities, we looked at patterns of the next three celebrities based on social media popularity. As depicted in Table 1, the increases observed following Lady Gaga's story were not observed for these stories.[2] Moreover, paired t-tests confirmed that pro-ED search volume changes for these lower profile celebrities were non-significant, $p > .05$.

Discussion

The current study was conducted to examine whether media coverage of celebrity ED disclosures corresponded with changes in Google searches for pro-ED terms. Findings suggest that pro-ED searches *may* increase soon after media coverage of high-profile celebrities who discuss past struggles with EDs. In the present study we

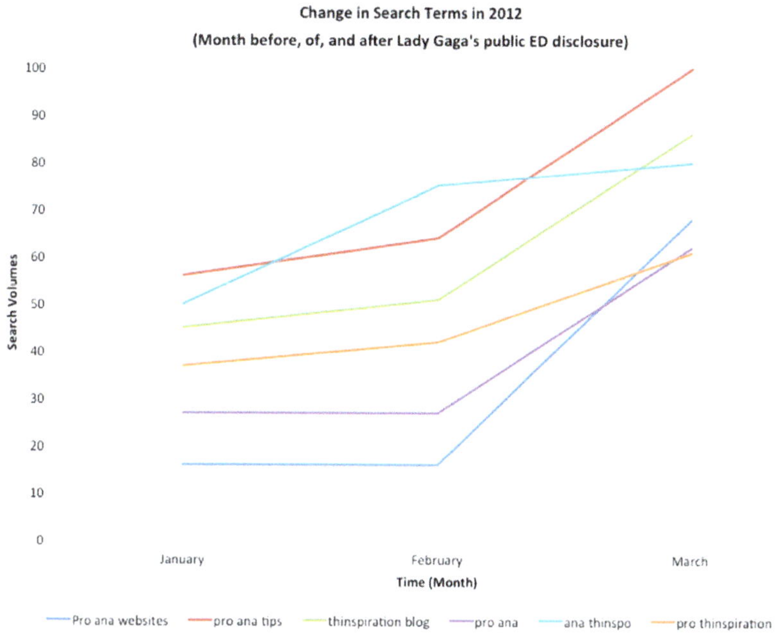

Fig. 1 Search volumes for pro-ED key words via Google from January to March 2012. Notes: Values represent normalized rather than absolute values of the number of online pro-ED searches for the month before (January, 2012), at the time of (February, 2012), and after (March, 2012) Lady Gaga's public ED disclosure via news media

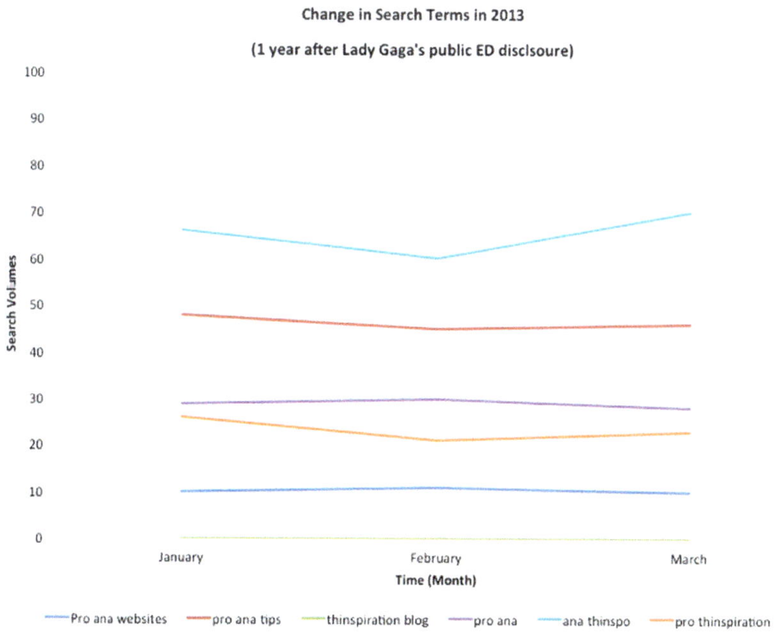

Fig. 2 Search volumes for pro-ED key words via Google from January to March 2013. Notes: Values represent normalized rather than absolute values of the number of online pro-ED searches 1 year following Lady Gaga's public ED disclosure via news media

Table 1 Mean search volumes for pro-ED search terms following public ED disclosures of top 4 celebrities based on social media following

Celebrity	Month *Before* ED Disclosure Publicized	Month *When* ED Disclosure Publicized	Month *After* ED Disclosure Publicized
Lady Gaga	38.50	45.83	76.17
Demi Lovato	42.33	38.83	37.67
Kesha	27.00	33.50	28.83
Snooki	49.33	50.00	59.00

Notes: Values presented represent average standardized search volumes derived from Google Trends across the following search terms: *Pro ana website, Pro Ana, Pro ana tips, Ana Thinspo, Thinspiration blog, Pro thinspiration*. The 4 celebrities presented had the largest following on social media, indexed by total number of likes on Facebook and followers on Twitter. *ED* eating disorder

found that in the month immediately following publication of one such story (i.e., Lady Gaga's) there was a significant increase in the search volumes for pro-ED search terms when compared to both the month before the story was published and the month during which the story was published. This was not observed for the same period of time in the subsequent year. An important caveat to the trend observed is that the potential change in pro-ED search patterns might be circumscribed to particularly high-profile celebrity stories versus media coverage of celebrity ED disclosures in general.

The current findings build on research demonstrating that media coverage may inadvertently influence potentially harmful search trends online [7] by suggesting that a similar effect may occur when high-profile celebrity ED disclosures are covered. Our findings also suggest that pro-ED search terms identified in past work [2] may be especially salient in this regard. Indeed, the terms used in this study have been identified as associating with more pernicious pro-ED material. As a growing body of research has shown that access to pro-ED material online may contribute to offline ED pathology [1, 3], this is worrisome.

As with any study, the present findings should be interpreted within the context of several limitations. We cannot assume a causal relation between media story coverage of high-profile celebrity ED disclosures and Google search patterns for pro-ED content. Additionally, we do not have access to data about *who* conducted the Google searches reported and the impact (if any) these searches have on body image or ED behaviour. We also acknowledge that not all news stories of celebrity eating disorder disclosures yielded changes in pro-ED searches; indeed, this was only observed in the case of a higher-profile celebrity. Thus, the trend observed in the current study may only apply to particular celebrity stories versus *any* celebrity story. Finally, given the nature of data obtained, and because we were looking at individual search terms (versus an aggregate of multiple terms), we were limited in the types of analyses we could perform.

While there is certainly merit in reporting celebrity ED disclosures (e.g., help-seeking encouragement, de-stigmatization of EDs), some reports may evoke increases in pro-ED search patterns. Given the link between exposure to pro-ED content and ED behaviour [1–3], it seems prudent to intervene *prior to the point of access* - that is, before individuals access pro ED websites. Hence, provision of recovery-oriented ED resources in search results following pro-ED searches may be warranted, similar to what is presently implemented for suicide-related searches on Google [6]. Likewise, providing pro-recovery resources within the reported news stories may be needed. Research-informed and supportive online ED resources are recommended in such efforts.

Endnotes

[1]Data were determined to have a normal distribution using the Shapiro-Wilk Statistic ($W = .96$; $p > .05$) prior to computing paired t-tests.

[2]Overall, the changes in pro-ED search volumes following Lady Gaga's news story were not observed for the other 3 celebrities depicted in Table 1. A similar pattern emerged for other lower-profile celebrity news stories not reported here.

Competing interest
The authors declare that they have no competing interests.

Authors' contributions
SPL conceived of the study, wrote the initial draft of the introduction and discussion, edited and approved the final manuscript, and supervised the study. LK managed data collection, analyzed the data, co-wrote the initial draft of the methods and results,and edited and approved the final manuscript. IM analyzed the data, contributed to methodological development, co-wrote the initial draft of the methods and results, and edited and approved the final manuscript.

References
1. Rouleau CR, von Ranson KM. Potential risks of pro-eating disorder websites. Clin Psych Rev. 2011;31:525–31.
2. Lewis SP, Arbuthnott AE. Searching for thinspiration: the nature of Internet searches for pro-eating disorder websites. Cyber Beh Soc Net. 2012;15(4):200–4.
3. Jett S, LaPorte DJ, Wanchisn J. Impact of exposure to pro-eating disorder websites on eating behaviour in college women. Eur Eating Dis Rev. 2010;18(5):410–6.
4. Lewis SP, Arbhuthnott AE. Non-suicidal self-injury, Eating Disorders: The Influence of the Internet and Social Media. In: Claes L, Muehlenkamp J, editors. Non-suicidal Self-injury in Eating Disorders. Berlin: Springer; 2014. Non-suicidal Self-injury in Eating Disorders.

5. Cohen N. 'Suicide' query prompts Google to offer hotline. New York Times; 2010. http://www.nytimes.com/2010/04/05/technology/05google.html. Accessed date July 15, 2015.
6. Google News.http://news.google.com Accessed September, 2014.
7. Chang S, Page A, Gunnell G. Internet searches for a specific suicide method follow its high-profile media coverage. Am J Psych. 2011;168(8):855–7.
8. Alexa.Worldwide Traffic Rank. Website. Updated daily. Accessed August 31, 2015. http://www.alexa.com/siteinfo/google.com
9. Google. Google Trends. https://www.google.com/trends/

Implicitly assessed attitudes toward body shape and food: the moderating roles of dietary restraint and disinhibition

Joanna Myriam Moussally[1,2*], Joël Billieux[1,3], Olivia Mobbs[1], Stéphane Rothen[4,5] and Martial Van der Linden[1,2,6]

Abstract

Background: Attitudes toward body shape and food play a role in the development and maintenance of dysfunctional eating behaviors. Nevertheless, they are rarely investigated together. Therefore, this study aimed to explore the interrelationships between implicitly assessed attitudes toward body shape and food and to investigate the moderating effect on these associations of interindividual differences in problematic and nonproblematic eating behaviors (i.e., flexible versus rigid cognitive control dimension of restraint, disinhibition).

Methods: One hundred and twenty-one young women from the community completed two adapted versions of the Affect Misattribution Procedure to implicitly assess attitudes toward body shape (i.e., thin and overweight bodies) and food (i.e., "permitted" and "forbidden" foods), as well as the Three-Factor Eating Questionnaire to evaluate restraint and disinhibition.

Results: The results revealed that an implicit preference for thinness was positively associated with a positive attitude toward permitted (i.e., low-calorie) foods. This congruence between implicitly assessed attitudes toward body shape and food was significant at average and high levels of flexible control (i.e., functional component of eating). Moreover, an implicit preference for thinness was also positively associated with a positive attitude toward forbidden (i.e., high-calorie) foods. This discordance between implicitly assessed attitudes was significant at average and high levels of rigid control and disinhibition (i.e., dysfunctional components of eating).

Conclusions: These findings shed new light on the influence of congruent or discordant implicitly assessed attitudes toward body shape and food on normal and problematic eating behaviors; clinical implications are discussed.

Keywords: Implicitly assessed attitudes, Food, Body shape, Restraint, Disinhibition

Background

Attitudes are representations stored in memory about the valence of a specific stimulus [1]. These valenced representations of body shape/weight and food seem to play an important role in the development and maintenance of dysfunctional eating behaviors [2, 3]. Indeed, in Western societies, thinness is valued and the thin-ideal body is promoted by the media, while excess weight is disapproved of [4]. Nevertheless, the thin-ideal body is difficult or impossible to achieve. Every woman has a minimum weight, defined by genetic and physiological influences (e.g., morphology); it is difficult to maintain a weight below that minimum and remain healthy [5]. Internalization of the thin-ideal, coupled with this divergence between cultural standards and biological constraints, promotes body dissatisfaction and problematic eating behaviors, such as inflexibly restrictive eating behaviors intended to lose weight [4]. In dietary restraint, foods are categorized as negative or positive, meaning that they are perceived as "forbidden" (usually high-calorie foods) or "permitted" (usually low-calorie foods) [6]. Thus, attitudes toward body shape/weight

* Correspondence: Joanna.Moussally@unige.ch
[1]Psychology Department, FPSE, Cognitive Psychopathology and Neuropsychology Unit, University of Geneva, Boulevard du Pont d'Arve 40, CH-1205 Geneva, Switzerland
[2]Swiss Center for Affective Sciences, Campus Biotech, University of Geneva, Case Postale 60, CH-1211 Geneva 20, Switzerland
Full list of author information is available at the end of the article

(i.e., valuing thinness) seem to influence attitudes toward foods (i.e., dichotomous categorization of foods), at least among women who are dissatisfied with their bodies and want to achieve their ideal thinness by dieting.

Attitudes have been extensively studied with two types of measurement – *explicit* and *implicit* – to better understand and predict behaviors. Explicit measures of attitudes (e.g., self-reports) tap into reflective processes activated with voluntary cognitive control, meaning that they depend on responses and behaviors that participants are aware of, willing to report, and able to modify. Conversely and complementarily, implicit measures of attitudes reflect automatic processes activated without awareness or the possibility of controlling or modifying them [1, 7]. It has been demonstrated that, in certain cases, implicitly and explicitly assessed attitudes predict different types of behaviors (spontaneous behaviors for implicitly assessed attitudes and intentional behaviors for explicitly assessed attitudes), but they can also interact to influence behaviors [8]. Indeed, implicitly assessed attitudes not only affect spontaneous behaviors but can also influence intentional behaviors [9], explaining a significant proportion of the variance in different behaviors (e.g., drinking) independently of explicitly assessed attitudes [10]. It has therefore been proposed that, under some conditions, implicitly assessed attitudes might predict behaviors better than explicitly assessed attitudes, due to the biases associated with explicit assessment [9, 10]. In the field of eating disorders, various researchers [11, 12] have promoted the examination of implicitly assessed cognitions to gain access to representations that participants feel uncomfortable about confessing (e.g., preference for emaciation) and to better understand how implicit representations (e.g., liking of high-calories foods) might influence the development and maintenance of problematic eating behaviors (e.g., overeating, rigid restraint).

Past studies of implicitly assessed attitudes toward body shape emphasized the existence of positive attitudes toward thinness and/or negative attitudes toward fatness in participants from the community [13, 14], restrained and unrestrained eaters [15], participants with a high drive for thinness [16], individuals with anorexia nervosa [17] and obese/overweight persons [18]. Studies that focused on implicitly assessed attitudes toward food produced more inconsistent results. Some studies observed positive attitudes toward low-calorie foods and/or negative attitudes toward high-calorie foods in participants from the community [19], obese persons [20], and restrained eaters [12]. Other studies, though, showed the reverse pattern: positive attitudes toward high-calorie foods and/or negative attitudes toward low-calorie foods. This effect has been found in normal-weight, overweight and obese persons [21], as well as in restrained and unrestrained eaters [22, 23].

A first explanation for these divergent results might be the influence of methodological factors, such as the type of task used. Almost all studies examining attitudes toward body shape employed a relative measure: the Implicit Association Task (IAT) [24]. In contrast, studies of attitudes toward food have used several tasks. Interestingly, studies that observed positive attitudes toward low-calorie foods and/or negative attitudes toward high-calorie foods used the IAT, while studies that obtained the reverse pattern of results used nonrelative measures. In relative measures, the strength of the association for a targeted concept (e.g., "thin and positive") is connected to the strength of the association for another targeted concept (e.g., "overweight and negative"), meaning that a positive attitude toward thinness necessarily also reflects a negative attitude toward fatness [25]. Conversely, a nonrelative measure can reveal independent attitudes toward two targeted stimuli, allowing exploration of the presence of similar attitudes toward different types of stimuli (e.g., positive attitudes toward both permitted and forbidden foods), which might explain some of the inconsistent findings about attitudes toward food.

A second explanation might be the influence of interindividual differences. Stimulus valuation, for example, could be related to the type of problematic eating behaviors or cognitions a person has. Based on their literature review, Roefs et al. [3] hypothesized that individuals with bulimia nervosa, restrained eaters and obese persons would have positive implicitly assessed attitudes toward high-calorie foods, given that these individuals present episodes of disinhibited overeating. In contrast, individuals with restrictive anorexia nervosa (who do not exhibit disinhibited overeating) would present negative attitudes toward similar foods. Furthermore, the effects observed in overall samples might hide subgroup profiles. Ahern et al. [16] observed that, unlike the negative attitudes toward thinness found in their overall sample of young women from the community, a subgroup of participants with an elevated drive for thinness had positive attitudes. Accordingly, interindividual differences in the domain of eating disorders should be explored.

Although, as mentioned above, attitudes toward body shapes seem to influence attitudes toward foods, few studies have tested their interrelationships when these attitudes were implicitly investigated. However, associations between food and body image have been studied extensively with both explicit and indirect behavioral measures. Mere exposure to food stimuli (e.g., high-calorie foods) or food consumption (e.g., having a milkshake) increases the explicitly reported state dissatisfaction with body or weight, especially among participants who display food, weight and shape concerns, such as restrained eaters [26, 27]. Furthermore, exposure to body-shape-related stimuli may also impact explicitly reported feelings and motivational states toward food (e.g., increase in guilt about chocolate consumption after exposure to images of thin women) [28]. Based on these results, it seems essential to explore the relationships between body shape/weight and food in the field of implicitly assessed attitudes.

Overview of the present study

This study had three objectives. We first wanted to reexamine, using a nonrelative measure, implicitly assessed attitudes toward body shape (i.e., thin versus overweight bodies) and food (i.e., "forbidden" high-calorie versus "permitted" low-calorie foods) among young women from the community in order to replicate previous consistent findings (studies about attitudes toward body shape) or to find possible explanations for inconsistent findings described in the literature (studies about attitudes toward food). Second and more importantly, we wanted to highlight relationships between attitudes toward body shape and food, given that both play an important role in dysfunctional eating behaviors [2, 3], but have rarely been investigated together. Finally, we wanted to explore the role of interindividual differences in eating behaviors as moderators of the relationships between attitudes to better understand implicit representation patterns (associations between body shape and food concepts) that might underline behaviors [12]. Specifically, we wished to examine variations in attitude association patterns (e.g., positive attitudes toward thinness and permitted foods; positive attitudes toward thinness and forbidden foods) depending on participants' levels (high versus low) of problematic and nonproblematic behaviors.

Regarding this third objective, we focused on two behavioral and cognitive components of eating: restraint and disinhibition. Restraint refers to the tendency to voluntarily restrict food intake by cognitively controlling eating behavior [29]. Westenhoefer [29] proposed dividing restraint into two manifestations: (a) flexible cognitive control (a nuanced attitude toward eating, where "forbidden" foods can be eaten in small quantities) is a more functional component, while (b) rigid cognitive control (a dichotomous, all-or-nothing attitude toward eating) is a more dysfunctional component. Disinhibition reflects the tendency to lose control over eating behaviors while experiencing adverse emotional states [29]. Consideration of restraint and disinhibition is relevant, as they are widely described as "characteristic features" of people with eating disorders and are transdiagnostic (found across different eating disorders) [30]. These components were described among restrained eaters and patients with bulimia or anorexia nervosa who tend to have episodes of disinhibited overeating between their restraint periods [30, 31]. Furthermore, these components are interconnected: rigid cognitive control was associated with high levels of disinhibition [29]. Finally, considering the two manifestations of restraint allows us to focus on the different mechanisms that underlie dieting behavior. Indeed, Westenhoefer [29] highlighted that the homogeneity of the restraint construct is questionable. He pointed out that all restrained eaters do not present episodes of disinhibited overeating; some succeed in restraint (probably because they have established more adaptive strategies). Therefore, assessing flexible and rigid cognitive controls might allow us to dissociate attitude patterns that underline the two different types of restraint.

Methods

Participants

One hundred and twenty-one young women took part in the study. All participants were volunteers and were recruited from the community in Geneva, Switzerland (41.32 % of the sample), and Liège, Belgium (58.68 %). Their ages ranged from 19 to 37 years old (M = 23.97, SD = 4.80) and their body mass indexes (BMI) from 15.73 to 35.86 (M = 21.38, SD = 3.40). All participants gave their consent prior to starting the experiment. The study protocol was approved by the Ethical Committee of the Psychology Department of the University of Geneva and carried out according to the 1964 Declaration of Helsinki.

Measures

Personal information

Various questions were asked about participants' sociodemographic and anthropometric data (e.g., age, height, weight). The self-reported height and weight were used to calculate the participants' BMI.

Implicitly assessed attitudes

Attitudes toward body shape and food were assessed with two versions of the Affect Misattribution Procedure (AMP), adapted from Payne et al. [32]. The AMP was chosen because it is a nonrelative measure. It thus allowed us to explore the presence of independent attitudes toward two targeted stimuli (thin versus overweight bodies; permitted versus forbidden foods). It has also increasingly been used in various research fields (e.g., drinking or eating behaviors) [10, 33] and is characterized by elevated internal consistency (Cronbach's alphas: .73 to .95). The construct validity of the AMP is supported by previous studies showing dissociations between implicit attitudes toward universally positive versus negative stimuli and associations with explicit attitude measures [10, 32]. Moreover, AMP-assessed attitudes predict judgments and behavioral outcomes even when explicit measures are controlled for, highlighting that AMP-assessed attitudes explain unique variance independently of explicit measures, which supports satisfactory predictive validity [10].

In AMP trials, an image (e.g., an emotional prime) appeared briefly (75 ms) in the center of the screen. Immediately following its disappearance, a blank screen appeared for 125 ms, and then an ambiguous pictograph (a Chinese character that is not familiar and therefore meaningless to participants)[1] for 100 ms. After the pictograph disappeared, a pattern mask appeared and remained on the screen until the participant indicated the pleasantness (valence judgment) of the Chinese character by pressing a key. Participants were instructed to press a key labeled "pleasant" if they evaluated the character to be more pleasant than average and a key labeled "unpleasant" if they evaluated it to be less pleasant than average. The outcome variables were the proportion of Chinese characters evaluated as pleasant in each prime condition.

The AMP is based on people's tendency, in ambiguous conditions, to erroneously attribute their feelings to one source (i.e., the pictograph) when they actually emanate from another one that is close in space and time (i.e., the emotional prime) [32]. Accordingly, judgment of the pictograph is influenced by the emotional prime preceding it. The participants were thus instructed that the picture preceding the Chinese character might influence their judgment of the pictograph and told that they should do their best not to let that happen.

The two created AMP versions were similar except for the stimuli (i.e., primes) used. They were composed of 72 randomly ordered trials consisting of three different types of primes; 72 different Chinese characters were used as targets in each task.

In the "body shape" version, the three types of primes consisted of (a) full-body pictures of thin women (*thin* primes; approximate BMIs located within the "moderate thinness" and "normal range" classes corresponding to 16.00–24.99 kg/m^2), (b) full-body pictures of overweight women (*overweight* primes; approximate BMIs located within the "overweight" and "moderate obesity" classes corresponding to 25.00–39.99 kg/m^2), and (c) pictures of shrubs (*control* primes). The pictures of thin and overweight women did not differ in clothing or skin color. Each prime condition contained 12 different pictures, which were presented twice. The images were evaluated, with 9-point Likert scales, in a pilot study of 40 women aged 20 to 35 years old. The results revealed that the pictures of thin and overweight women differed in fatness (median diff. = 3.80; Mann–Whitney U-test; z = 4.13, $p < .001$),[2] but not in beauty (mean diff. = 0.25, 95 % CI = [−.40, .89], $t(22) = .80$, $p = .434$, $d = .325$).

In the "food" version, the three types of primes consisted of (a) pictures of "low-calorie" foods (*permitted* primes; e.g., vegetables), (b) pictures of "high-calorie" foods (*forbidden* primes; e.g., hamburger), and (c) pictures of everyday objects (*control* primes; e.g., bucket). Once again, each prime condition contained 12 different pictures. The pilot study mentioned above showed that permitted and forbidden foods differed significantly in the "forbidden" value they conveyed (median diff. = 6.90; Mann–Whitney U-test; z = 4.13, $p < .001$).[2]

The decision to use control stimuli other than the neutral gray square used by Payne et al. [32] was made to avoid repetition of the same stimulus throughout the task, which might lead to a habituation effect. In our study, each control stimulus appeared the same number of times as an emotional stimulus (*thin, overweight, permitted* and *forbidden* primes). Moreover, the use of images for the control stimuli increased the task's ecological validity.

Eating behaviors

Restraint and disinhibition were measured with the French version [34] of the Three-Factor Eating Questionnaire (TFEQ) [35]. Restraint is measured with 21 items scored 0 (false) or 1 (true) and disinhibition is assessed with 16 items.[3] The internal reliability of the two dimensions in the present sample was satisfactory (Cronbach's alphas were respectively .88 and .74). As the objective of this study was to examine the roles of the different restraint manifestations, we calculated the scores for the rigid (7 items) and flexible (7 items) cognitive control dimensions proposed by Westenhoefer [29]. The internal reliability of the two subdimensions was acceptable (Cronbach's alphas were respectively .76 and .65).

Procedure

After giving their informed consent, participants completed the personal information sheet. Then they were randomly assigned to an order for the AMP versions: half of the participants started with the body shape version and the other half with the food version. Afterward, participants completed the TFEQ and were subsequently debriefed.

Hypotheses and statistical analyses

Attitudes in the overall sample

Our first objective was to examine attitudes in the overall sample (i.e., mean level of AMP performances). Concerning attitudes toward body shape, we expected to replicate the findings obtained in community samples (i.e., positive attitudes toward thinness and negative toward fatness) [13]. For attitudes toward food, given that previous findings from community samples are inconsistent [19, 21], we had no a priori hypothesis. Indeed, the inconsistent findings described in the literature might suggest either dissimilar attitudes (positive attitudes toward permitted foods and negative toward forbidden foods) or similar attitudes (positive attitudes toward permitted and forbidden foods).

To meet this objective, we computed repeated measures analyses of variance (ANOVAs) on the AMP performances (proportion of pleasant judgments in each prime condition) separately for the "body shape" and "food" versions. We used Tukey's post hoc tests to test the differences in evaluative responses between the conditions. All mean levels of AMP performances were then compared with the chance level of .50 to reinforce findings from prior Tukey's post hoc tests. Indeed, in determining the valence of an attitude, two conditions are required. First, the proportion of pleasant judgements in the emotional conditions has to significantly differ from the control condition (highlighted by Tukey's post hoc tests). Second, the proportion of pleasant judgements has to differ from .50. Conversely, it is expected that the pleasant judgements in the control condition are about .50 [10, 32]. For these analyses, the conventional significance level was adjusted for multiple comparisons with the Bonferroni correction.

Relationships between attitudes

Concerning our second objective of highlighting relationships between attitudes toward body shape and food, we were particularly interested in the valuing of thinness (compared with fatness), given the antagonist valences assigned to thinness and excess weight in Western societies and the central role of thin-ideal internalization (preference for thinness) in food categorization and eating behaviors [4, 6]. We therefore posited that attitudes toward thinness would be positively related to attitudes toward "permitted" foods and negatively related to attitudes toward "forbidden" foods. Indeed, in order to lose weight, an individual will categorize foods as "positive/permitted" and "negative/forbidden" [6].

Interrelationships among attitudes were explored with Pearson correlations. For these analyses, we computed AMP scores corresponding to the guidelines provided by Payne et al. [10, 32, 36]: the AMP can be scored either as a relative preference score (relative preference for a type of stimuli over another) or as an independent attitude score (positivity toward a type of stimuli).

In the "body shape" version, we were interested in the relative preference for thin or overweight bodies (*AMP-assessed attitude toward body shape*), given that we particularly wanted to examine the valuing of thinness. Therefore, the proportion of pleasant responses on *overweight* trials was subtracted from the proportion of pleasant responses on *thin* trials. A positive score indicates a preference for thin bodies.

For the "food" version, we created three different scores because, as mentioned above, unlike studies in the domain of implicitly assessed attitudes toward body shape, which present quite consistent findings, studies in the field of attitudes toward food have produced more inconsistent results. Therefore, we computed (a) a score of relative preference for permitted or forbidden foods (*AMP-assessed attitude toward food*), and (b) two independent scores of attitudes (i.e., *AMP-assessed attitude toward permitted foods* and *AMP-assessed attitude toward forbidden foods*) since we expected that different types of foods might receive the same implicit judgment. For the AMP-assessed attitude toward food, responses on *forbidden* trials were subtracted from responses on *permitted* trials. A positive score indicates a relative preference for permitted foods. For the AMP-assessed attitude toward permitted foods, responses on *control* trials were subtracted from responses on *permitted* trials. A positive score indicates a preference for permitted foods. Finally, for the AMP-assessed attitude toward forbidden foods, responses on *control* trials were subtracted from responses on *forbidden* trials. The consideration of *control* trials in the creation of independent attitude scores allows interindividual differences in responses to be taken into account (e.g., tendency to respond in a similar way through prime conditions, such as showing "pleasant responses").

Pearson correlations were run between the relative preference score obtained for the "body shape" version and the three scores obtained for the "food" version. To take multiple testing into account, we used the Bonferroni correction. Moreover, as responses on *control* trials in the "body shape" version were not included in any of the AMP scores, their effect was controlled for (by being holding constant) in order to take into account interindividual differences in responses. Therefore, in the Results section, we report partial correlations.

Interindividual differences in eating behaviors

Regarding this last objective of exploring the role of eating behaviors as moderators of the relationships between attitudes toward body shape and food, two divergent assumptions might be proposed. First, in line with the hypothesized interrelationships postulated above (positive association between attitudes toward thinness and permitted foods; negative association with forbidden foods), the strength of associations between attitudes might be higher at high levels of dysfunctional components of eating (rigid restraint and disinhibition) than at low levels. Nevertheless, our hypothesized interrelationships describe congruent attitudes. Therefore, it is also conceivable that, at high levels of dysfunctional components, the interrelationships would illustrate discordance between attitude patterns. More specifically, Roefs et al. [3] proposed that people who alternated between restraint and disinhibition would present positive implicitly assessed attitudes toward high-calorie foods. Because these persons probably also display positive implicitly assessed attitudes toward thinness [12], their attitudes can be considered to be discordant.

For this objective, several multiple linear regression models were performed. The dependent variable was one of the scores obtained on the "food" version (see Results section for details). This choice was based on the assumption that attitudes toward foods might be influenced by attitudes toward body shapes. Therefore, the independent variables were (a) AMP-assessed attitude toward body shape; (b) the potential moderating variable (flexible or rigid control dimension of restraint, or disinhibition);[4] and (c) the interaction term.[5] Once again, performance on *control* trials in the "body shape" version was taken into account by entering this variable in the regression models as a control variable. When an interaction term was significant, it was further analyzed by using the method proposed by Aiken and West [37] in order to check whether high versus low levels of problematic or nonproblematic behaviors influence attitude associations (see Results section for details). The normality, linearity and homoscedasticity assumptions of residuals were satisfied for all regression models and no multicollinearity problems were detected (smallest tolerance value = .82).

Results

Attitudes in the overall sample

Body shape AMP

A significant main effect of prime type was observed ($F(1.92, 230.75) = 4.37$, $p = .015$, $\eta^2 = .035$).[6] Post hoc tests showed that participants judged the pictographs to be significantly ($p = .011$) more "pleasant" on *control* trials ($M = 0.54$, $SD = 0.19$) than on *overweight* trials ($M = 0.48$, $SD = 0.18$). Responses on *thin* trials ($M = 0.50$, $SD = 0.18$) did not differ significantly from either responses on *control* trials or responses on *overweight* trials (both *p*s > .05). Mean levels of AMP performance were then compared with the chance level of .50 (corrected alpha error level resulting from the Bonferroni correction: $p = .017$). Neither responses on *thin* trials nor responses on *overweight* trials nor responses on *control* trials differed significantly from the chance level (all *p*s > .017). Two differences are necessary to reach a conclusion about the valence of attitudes (i.e., positive or negative): a significant difference between emotional and control stimuli, and a difference from chance level. Thus, overweight and thin bodies seemed to be implicitly considered as ambiguous (i.e., without a defined valence) by our sample, even though the overweight bodies showed an interstimulus tendency to be judged as more negative than control primes.

Food AMP

A significant main effect of prime type was obtained ($F(1.92, 230.08) = 3.23$, $p = .044$, $\eta^2 = .026$).[6] Post hoc tests showed that participants judged the pictographs to be significantly ($p = .034$) more "pleasant" on *permitted* trials ($M = 0.57$, $SD = 0.18$) than on *control* trials ($M = 0.53$, $SD = 0.18$). Responses on *forbidden* trials ($M = 0.56$, $SD = 0.21$) did not differ significantly from either responses on *permitted* trials or responses on *control* trials (both *p*s > .05). Mean performance levels were then compared with the chance level of .50 (corrected alpha error level for multiple comparisons: $p = .017$). Responses on *permitted* trials ($t(120) = 4.10$, $p < .001$) and responses on *forbidden* trials ($t(120) = 2.94$, $p = .004$) differed significantly from the chance level, but responses on *control* trials did not ($t(120) = 1.65$, $p = .102$). Therefore, the sample's attitudes toward permitted foods could be considered as positive. Attitudes toward forbidden foods must be considered as ambiguous, given that they did not differ from responses in the control condition; still, they showed a tendency to be positive as they differed from the chance level.

Relationships between attitudes

Pearson correlations between the different AMP scores – after partialing out the effect of responses on *control* trials in the "body shape" AMP – are shown in Table 1. Interestingly, the AMP-assessed attitude toward body shape was not significantly correlated with the AMP-assessed attitude toward food. However, it was positively correlated with the AMP-assessed attitude toward permitted foods and the AMP-assessed attitude toward forbidden foods. Finally, these two independent scores were also positively correlated.

These results mean that the stronger participants' relative implicit preference was for *thin* bodies (over *overweight* bodies), the stronger their positive implicitly

Table 1 Partial correlations between attitudes toward body shape and food

	1	2	3	4
1. AMP: "body shape"	–			
2. AMP: "food"	–.119	–		
3. AMP: "permitted foods"	.287*	.421*	–	
4. AMP: "forbidden foods"	.361*	–.643*	.424*	–

Note. $N = 121$. * $p \le .001$. The Bonferroni correction was used in these analyses, resulting in a corrected alpha error level of $p = .008$. The partial variable is the proportion of "pleasant" responses on *control* trials in the "body shape" AMP. AMP: "body shape" = relative preference for thin or overweight bodies; AMP: "food" = relative preference for permitted or forbidden foods; AMP: "permitted foods" = preference for permitted foods over control images in the "food" AMP; AMP: "forbidden foods" = preference for forbidden foods over control images in the "food" AMP assessed attitudes toward both *permitted* and *forbidden* foods also were. Moreover, the more positive the participants' attitude toward *permitted* foods was, the more positive their attitude also was toward *forbidden* foods. Taken together with performance in the "food version" of the AMP (i.e., positive attitudes toward permitted foods and a tendency to make pleasant responses on forbidden trials), this finding shows that the different types of foods seemed to elicit similar (i.e., positive) attitudes in the overall sample. This could explain why the correlation between the two relative preference scores was not significant, and suggests that the use of a relative preference score toward food is not appropriate. This AMP score (*AMP-assessed attitude toward food*) will therefore not be included in further analyses.

Interindividual differences in eating behaviors

To examine interindividual differences in eating behaviors, we thus focused on the relationships between the AMP-assessed attitude toward body shape and the two independent AMP-assessed attitudes toward foods. The dependent variable of the regression models was therefore the AMP-assessed attitude toward either permitted foods or forbidden foods. The results of the regression models for the mean levels of eating behaviors are displayed in Table 2.

Flexible cognitive control dimension of restraint

At the mean level of flexible control, the AMP-assessed attitude toward body shape, the flexible control dimension and the interaction term "AMP body shape × flexible control" were significant predictors of the AMP-assessed attitude toward permitted foods (see Table 2). The overall model fit had a medium effect size (R^2 = .154, 95 % CI = [.041, .267]). To further analyze this significant two-way interaction and determine when the AMP-assessed attitude toward body shape is a significant predictor of the AMP-assessed attitude toward permitted foods, we checked whether the main effect of the AMP-assessed attitude toward body shape was significant at high and low levels (i.e., ±1 *SD*) of the moderator [37].[7] The AMP-assessed attitude toward body shape was a significant predictor of the AMP-assessed attitude toward permitted foods at a high level of flexible control (b^* = .469, *SE* = .136, $t(116)$ = 3.45, p = .001),[8] but not at a low level (b^* = .122, *SE* = .111, $t(116)$ = 1.10, p = .274). Therefore, when flexible control was average or high, the more the participants presented a relative implicit preference for *thin* bodies, the more positive their attitude was toward *permitted* foods. The intensity of the relationship between attitudes was stronger when flexible control was high than when it was average (i.e., increased *standardized beta coefficient*). The two-way interaction is illustrated in Additional file 1. The AMP-assessed attitude toward body shape was also a significant predictor of the AMP-assessed attitude toward forbidden foods; nonetheless, the interaction term "AMP body shape × flexible control" was not (see Table 2).

Rigid cognitive control dimension of restraint

At the mean level of rigid control, the AMP-assessed attitude toward body shape was a significant predictor of

Table 2 Linear regressions between attitudes toward body shape and food at mean level of eating behaviors

	Permitted foods				Forbidden foods			
Regression models 1 and 2	b^{*a}	SE^b	$t(116)$	p	b^{*a}	SE^b	$t(116)$	p
AMP-assessed attitude toward body shape	.296	.090	3.29	< .01	.370	.087	4.24	< .001
Flexible cognitive control	−.175	.088	−1.98	< .05	−.107	.086	−1.25	ns
Interaction term	.178	.087	2.03	< .05	.147	.085	1.74	ns
Regression models 3 and 4	b^{*a}	SE^b	$t(115)^c$	p	b^{*a}	SE^b	$t(116)$	p
AMP-assessed attitude toward body shape	.192	.091	2.10	< .05	.318	.084	3.77	< .001
Rigid cognitive control	−.135	.094	−1.43	ns	−.086	.085	−1.00	ns
Interaction term	−.035	.091	−.38	ns	.230	.083	2.76	< .01
Regression models 5 and 6	b^{*a}	SE^b	$t(115)^c$	p	b^{*a}	SE^b	$t(116)$	p
AMP-assessed attitude toward body shape	.195	.093	2.09	< .05	.251	.086	2.94	< .01
Disinhibition	.088	.096	.92	ns	.035	.086	.41	ns
Interaction term	.067	.097	.70	ns	.352	.087	4.03	< .001

Note. N = 121. In the six multiple regression models, the proportion of "pleasant" responses on *control* trials in the "body shape" AMP was entered as a control variable. The moderating variable was respectively (1) flexible cognitive control dimension of restraint, (2) rigid cognitive control dimension of restraint, and (3) disinhibition, resulting in the creation of three interaction terms: (1) "AMP-assessed attitude toward body shape × flexible control", (2) "AMP-assessed attitude toward body shape × rigid control", and (3) "AMP-assessed attitude toward body shape × disinhibition". [a]Standardized regression coefficients. [b]Standard errors of b^*. [c]Degrees of freedom = 115, because of the exclusion of a participant with a Cook's distance > 1.00

the AMP-assessed attitude toward permitted foods, but the interaction term "AMP body shape × rigid control" was not. However, both were significant predictors of the AMP-assessed attitude toward forbidden foods (see Table 2). The AMP-assessed attitude toward body shape was significant at a high level of rigid control ($b^* = .559$, $SE = .111$, $t(116) = 5.05$, $p < .001$), but not at a low level ($b^* = .076$, $SE = .131$, $t(116) = .58$, $p = .563$). Thus, when rigid control was average or high, the more the participants presented a relative implicit preference for *thin* bodies, the more positive their attitude was toward *forbidden* foods. The intensity of the relationship between attitudes was stronger when rigid control was high. The overall model fit had a medium effect size ($R^2 = .228$, 95 % CI = [.103, .354]). The two-way interaction is illustrated in Additional file 1.

Disinhibition

At the mean level of disinhibition, the AMP-assessed attitude toward body shape was a significant predictor of the AMP-assessed attitude toward permitted foods, but the interaction term "AMP body shape × disinhibition" was not. However, once again, both were significant predictors of the AMP-assessed attitude toward forbidden foods (see Table 2). The AMP-assessed attitude toward body shape was significant at a high level of disinhibition ($b^* = .504$, $SE = .091$, $t(116) = 5.54$, $p < .001$), but not at a low level ($b^* = -.001$, $SE = .119$, $t(116) = -.01$, $p = .991$). Therefore, when disinhibition was average or high, the more the participants presented a relative implicit preference for *thin* bodies, the more positive their attitude was toward *forbidden* foods. The intensity of the relationship between attitudes was stronger when disinhibition was high. The overall model fit had a large effect size ($R^2 = .273$, 95 % CI = [.144, .403]). The two-way interaction is illustrated in Additional file 1.

Discussion

This study reexamined implicitly assessed attitudes toward body shape and food in a sample of young women from the community; more importantly, it also investigated the interrelationships between attitudes toward body shape and food as well as the moderating role of the flexible and rigid cognitive control dimensions of restraint, and disinhibition. Given the lack of studies investigating implicitly assessed attitudes toward body shape and food together, the main contribution of the present study is the examination of congruence and discordance in patterns of implicitly assessed attitudes in the understanding of problematic and nonproblematic eating behaviors.

The current study did not replicate earlier findings of positive attitudes toward thinness and negative attitudes toward fatness [13]. We found that both overweight and thin bodies were perceived as implicitly ambiguous (without a defined valence). As for attitudes toward food, a positive implicitly assessed attitude toward permitted foods was detected, replicating some previous findings [19]. Attitudes toward forbidden foods did not present a defined valence. However, these results are not surprising. First, it is conceivable that interindividual differences masked effects in the overall sample. Indeed, AMP performances in our sample presented considerable variability. The undefined valences obtained for attitudes toward forbidden foods and both body types could therefore be explained by the presence of incompatibly valenced attitudes (i.e., positive and negative) toward a single type of stimuli among participants, which canceled out the overall effects. The consideration of interindividual differences in the present sample highlighted some specific attitude patterns in subgroups of participants, as past studies had also found. For example, Ahern et al. [16] reported that participants could be characterized by either negative or positive attitudes toward thin bodies depending on their level of drive for thinness. Second, as mentioned, past studies obtained inconsistent results concerning forbidden foods [20, 23]; the same was also true of body shape. Roddy et al. [14], for instance, also failed to detect anti-overweight attitudes using a nonrelative measure like the AMP, underlying the influence of the task. Finally, in our overall sample, the different types of food seemed to elicit similar (positive) implicitly assessed attitudes rather than dissimilar attitudes. This result could account for some previous inconsistent findings. Indeed, the use of the IAT (relative measure) in several studies made it impossible to identify a similar pattern of attitudes for two targeted stimuli.

Regarding interrelationships between attitudes, the positive correlation observed between attitudes toward thinness and permitted foods supports our hypothesis. However, we did not expect that attitudes toward thinness would be positively – and not negatively – correlated with attitudes toward forbidden foods. This discordance between attitudes (i.e., positive association, whereas forbidden foods should be devalued to promote thinness) became meaningful when interindividual differences were considered. Indeed, their exploration revealed different patterns of attitudes toward body shape and food at average and high levels of problematic versus nonproblematic eating behaviors. More specifically, the functional component of restraint (i.e., flexible cognitive control) contributes to a positive relationship between attitudes toward thinness and permitted foods (*congruent* attitudes), whereas dysfunctional eating behaviors (i.e., rigid component of restraint and disinhibition) contribute to a positive relationship between attitudes toward thinness and forbidden foods (*discordant* attitudes). Therefore, the discordance between attitudes observed in the overall sample (i.e., positive association between attitudes toward thinness and forbidden foods) seemed to characterize primarily participants with problematic eating behaviors (rigid restraint and disinhibition), given that women whose eating behaviors were not problematic (flexible restraint) were characterized by congruent attitudes.

To our knowledge, the congruence or discordance between implicitly assessed attitudes had not previously been explored. However, one study that also used a nonrelative measure to implicitly assess attitudes explored discrepancies between explicitly and implicitly assessed attitudes in the field of dietary restraint and observed that restrained eaters, and not unrestrained eaters, exhibited discordant attitudes toward high caloric foods (negative explicitly assessed attitudes, positive implicitly assessed attitudes) [22]. In line with our results, these findings suggest that a conflict between attitudes might influence the development and/or maintenance of problematic eating behaviors. It is indeed likely that discordant attitudes toward relevant goal-related constructs (e.g., a positive implicit attitude toward high-calorie foods in someone who is dieting to become thinner) will promote aversive emotional states and, ultimately, disordered eating (e.g., overeating, rigid restraint). In contrast, when attitudes are congruent, there is less internal tension, which allows for more flexible food control and intake (e.g., forbidden foods can be eaten in small quantities). Nevertheless, because our study is correlational in nature, the causal role of discordant implicitly assessed attitudes in the onset and maintenance of problematic eating remains tentative and should be addressed in future longitudinal studies.

It has been suggested that attitudes toward forbidden foods need to be negative in order to be congruent with positive attitudes toward thinness and the goal of losing weight [6]. However, the opposite relationship (i.e., discordance between attitudes) was observed in our sample. Therefore, it is possible that congruent attitudes exist only at the explicit level, at least among restrained eaters, who will disparage forbidden foods to promote their goal of dieting [6, 22]. Future studies should address this hypothesis.

Finally, although the investigation of interindividual differences make a substantial contribution by providing some explanations of the unpredicted results obtained for the overall sample, we cannot reach a conclusion regarding the nonsignificant results we obtained. In this sample, dysfunctional components of eating were related only to the link between attitudes toward thinness and forbidden foods (causing us to hypothesize that discordant attitudes existed), while the functional component was related only to the association with permitted foods (i.e., hypothesized congruent attitudes). However, the nonsignificant effects obtained for the other regression models do not necessarily mean that such effects were not present. Replication studies are necessary in order to draw more firmly based conclusions.

Limitations

Some limitations on this study warrant further discussion. First, while this study focused on implicitly assessed attitudes, explicit measures of attitudes would also have been valuable. The consideration of explicitly assessed attitudes could lead to a better understanding of interindividual differences, given that, in certain cases, implicit and explicit measures of attitudes provide different information [8–10]. Moreover, explicit measures of attitudes would have allowed us to explore the discordance between explicitly and implicitly assessed attitudes toward similar stimuli (e.g., positive implicitly assessed attitudes and negative explicitly assessed attitudes toward forbidden foods), as well as the discordance between explicitly assessed attitudes and their links to symptoms of disordered eating.

Second, we used pictorial control stimuli in the two AMP versions to avoid a habituation effect due to the repetition of the same neutral stimulus (e.g., a gray square like the one used by Payne et al. [32]) and to increase the ecological validity of the tasks. These control stimuli had no connection with the concepts of interest for the AMP versions (respectively, body shape and food) and should therefore be irrelevant to the participants. Although they allowed us to take interindividual differences in responses into account (e.g., a general tendency to respond "pleasant"), we cannot exclude the possibility that relevant (thin and overweight bodies, high- and low-calorie foods) and irrelevant (shrubs, objects) stimuli were processed differently. Hence, the use of control stimuli related to the concept of interest might improve the methodology. For example, in the field of body image, in addition to positive (thin bodies) and negative (overweight bodies) "emotional" stimuli, the control stimuli could be "nonemotional" body-related stimuli, namely bodies evaluated as neither "thin" nor "overweight", neither "positive" nor "negative", but with a median judgment between the two poles (i.e., "zero-value" judgments).

Third, a general bias to respond "pleasant" might exist in AMP performances. Nevertheless, interindividual differences relativized this: some people might respond positively to a range of situations, whereas others might present the opposite tendency (to respond negatively) for the same situations [38]. Moreover, our findings showed that, as expected, responses in *control* trials did not significantly differ from chance level, highlighting that if such a bias exists, it was not present in all AMP conditions. Finally, interindividual differences in responses were taken into account in the statistical analyses to reduce the impact of such a bias.

Fourth, we did not use the classic TFEQ restraint scale, given that we wanted to explore the processes that underlie restraint (rigid and flexible cognitive controls). However, this choice makes our findings difficult to compare with previous studies that used the classic scale. Moreover, even if the internal reliability of the subscales was acceptable, it was lower than that of the classic scale, given the smallest number of items in the subscales (which have negatively influenced internal consistency) [39].

Finally, participants' BMIs were based on self-reported measures. Estimation biases could therefore have influenced the measures. Nonetheless, previous research demonstrated that estimation biases are more likely to appear among people with "extreme" BMI [40, 41]. Given that such BMIs are rare in the current sample (nine participants have a BMI < 17.00 kg/m^2 or > 30.00 kg/m^2), we assume that estimation biases are minimal. Moreover, as BMI did not significantly correlate with the main AMP variables (i.e., AMP-assessed attitude toward body shape, permitted foods, or forbidden foods), it was not entered in the statistical analyses. Thus, our findings could not have been affected by such potential biases.

Conclusions

Our results highlighted the importance of taking into account the congruence or discordance in patterns of attitudes toward body shape and food, as well as interindividual differences, in understanding problematic and nonproblematic eating behaviors. Focusing on interindividual differences seems essential to investigate the existence of different psychological patterns in a sample and highlight the mechanisms that may underlie a given subgroup's behaviors. Further studies are nevertheless required to pursue the investigation of interrelationships between implicitly assessed attitudes toward body shape and food and obtain a more detailed picture of their influences on the onset and maintenance of eating behaviors.

These results have some critical clinical implications. Nowadays, in the field of eating disorders, schemas and implicit cognitions have been proposed to be a key focus for interventions [12, 30]. But our findings suggest a further step. First and foremost, given that discordance between implicitly assessed attitudes was found to be associated with problematic eating behaviors, the assessment of implicit representations toward body shape and food and their characterization in terms of congruent or discordant patterns seems necessary. Afterwards, interventions could target discordant implicit cognitions in order to treat problematic eating behaviors. For instance, Martijn et al. [42] proposed modifying positive implicit associations toward thinness (e.g., "thin – good") through a conditioning procedure in which pictures of thin-ideal models were followed by a negative adjective (e.g., "fake"), emphasizing that models' images are often retouched. By making thinness less positive, this intervention could reduce the internal attitudinal conflict among women who present positive implicitly assessed attitudes toward thinness and forbidden foods and perhaps allow them to engage in more flexible food control and intake, decreasing the frequency of problematic eating behaviors.

For definitions of specific terms, see Additional file 2.

Endnotes

[1]In the present sample, no participant spoke Chinese or was familiar with this language, thereby fulfilling the inclusion criteria for the AMP.

[2]The Mann–Whitney *U*-test was performed because the assumption of normality was not met.

[3]Since this study focuses on restraint and disinhibition, the third dimension evaluated by the TFEQ (susceptibility to hunger, namely the perception of hunger and its impact on eating behaviors) was not used in the study.

[4]The two manifestations of restraint and disinhibition did not significantly correlate with the predictor (AMP-assessed attitude toward body shape), respecting the criteria recommended by Kraemer et al. [43] for moderating variables. These variables were therefore considered as moderators when the interaction with the predictor had a significant effect on the outcome.

[5]As BMI and age did not significantly correlate with the three main variables in the regression models (i.e., AMP-assessed attitude toward body shape, AMP-assessed attitude toward permitted foods and AMP-assessed attitude toward forbidden foods), they were not entered as control variables in the regression models to avoid reducing the statistical power.

[6]As the Mauchly's sphericity test (which evaluates whether the sphericity assumption associated with the repeated measures ANOVAs is met) was significant, the *F*-test was adjusted by the Huynh-Feldt correction, as needed.

[7]Variables entered in the regression models were centered and the interaction term was computed with the centered variables. To test whether the main effect of the AMP-assessed attitude toward body shape was significant at a low level of flexible control, we reran the same regression model, except that the centered moderating variable was replaced by "centered flexible control +1 *SD*". To explore whether the main effect was significant at a high level of flexible control, we replaced the centered moderating variable by "centered flexible control −1 *SD*".

[8]b^* corresponds to the standardized regression coefficient. *SE* corresponds to the standard error of b^*.

Additional files

Additional file 1: Figures representing associations between attitudes toward body shape and food at different levels of eating behaviors. Three figures showing the regression lines illustrating the relations between AMP-assessed attitude toward body shape and (1) AMP-assessed attitude toward permitted foods at high, average, and low levels of the flexible cognitive control dimension of restraint; (2) AMP-assessed attitude toward forbidden foods at high, average, and low levels of the rigid cognitive control dimension of restraint; and (3) AMP-assessed attitude toward forbidden foods at high, average, and low levels of disinhibition. (PDF 474 kb)

Additional file 2: Definitions of specific terms. Table in which all definitions of specific terms are presented in order to facilitate the reader's understanding. (PDF 178 kb)

Abbreviations

AMP: Affect Misattribution Procedure; ANOVAs: analyses of variance; BMI: body mass index; IAT: Implicit Association Task; TFEQ: Three-Factor Eating Questionnaire.

Competing interests

The authors declare that they have no competing interests.

Authors' contributions

JMM supervised the data acquisition, conducted data analyses and interpretation, and wrote the manuscript. JB participated in the conceptualization of the study, the data acquisition and analyses, and the writing of the manuscript. OM designed the study, participated in the data acquisition, and assisted in the writing of the manuscript. SR participated in the data analyses and assisted in the writing of the manuscript. MVdL participated in the conceptualization of the study, supervised the data acquisition, and participated in the results interpretation and the writing of the manuscript. All authors read and approved the final manuscript.

Acknowledgments

We would like to thank Fanny Delorme and Lan-Anh Nguyen for their help with the data acquisition.

Author details

[1]Psychology Department, FPSE, Cognitive Psychopathology and Neuropsychology Unit, University of Geneva, Boulevard du Pont d'Arve 40, CH-1205 Geneva, Switzerland. [2]Swiss Center for Affective Sciences, Campus Biotech, University of Geneva, Case Postale 60, CH-1211 Geneva 20, Switzerland. [3]Psychological Sciences Research Institute, Laboratory for Experimental Psychopathology, Catholic University of Louvain, Place Cardinal Mercier 10, B-1348 Louvain-la-Neuve, Belgium. [4]Mental Health and Psychiatry Department, Addictology Division, Geneva University Hospitals, Rue Grand-Pré 70C, CH-1202 Geneva, Switzerland. [5]Geneva School of Economics and Management, Research Center for Statistics, University of Geneva, Boulevard du Pont d'Arve 40, CH-1205 Geneva, Switzerland. [6]Cognitive Sciences Department, Cognitive Psychopathology Unit, University of Liège, Boulevard du Rectorat B33 (TriFacultaire), 4000 Liège, Belgium.

References

1. Cunningham WA, Zelazo PD, Packer DJ, Van Bavel JJ. The iterative reprocessing model: a multilevel framework for attitudes and evaluation. Soc Cogn. 2007;25:736–60.
2. Juarascio AS, Forman EM, Timko CA, Herbert JD, Butryn M, Lowe M. Implicit internalization of the thin ideal as a predictor of increases in weight, body dissatisfaction, and disordered eating. Eat Behav. 2011;12:207–13.
3. Roefs A, Huijding J, Smulders FT, MacLeod CM, de Jong PJ, Wiers RW, et al. Implicit measures of association in psychopathology research. Psychol Bull. 2011;137:149–93.
4. Stice E, Shaw HE. Role of body dissatisfaction in the onset and maintenance of eating pathology: a synthesis of research findings. J Psychosom Res. 2002;53:985–93.
5. Brownell KD. Dieting and the search for the perfect body: where physiology and culture collide. Behav Ther. 1991;22:1–12.
6. Francis JA, Stewart SH, Hounsell S. Dietary restraint and the selective processing of forbidden and nonforbidden food words. Cogn Ther Res. 1997;21:633–46.
7. De Houwer J, Teige-Mocigemba S, Spruyt A, Moors A. Implicit measures: a normative analysis and review. Psychol Bull. 2009;135:347–68.
8. Perugini M. Predictive models of implicit and explicit attitudes. Br J Soc Psychol. 2005;44:29–45.
9. Rudman LA. Sources of implicit attitudes. Curr Dir Psychol Sci. 2004;13:79–82.
10. Payne BK, Govorun O, Arbuckle NL. Automatic attitudes and alcohol: does implicit liking predict drinking? Cogn Emot. 2008;22:238–71.
11. Smith AR, Joiner TE, Dodd DR. Examining implicit attitudes toward emaciation and thinness in anorexia nervosa. Int J Eat Disord. 2013;47:138–47.
12. Vartanian LR, Polivy J, Herman CP. Implicit cognitions and eating disorders: their application in research and treatment. Cogn Behav Pract. 2004;11:160–7.
13. Ahern AL, Hetherington MM. The thin ideal and body image: an experimental study of implicit attitudes. Psychol Addict Behav. 2006;20:338–42.
14. Roddy S, Stewart I, Barnes-Holmes D. Anti-fat, pro-slim, or both? Using two reaction-time based measures to assess implicit attitudes to the slim and overweight. J Health Psychol. 2010;15:416–25.
15. Vartanian LR, Herman CP, Polivy J. Implicit and explicit attitudes toward fatness and thinness: the role of the internalization of societal standards. Body Image. 2005;2:373–81.
16. Ahern AL, Bennett KM, Hetherington MM. Internalization of the ultra-thin ideal: positive implicit associations with underweight fashion models are associated with drive for thinness in young women. Eat Disord. 2008;16:294–307.
17. Cserjési R, Vermeulen N, Luminet O, Marechal C, Nef F, Simon Y, et al. Explicit vs. implicit body image evaluation in restrictive anorexia nervosa. Psychiatry Res. 2010;175:148–53.
18. Schwartz MB, Vartanian LR, Nosek BA, Brownell KD. The influence of one's own body weight on implicit and explicit anti-fat bias. Obesity. 2006;14:440–7.
19. Maison D, Greenwald AG, Bruin R. The Implicit Association Test as a measure of implicit consumer attitudes. Pol Psychol Bull. 2001;32:61–9.
20. Roefs A, Jansen A. Implicit and explicit attitudes toward high-fat foods in obesity. J Abnorm Psychol. 2002;111:517–21.
21. Czyzewska M, Graham R. Implicit and explicit attitudes to high- and low-calorie food in females with different BMI status. Eat Behav. 2008;9:303–12.
22. Hoefling A, Strack F. The tempting effect of forbidden foods: high calorie content evokes conflicting implicit and explicit evaluations in restrained eaters. Appetite. 2008;51:681–9.
23. Papies EK, Stroebe W, Aarts H. Who likes it more? Restrained eaters' implicit attitudes towards food. Appetite. 2009;53:279–87.
24. Greenwald AG, McGhee DE, Schwartz JL. Measuring individual differences in implicit cognition: the implicit association test. J Pers Soc Psychol. 1998;74:1464–80.
25. Houben K, Roefs A, Jansen A. Guilty pleasures: implicit preferences for high calorie food in restrained eating. Appetite. 2010;55:18–24.
26. Fett A-K, Lattimore P, Roefs A, Geschwind N, Jansen A. Food cue exposure and body image satisfaction: the moderating role of BMI and dietary restraint. Body Image. 2009;6:14–8.
27. Vocks S, Legenbauer T, Heil A. Food intake affects state body image: impact of restrained eating patterns and concerns about eating, weight and shape. Appetite. 2007;49:467–75.
28. Durkin K, Rae K, Stritzke WGK. The effect of images of thin and overweight body shapes on women's ambivalence towards chocolate. Appetite. 2012;58:222–6.
29. Westenhoefer J. Dietary restraint and disinhibition: is restraint a homogeneous construct? Appetite. 1991;16:45–55.
30. Fairburn CG. Eating disorders: the transdiagnostic view and the cognitive behavioral theory. In: Fairburn CG, editor. Cognitive behavior therapy and eating disorders. New York: The Guilford Press; 2008. p. 7–22.
31. Heatherton TF, Herman CP, Polivy J, King GA, McGree ST. The (mis) measurement of restraint: an analysis of conceptual and psychometric issues. J Abnorm Psychol. 1988;97:19–28.
32. Payne BK, Cheng CM, Govorun O, Stewart BD. An inkblot for attitudes: affect misattribution as implicit measurement. J Pers Soc Psychol. 2005;89:277–93.
33. Bar-Anan Y, Nosek BA. Reporting intentional rating of the primes predicts priming effects in the Affective Misattribution Procedure. Pers Soc Psychol Bull. 2012;38:1194–208.

34. Lluch A. Identification des conduites alimentaires par approches nutritionnelles et psychométriques: Implications thérapeutiques et préventives dans l'obésité humaine [Identification of eating patterns by nutritional and psychometric approaches: implications for the prevention and treatment of human obesity] [Doctoral thesis]. Nancy, France: Henri Poincaré University, Nancy I; 1995.
35. Stunkard AJ, Messick S. The three-factor eating questionnaire to measure dietary restraint, disinhibition and hunger. J Psychosom Res. 1985;29:71–83.
36. Payne BK, McClernon FJ, Dobbins IG. Automatic affective responses to smoking cues. Exp Clin Psychopharmacol. 2007;15:400–9.
37. Aiken LS, West SG. Multiple regression: testing and interpreting interactions. London, UK: Sage Publications; 1991.
38. Aiken LR. Attitudes toward mathematics. Rev Educ Res. 1970;40:551–96.
39. Field A. Discovering statistics using SPSS. 3rd ed. London, UK: Sage Publications; 2009.
40. Connor Gorber S, Tremblay M, Moher D, Gorber B. A comparison of direct vs. self-report measures for assessing height, weight and body mass index: a systematic review. Obes Rev. 2007;8:307–26.
41. Tovée MJ, Emery JL, Cohen-Tovée EM. The estimation of body mass index and physical attractiveness is dependent on the observer's own body mass index. Proc R Soc B Biol Sci. 2000;267:1987–97.
42. Martijn C, Alleva JM, Jansen A. Improving body satisfaction: do strategies targeting the automatic system work? Eur Psychol. 2015;20:62–71.
43. Kraemer HC, Stice E, Kazdin A, Offord D, Kupfer D. How do risk factors work together? Mediators, moderators, and independent, overlapping, and proxy risk factors. Am J Psychiatry. 2001;158:848–56.

Permissions

All chapters in this book were first published in JED, by BioMed Central; hereby published with permission under the Creative Commons Attribution License or equivalent. Every chapter published in this book has been scrutinized by our experts. Their significance has been extensively debated. The topics covered herein carry significant findings which will fuel the growth of the discipline. They may even be implemented as practical applications or may be referred to as a beginning point for another development.

The contributors of this book come from diverse backgrounds, making this book a truly international effort. This book will bring forth new frontiers with its revolutionizing research information and detailed analysis of the nascent developments around the world.

We would like to thank all the contributing authors for lending their expertise to make the book truly unique. They have played a crucial role in the development of this book. Without their invaluable contributions this book wouldn't have been possible. They have made vital efforts to compile up to date information on the varied aspects of this subject to make this book a valuable addition to the collection of many professionals and students.

This book was conceptualized with the vision of imparting up-to-date information and advanced data in this field. To ensure the same, a matchless editorial board was set up. Every individual on the board went through rigorous rounds of assessment to prove their worth. After which they invested a large part of their time researching and compiling the most relevant data for our readers.

The editorial board has been involved in producing this book since its inception. They have spent rigorous hours researching and exploring the diverse topics which have resulted in the successful publishing of this book. They have passed on their knowledge of decades through this book. To expedite this challenging task, the publisher supported the team at every step. A small team of assistant editors was also appointed to further simplify the editing procedure and attain best results for the readers.

Apart from the editorial board, the designing team has also invested a significant amount of their time in understanding the subject and creating the most relevant covers. They scrutinized every image to scout for the most suitable representation of the subject and create an appropriate cover for the book.

The publishing team has been an ardent support to the editorial, designing and production team. Their endless efforts to recruit the best for this project, has resulted in the accomplishment of this book. They are a veteran in the field of academics and their pool of knowledge is as vast as their experience in printing. Their expertise and guidance has proved useful at every step. Their uncompromising quality standards have made this book an exceptional effort. Their encouragement from time to time has been an inspiration for everyone.

The publisher and the editorial board hope that this book will prove to be a valuable piece of knowledge for researchers, students, practitioners and scholars across the globe.

List of Contributors

Yael Latzer
Faculty of Social Welfare & Health Sciences, Haifa University, Haifa, Israel
Eating Disorders Clinic, Psychiatric Division, Rambam Medical Center, Haifa, Israel

Daniel Stein
Pediatric Psychosomatic Department, the Edmond and Lily Safra Children's Hospital, The Chaim Sheba Medical Center, Tel Hashomer, affiliated with The Sackler Faculty of Medicine, Tel Aviv University, Tel Aviv, Israel

Loa Clausen
Centre of Child- and Adolescent Psychiatry, Aarhus University Hospital, Skovagervej 2, DK-8240 Risskov, Denmark

Allan Jones
Institute of Psychology, University of Southern Denmark, Campusvej 55, DK-5230 Odense M, Denmark

Lisa Bloom
School of Health Sciences, RMIT University, Melbourne, Australia

Beth Shelton
Monash Link Community Health Service, Melbourne, Australia
Southern Health Wellness Recovery Adult Outpatient Eating Disorder Service, Melbourne, Australia

Melissa Bengough
Southern Health Wellness Recovery Adult Outpatient Eating Disorder Service, Melbourne, Australia

Leah Brennan
School of Psychology, Australian Catholic University, Melbourne, Australia

David H Gleaves
School of Psychology, Social Work and Social Policy, University of South Australia, Magill Campus, GPO Box 2471, Adelaide, SA 5001, Australia

Crystal A Pearson and Leslie C Morey
Texas A&M University, College Station, TX, USA

Suman Ambwani
Dickinson College, Carlisle, PA, USA

Ned Scott
Clinical Psychology Program, School of Behavioural, Cognitive and Social Sciences, University of New England, Armidale, NSW 2351, Australia
School of Psychology, University of Newcastle, Callaghan, NSW 2308, Australia

Tanya L Hanstock
Clinical Psychology Program, School of Behavioural, Cognitive and Social Sciences, University of New England, Armidale, NSW 2351, Australia
School of Psychology, University of Newcastle, Callaghan, NSW 2308, Australia

Chris Thornton
The Redleaf Practice, Wahroonga, NSW 2076, Australia

Alix Vann
Queensland University of Technology School of Psychology & Counselling, Level 5, O Block, B Wing, QUT Kelvin Grove Campus, Victoria Park Road, Kelvin Grove Queensland 4059, Brisbane, Australia

Esben Strodl
Queensland University of Technology School of Psychology & Counselling, Level 5, O Block, B Wing, QUT Kelvin Grove Campus, Victoria Park Road, Kelvin Grove Queensland 4059, Brisbane, Australia

Erin Anderson
Eating Disorders Outreach Service, 14 Cartwright Street, Herston Queensland 4029, Brisbane, Australia

Jeremy Alman, Kimberley J Hoiles, Matthew Hamilton and Chloe Shu
Eating Disorders Program, Child and Adolescent Mental Health Service, Child and Adolescent Health Service, Roberts Road, Subiaco, Western Australia, Australia
School of Psychology and Speech Pathology, Division of Health Sciences, Curtin University, Kent St, Bentley, Western Australia, Australia
School of Paediatrics and Child Health, Faculty of Medicine, Dentistry and Health Sciences, The University of Western Australia, 35 Stirling Highway, Crawley, Western Australia, Australia
UNC Center of Excellence for Eating Disorders, Department of Psychiatry, Neurosciences Hospital, 101 Manning Drive, Chapel Hill, North Carolina, USA
Princess Margaret Hospital for Children Eating Disorders Program, GPO Box D184, Perth 6840, Western Australia, Australia

Hunna J Watson
Eating Disorders Program, Child and Adolescent Mental Health Service, Child and Adolescent Health Service, Roberts Road, Subiaco, Western Australia, Australia
School of Psychology and Speech Pathology, Division of Health Sciences, Curtin University, Kent St, Bentley, Western Australia, Australia
School of Paediatrics and Child Health, Faculty of Medicine, Dentistry and Health Sciences, The University of Western Australia, 35 Stirling Highway, Crawley, Western Australia, Australia
UNC Center of Excellence for Eating Disorders, Department of Psychiatry, Neurosciences Hospital, 101 Manning Drive, Chapel Hill, North Carolina, USA
Princess Margaret Hospital for Children Eating Disorders Program, GPO Box D184, Perth 6840, Western Australia, Australia

Sarah J Egan
School of Psychology and Speech Pathology, Division of Health Sciences, Curtin University, Kent St, Bentley, Western Australia, Australia

Julie McCormack and Julie Potts
Eating Disorders Program, Child and Adolescent Mental Health Service, Child and Adolescent Health Service, Roberts Road, Subiaco, Western Australia, Australia

David A Forbes
Eating Disorders Program, Child and Adolescent Mental Health Service, Child and Adolescent Health Service, Roberts Road, Subiaco, Western Australia, Australia
School of Paediatrics and Child Health, Faculty of Medicine, Dentistry and Health Sciences, The University of Western Australia, 35 Stirling Highway, Crawley, Western Australia, Australia

Manfred Maximilian Fichter
Department of Psychiatry and Psychotherapy, University of Munich (LMU), Nussbaumstraße 7, 80336 München, Germany
Schön Klinik Roseneck affiliated with the Medical Faculty of the University of Munich (LMU), 83209 Prien, Germany

Norbert Quadflieg and Susanne Lindner
Department of Psychiatry and Psychotherapy, University of Munich (LMU), Nussbaumstraße 7, 80336 München, Germany

Laurel M Wallace, Philip C Masson and Kristin M von Ranson
Department of Psychology, University of Calgary, 2500 University Drive NW, Calgary, Alberta, Canada

Debra L Safer
Department of Psychiatry and Behavioral Sciences, Stanford University, Stanford, California, USA

Eric M Stephen, Jennifer Rose, Lindsay Kenney and Ruth Striegel Weissman
Department of Psychology, Wesleyan University, 207 High Street, Middletown, CT 06459, USA

Francine Rosselli-Navarra
Department of Psychology, Manchester Community College, Great Path MS#4, Manchester, CT, USA

Deborah Mitchison
School of Psychology and Social Science, University of Western Sydney, Sydney, NSW, Australia

Rocco Crino
School of Psychology, Charles Sturt University, Bathurst, NSW, Australia

Phillipa Hay
School of Medicine and Centre for Health Research, University of Western Sydney, Sydney, NSW, Australia
School of Medicine, James Cook University, Townsville, QLD, Australia

Chengyuan Zhang
Imperial College London; South Kensington Campus, SW7 2AZ, Exhibition Road, London, UK

Alan P Bailey, Alexandra G Parker, Lauren A Colautti, Ping Liu and Sarah E Hetrick
Orygen Youth Health Research Centre, Centre for Youth Mental Health, The University of Melbourne, Locked Bag 10, Parkville, Melbourne, Victoria 3052, Australia
Centre of Excellence in Youth Mental Health, headspace National Youth Mental Health Foundation Ltd, Level 2, South Tower, 485 La Trobe Street, Melbourne, Victoria 3000, Australia

Laura M Hart
Melbourne School of Population Health, The University of Melbourne, Level 3, 207 Bouverie Street, Melbourne, Victoria 3010, Australia

Lois J Surgenor
Department of Psychological Medicine, University of Otago at Christchurch, 4 Oxford Terrace, Christchurch 8140, New Zealand

Sarah Maguire
Centre for Eating and Dieting Disorders, University of Sydney, 92-94 Parramatta Road, Camberdown, New South Wales 2050, Australia

Carolyn Black Becker, Maribel Plasencia, Lisa Smith Kilpela and Morgan Briggs
Department of Psychology, Trinity University, San Antonio, TX 78212, USA

Tiffany Stewart
Pennington Biomedical Research Center, 6400 Perkins Rd, Baton Rouge, LA 70808, USA

Carmen V Weiss
Department of Psychiatry, St. Joseph's Healthcare, Hamilton, Ontario, Canada

Henny A Westra and Jennifer S Mills
Department of Psychology, York University, Toronto, Ontario, Canada

Jacqueline C Carter
Department of Psychology, Memorial University of Newfoundland, St. John's, Newfoundland, Canada

Myra Cooper and Hannah Kelland
Isis Education Centre, University of Oxford, Warneford Hospital, Oxford OX3 7JX, UK

Franzisca V. Froreich, Lenny R. Vartanian and Jessica R. Grisham
School of Psychology, UNSW Australia, Sydney, New South Wales 2052, Australia

Stephen W. Touyz
School of Psychology, University of Sydney, Sydney 2006, New South Wales, Australia

Melissa Noetel
School of Psychology, The University of Sydney, Sydney, Australia

Jane Miskovic-Wheatley
Eating Disorder Service at The Sydney Children's Hospitals Network, Westmead, Australia
Westmead Clinical School, The University of Sydney, Sydney, Australia

Ross D. Crosby
Department of Psychiatry and Behavioral Science, University of North Dakota School of Medicine and Health Sciences, Fargo, USA
Neuropsychiatric Research Institute, Fargo, USA

Phillipa Hay
Centre for Health Research, School of Medicine, Western Sydney University, Penrith, Australia

Sloane Madden
Eating Disorder Service at The Sydney Children's Hospitals Network, Westmead, Australia
Discipline of Pediatrics, Faculty of Medicine, The University of Sydney, Sydney, Australia

Stephen Touyz
School of Psychology, The University of Sydney, Sydney, Australia

Maciej Wojciech Pilecki
Department of Child and Adolescent Psychiatry, Jagiellonian University Medical College, ul. Kopernika 21a, 31-501 Kraków, Poland
Jagiellonian University Medical College, ul. Kopernika 21a, 31-501 Kraków, Poland

Kinga Sałapa
Department of Bioinformatics and Telemedicine, Jagiellonian University Medical College, ul. Św. Łazarza 16, 31-530 Kraków, Poland

Barbara Józefik
Department of Child and Adolescent Psychiatry, Laboratory of Psychology and Systemic Psychotherapy

Stephen P. Lewis, Laura Klauninger and Ivana Marcincinova
University of Guelph, Guelph, ON N1G 2W1, Canada

Joanna Myriam Moussally
Psychology Department, FPSE, Cognitive Psychopathology and Neuropsychology Unit, University of Geneva, Boulevard du Pont d'Arve 40, CH-1205 Geneva, Switzerland
Swiss Center for Affective Sciences, Campus Biotech, University of Geneva, Case Postale 60, CH-1211 Geneva 20, Switzerland

Joël Billieux
Psychology Department, FPSE, Cognitive Psychopathology and Neuropsychology Unit, University of Geneva, Boulevard du Pont d'Arve 40, CH-1205 Geneva, Switzerland
Psychological Sciences Research Institute, Laboratory for Experimental Psychopathology, Catholic University of Louvain, Place Cardinal Mercier 10, B-1348 Louvain-la-Neuve, Belgium

Olivia Mobbs
Psychology Department, FPSE, Cognitive Psychopathology and Neuropsychology Unit, University of Geneva, Boulevard du Pont d'Arve 40, CH-1205 Geneva, Switzerland

Stéphane Rothen
Mental Health and Psychiatry Department, Addictology Division, Geneva University Hospitals, Rue Grand-Pré 70C, CH-1202 Geneva, Switzerland
Geneva School of Economics and Management, Research Center for Statistics, University of Geneva, Boulevard du Pont d'Arve 40, CH-1205 Geneva, Switzerland

Martial Van der Linden
Psychology Department, FPSE, Cognitive Psychopathology and Neuropsychology Unit, University of Geneva, Boulevard du Pont d'Arve 40, CH-1205 Geneva, Switzerland
Swiss Center for Affective Sciences, Campus Biotech, University of Geneva, Case Postale 60, CH-1211 Geneva 20, Switzerland
Cognitive Sciences Department, Cognitive Psychopathology Unit, University of Liège, Boulevard du Rectorat B33 (TriFacultaire), 4000 Liège, Belgium

Index